JOHN A. PUPILLO, M.D.

THE ECG OF ARTIFICIAL PACEMAKER

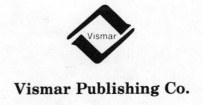
Vismar

Vismar Publishing Co.

*In memory of my father
Renzo Pupillo, M.D.*

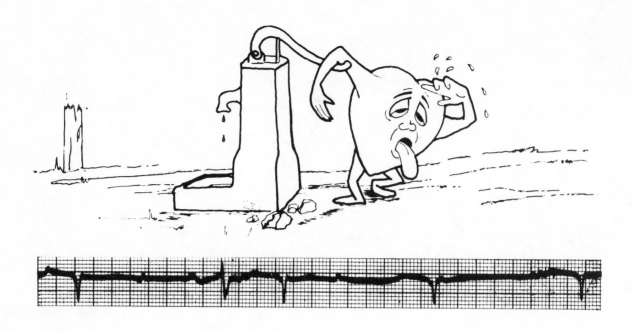

. . . in the field of observation, chance favors only the prepared minds. (Pasteur)

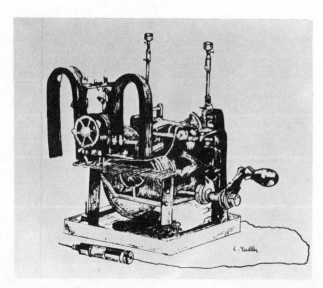

First "Artificial Pacemaker" (8.5 Kg)
Hyman 1932

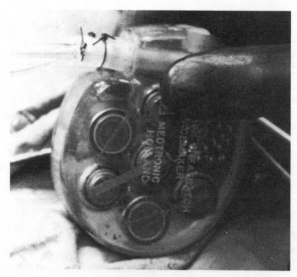

A Modern Pacemaker

PREFACE

This book is not for the "electronic elite" but rather for the practitioner interested in understanding the ECG aspect of cardiac pacemakers. Its main purpose is to be a practical guide in the ECG examination of the most commonly used pacing modalities.

The introduction of artificial pacemakers in the treatment of chronic heart block, has been one of the most dramatic events in medicine of the past 20 years. The common effort of investigators in medicine and electronics has resulted in the manufacture of totally implantable and miniaturized pacing units. The enormous quantity of data obtained in the prolonged use of artificial pacemakers has profoundly changed the concepts of pathophysiology and therapy of cardiac conduction abnormalities. Furthermore, cardiac pacing has permitted a better understanding of electrophysiological events which occur in the human heart and which are at the base of complex cardiac arrhythmias. In the light of the accumulated knowledge it is possible to stop for a moment, look back and reflect on what has been learned in the field. This book, so motivated, unifies an apparently etherogeneous material which has been derived from my personal experience with electrical pacing of the heart.

It is a common opinion that a patient with an artificial pacemaker must be periodically examined in highly specialized centers which need to be equipped with highly sophisticated machinery. This may be true only for some electrinic parameters, which represent the least important part of the periodical examination of a pacemaker function. The centralized control of patients with artificial pacemakers may be useful for research studies and statistical analysis, but it monopolizes the experience and may bring discomfort to the patient and to the doctor-patient relationship.

In the past few years the evolution of pacing modalities has been so rapid to leave many physicians uneasy when examining a patient with an artificial pacemaker. This fact may sometimes lead one to forget that a patient with a cardiac electrical prosthesis necessitates the same attentions and cures common to other heart patients.

A good knowledge of the different mechanisms of action of the most commonly used artificial pacemakers, the radiological examination of the patient, the use of provocative tests and, most of all, a careful analysis of an ECG tracing, are the basis of the routine control of an artificial pacemaker function and of its interaction with the patient's own rhythm. Pacemaker spikes are becoming familiar artifacts in the daily electrocardiography. It is, therefore, important to recognize a new "iatrogenic" artificial rhythm and separate it from a spontaneous one, to differentiate a symbiotic from a competitive rhythm and from those secondary to a pacemaker malfunction.

This volume presents and discusses the most commonly used pacing modalities: the Asynchronous Pacemaker, the P-wave synchronous Pacemaker, and the "Demand" Pacemaker, in both varieties: QRS-synchronous and QRS-inhibited. Since an official and universally accepted terminology is not yet available, it is possible to find the term "stand-by" and "demand", used in a slightly different way by other Authors. To avoid semantic confusions in this book they are synonymous and refer to both QRS-synchronous and QRS-inhibited type of units. However, the terminology and an individual familiarity with the multitude of commercially available stimulators, are not very important. What is necessary is that the reader understands the fundamental electrophysiologic differences between pacing modalities. Because of the great usefulness of visual aids in teaching, the illustrations are the essential part of this book. The ECG strips are lifesize and are accompanied by appropriate ladder diagrams. They offer a panoramic vision of this new aspect of cardiology and will guide in the discovery of the mechanism of action of artificial pacemakers and their interaction with spontaneous cardiac rhythms.

The inevitable and rapid evolution of learning in this field limits the purpose of this publication. The dogmatic presentation of the contents is deliberate and wants to offer a guide to the beginner in this new field of cardiology. The Author is indebted to the Ciba Pharmaceutical Company for having allowed the reproduction of figures 6-A and 7-A of the volume "The Heart" from the Ciba Collection of Medical Illustrations.

ACKNOWLEDGMENTS

It gives me great pleasure to acknowledge my indebtedness to those who inspired and taught me:

Dr. Henry Zimmerman	Dr. John Lister
Dr. Serge Barold	Dr. Lawrence Cohen
Dr. Philip Samet	Dr. Henry Marriott
Dr. Onkar Narula	Dr. Louis Bruno
Dr. Joseph Linhart	

TABLE OF CONTENTS

THE ECG OF ARTIFICIAL PACEMAKERS

Chapter I

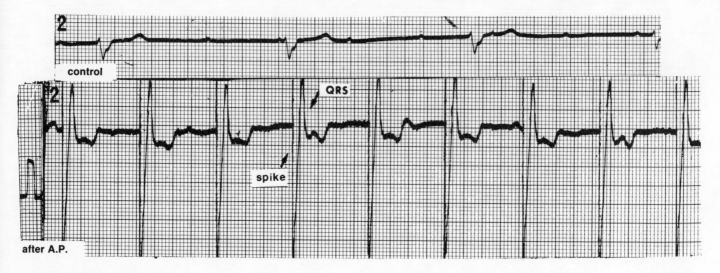

Fig. 1-A - Unipolar pacing. Notice the high amplitude, biphasic stimulus-artifact (spike) which alters the pacemaker QRS morphology.

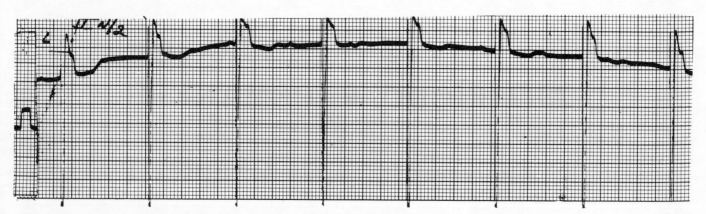

Fig. 1-B - Unipolar pacing. The spike has an amplitude of about 100 mV.

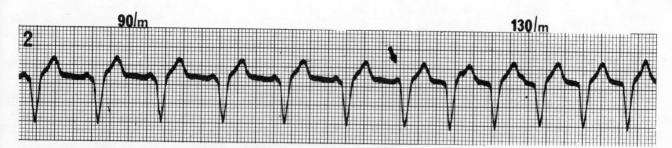

Fig. 1-C - Bipolar pacing. The increase of cardiac rate (from 90-130 beats/min.) is intentional through an increase of the artificial stimulation. Notice the lack of visibility of pacemaker spikes in L2 while the QRS morphology is clearly delineated.

THE STIMULUS-ARTIFACT (SPIKE)

The first step in the examination of an ECG of a patient with an artificial pacemaker (A.P.) is to recognize the *stimulus-artifact* or *spike* and to separate it from the corresponding ventricular response. The *stimulus-artifact* or *spike* recorded on the surface ECG appears as a sharp and clear deflection over the isoelectric baseline. Depending on whether the stimulation performed is of bipolar or unipolar type, the spike is very short in duration and quite different in amplitude. The great majority of artificial pacemakers (A.P.) available produce biphasic impulses with a duration of 1-2 msec. Therefore, the spike appears as a sharp vertical line when the ECG recording speed is the usual 25mm/sec. The spike of a unipolar stimulation usually has a remarkable amplitude (up to 100mV) and a biphasic configuration (fig. 1-A and 1-B), since the two poles are considerably distant from each other. Because of the short distance between the two poles, a bipolar spike is usually small, and at times may even be invisible in some leads. This is shown in L2 of Fig. 1-C where a ventricular pacing (90/m) simulates to perfection a spontaneous ventricular tachycardia. To demonstrate that the rhythm is artificially induced, the stimulation rate of the external pacer is intentionally increased in the second half of the tracing (130/m). The *amplitude* of the spike may vary from 1 to 100mV and does not give information on the amount of current applied to the heart. As explained later, it is only related to the dipole magnitude. The spike *direction* depends on the position of the stimulus-vector in relation to the particular ECG lead being recorded and must not be used in differentiating stimulation sites.

UNIPOLAR AND BIPOLAR PACING

The two systems are almost equivalent. Each one has its own features with advantages and disadvantages.

In *the unipolar stimulation* one electrode is in contact with the endocardium (or epicardium) and the "indifferent" electrode is located elsewhere in the body. In the *bipolar stimulation* both electrodes are in contact with the heart (epicardium or endocardium). Usually the indifferent electrode, which is always the positive one, is a metallic plate of the impulse generator in direct contact to the subcutaneous tissues of the pectoral or abdominal wall. The negative, stimulating electrode, is the tip of the catheter in direct contact either with the endocardium or the epicardium. The negative electrode is preferred as the stimulating pole because it appears that:

a) cardiac activation can be obtained with impulses of much lower intensity in a cathodic (negative) stimulation. To obtain the same results with anodic (positive) stimuli, it is necessary to use intensities 10-15 times higher.

b) the cathodic stimulation determines depolarization potentials similar to the spontaneous one.

The following paragraphs list some of the positive and negative aspects of unipolar and bipolar stimulation.

Unipolar Pacing

a) The epicardial implantation through a thoracotomy requires only one electrode on the heart and therefore decreases the chances of post-implant complications.

b) Since the indifferent electrode is far from the heart, the dipole is usually of considerable size and the resulting stimulus-artifact is usually more evident on the ECG than the one from a bipolar stimulation. Therefore, although the spike amplitude permits a better analysis of the pacemaker impulses it also partially obscures the morphology of the QRS which follows each impulse.

c) Because it involves a greater circuit area, the greater dipole of the unipolar system has the disadvantage of offering a wider penetration field to external electro-magnetic interference. This is especially true when demand pacemakers are used. External radiations have less influence on a bipolar system because of the small dipole and the narrower circuit.

Bipolar Pacing

a) A bipolar stimulation is usually applied in the emergency treatment of a conduction abnormality when urgent and reliable pacing is needed. With a bipolar pacing "the ventricular capture" (ventricular activation) can be obtained even if the tip of the catheter is in a non-perfect position (for example floating in the middle of the ventricular chamber). This can be accomplished by simply increasing the stimulus intensity. A perfect contact of the tip of the catheter with the endocardium is not as important for a bipolar as for the unipolar stimulation.

b) With a permanent pacemaker, the bipolar stimulation obtains an earlier stabilization of the cardiac excitability threshold and usually does so at lower levels.

c) If one of the cables or electrodes breaks down, there is another pole available and pacing can easily be transformed into the unipolar type.

d) With the bipolar system there seems to be a higher incidence of clot formation around the positive electrode. (This event, however, is rarely encountered in clinical practice.)

e) Bipolar stimulation offers a better electrophysiologic mechanism for the "re-entry phenomenon" and is accompanied by a higher incidence of ventricular arrhythmias. (This is also rarely encountered in clinical practice).

In short, there is not a clear-cut preference of one system over the other; patients with artificial pacemakers equally share the two stimulation techniques.

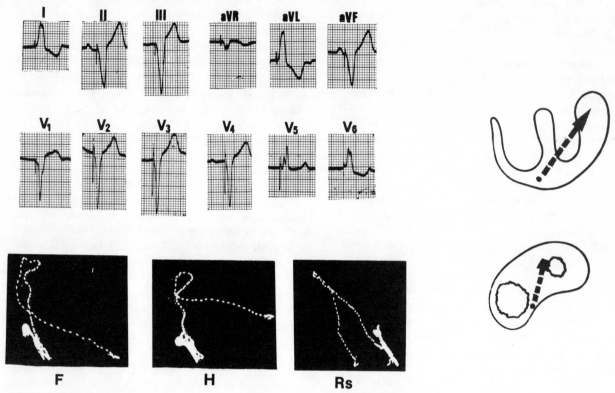

Fig. 2-A - Right ventricular pacing. The electrical axis is markedly deviated to the left and the QRS's have an LBBB morphology. The vectocardiogram shows QRS's oriented superiorly, to the left and posteriorly (F = frontal; H = horizontal; Sr = sagital rt.).

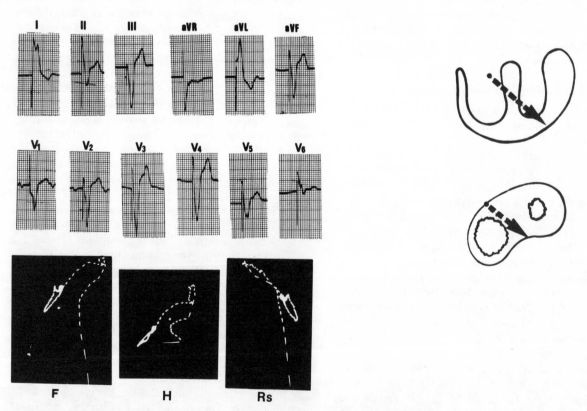

Fig. 2-B - Right ventricular pacing. The QRS's are of LBBB type but the electrical axis does not go beyond -30°. The direction of the electrical forces is counterclockwise and have a "figure of 8-inch configuration.

The morphology and spatial orientation of pacemaker-induced QRS complexes allow for a better location of the stimulation site than the analysis of the direction and amplitude of pacemaker spikes. QRS complexes induced by artificial impulses differ substantially from spontaneous supraventricular impulses normally conducted to the ventricles. A "pacemaker QRS" is due to an artificial impulse which *captures the ventricles*. Its morphology may vary according to the point of origin of ventricular activation as well as to the impulse propagation which does not follow the normal pathway of intraventricular conduction.

The morphology of a *pacemaker QRS* is always bizzare and anomalous compared to that of sinus beats. It resembles the morphology of ventricular extrasystoles or of supraventricular beat with left bundle branch (LBBB) or right bundle branch block (RBBB) patterns. The RBBB or LBBB morphology depends on whether the stimulation site is in the right or left ventricle.

RIGHT VENTRICULAR PACING

Right ventricular pacing performed at the apex (endo or epicardial) appears on the surface ECG as *QRS complexes with a left bundle branch block type configuration and it is usually associated with an electrical axis markedly deviated to the left* (between -30° and -90°). Right ventricular pacing = LBBB + LAD.

Since the right ventricle is the preferred site of stimulation, both for temporary and permanent pacemakers, this is the most commonly found ECG pattern. Therefore, when the tip of the catheter is in good contact with the endo or epicardium of the right ventricular apex, the right precordial leads (VI through V3) will record negative complexes of the QRS type. This indicates an activation front which goes away from those leads and is directed posteriorly and to the left.

The left axis deviation also suggests a propagation front from right to left and inferosuperior. This means it is from the apex to the postero-basal wall of the heart. V5 and V6 will usually record positive QRS complexes (figure 2-A and 2-B).

The vectocardiographic findings usually show a QRS loop spatially oriented posteriorly and to the left with a mean instantaneous vector directed either superiorly or inferiorly. A delay in the initial and terminal forces, with a left orientation, can be present in the efferent branch and in the terminal portion of the afferent branch of the QRS loop. The direction of forces can be clockwise, counterclockwise or, more frequently, may have a figure of S configuration.

The beginning of the QRS loop does not coincide with the point of origin of the stimulus-artifact. A transition between the spike and the beginning of a relatively slow ventricular activation is recognizable. Although it is particularly difficult to determine when the ventricular activation begins, it is thought that the rapid transition between the spike and the beginning of the myocardial activation is, in part, related to the biphasic characteristics of the stimulus-artifact. This is more evident in the unipolar stimulation.

The delay in the initial forces of the QRS loop, particularly evident with the use of epicardial electrodes, recalls to mind the Wolff-Parkinson-White syndrome. In both situations the initial vectorial changes are secondary to a "ventricular pre-excitation" which originates in one of the ventricles and spreads through non-specific muscular fibers. A common finding, in the vectocardiogram of right ventricular stimulation, is the presence of spatial opposition of QRS and ST-T loops. The ST-T loop may also show a delay in the terminal forces.

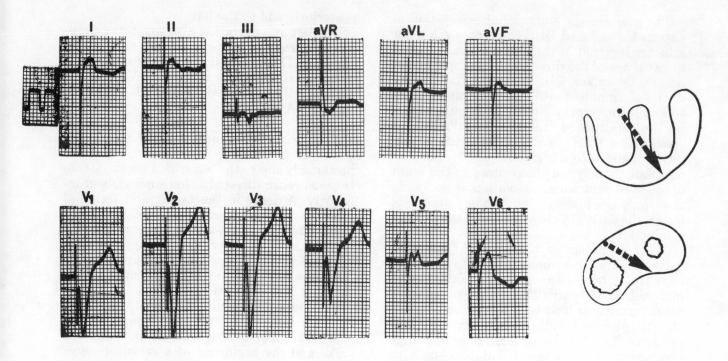

Fig. 3-A - Right ventricular pacing. The postero-basal position of the stimulating electrode determines QRS's of LBBB type but a normal electrical axis.

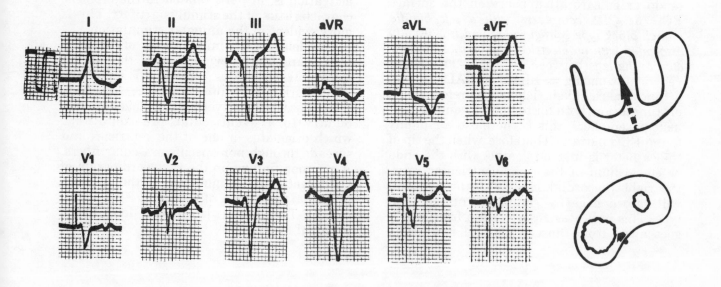

Fig. 3-B - Right ventricular pacing. The electrical axis is deviated to the left while V-5 and V-6 record predominately negative deflections.

Left axis deviation and QRS complexes with left bundle branch block configuration usually indicate a right apical stimulation. Occasionally, the tip of the intravenous catheter (or the implanted epicardial electrode) may not be in a perfect location at the right ventricular apex. For instance, it may be in closer contact with the wall of the inflow tract of the right ventricle (at the level of the tricuspid valve), or with the postero-basal wall or the pulmonary outflow tract. The electrical stimuli may determine QRS complexes with a left bundle branch block configuration but with a normal electrical axis.

The ECG of fig. 3-A is of a patient with a permanent pacemaker whose electrodes were implanted, after thoracotomy, in the postero-basal area of the right ventricle. The QRS complexes are of LBBB type and the electrical axis is within normal limits. The stimulus-artifact is of a unipolar type. The activation front propagates anteriorly and is particularly influenced by the supero-inferior position of the stimulating electrode.

A normal electrical axis, during right ventricular pacing, is a normal ECG finding. It indicates the site of the stimulating electrode in the postero-basal wall or in the pulmonary out-flow tract. In the latter situation, the tip of the intracavitary catheter is not very stable (compared with the more reliable apical site), and it calls for a closer observation of the patient. On the other hand a *sudden shift of the electrical axis from a left axis deviation to a normal axis is suggestive of a dislocation of the catheter tip from the right ventricular apex toward the tricuspid valve or the pulmonary outflow tract.*

Occasionally, it is possible to find patients with tracings similar to that of fig. 3-B. Here the surface ECG records QRS complexes with left bundle branch block (as it appears from L1 and aVL) while the left precordial leads are predominantly negative. The axis is deviated markedly to the left. Without a vectorcardiographic evaluation, it is difficult to locate the exact stimulation site from this tracing.

It must be kept in mind, that in the presence of a marked left axis deviation, either V6 or the X electrocardiographic plane may show predominantly negative deflection. This will indicate that the mean instantaneous vector in the frontal plane is oriented superiorly and to the right. The main forces, therefore, move away and superiorly from the X plane and the V5 and V6 leads. The patient of fig. 3-B had, in fact, a bipolar catheter in the right ventricular apex.

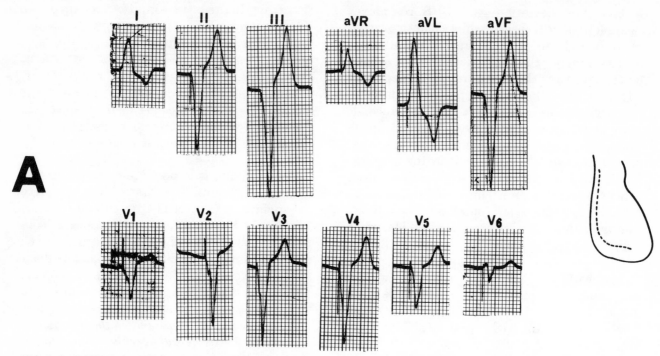

Fig. 4-A - Right ventricular pacing. The catheter tip is located at the apex of the right ventricle. The electrical axis is deviated to the left.

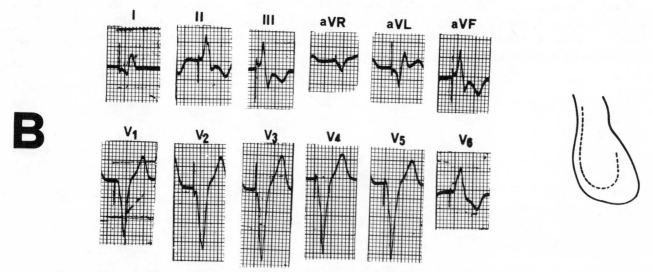

Fig. 4-B - Right ventricular pacing. Ventricular pacing starts in the septal wall of the pulmonary outflow tract. Notice the normalization of the electrical axis in the presence of QRS's of LBBB type.

A change in the electrical axis and in the QRS morphology (from one type of bundle branch block to another), is most of the time, due to a change of the stimulation site. Since endocardial stimulation is the preferred method of pacing and it is performed with catheters inserted into a cardiac chamber an axis shift may occasionally be found on serial ECG recordings. It must be kept in mind that on rare occasions, even right apical stimulation may determine QRS complexes very similar to those present when pacing the anterior wall of the left ventricle. Furthermore, the pacing of the anterior wall of the heart, on both sides of the intraventricular septum, may result in forces with a right and posterior orientation.

More often dislocation of the tip of the catheter into the right ventricular chamber may cause marked alteration of the QRS morphology and a shift of the electrical axis. This is shown in the tracings of fig. 4-A and 4-B which are taken from the same patient. The artificial stimulation is intentionally performed first at the apex of the right ventricle (A), and later in the outflow tract of the right ventricle (B).

During apical pacing (A), the surface ECG shows an electrical axis with a marked deviation to the left and QRS complexes with a left bundle branch block configuration. As it appears from L1 and AVL, the activation front is directed to the left and superiorly, while predominantly negative complexes are recorded in the left precordial leads.

When pacing is performed in the outflow tract of the right ventricle, just below the semilunar valves (B), a normalization of the electrical axis is obtained. The morphology of LBBB also becomes more evident.

These tracings show that it is necessary to proceed with caution in locating a site of stimulation when using only the examination of single frontal or precordial leads.

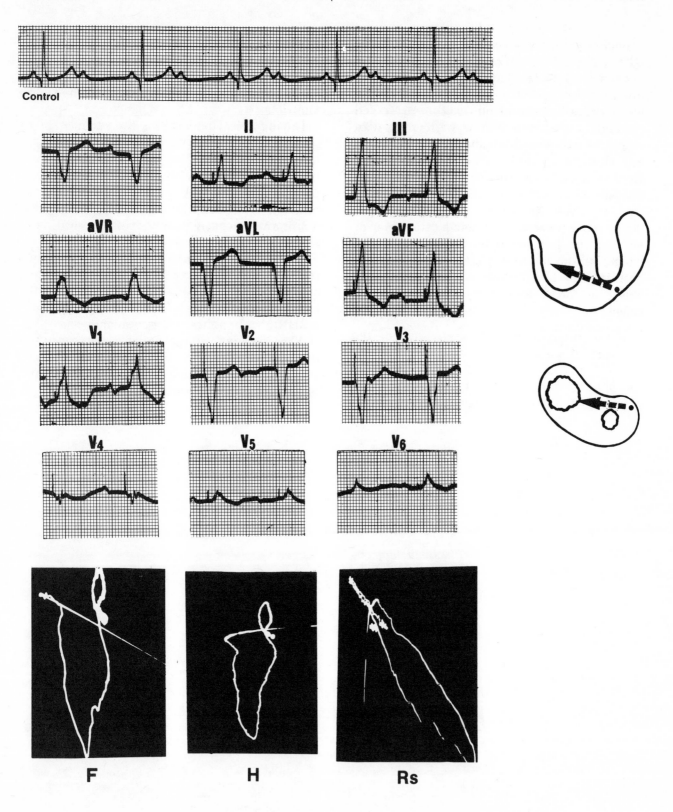

Fig. 5-A - Left ventricular pacing. The control tracing shows a second degree A-V block. The post-implant ECG shows an electrical axis deviated to the right and QRS complexes with a RBBB configuration (V1). The QRS loop is oriented to the right, anteriorly and inferiorly (F = frontal; H = horizontal; Sr = Sagital right).

LEFT VENTRICULAR PACING

Left ventricular pacing is usually performed through the implantation of one or two electrodes in the free left ventricular wall. The preferred area is usually the antero-lateral wall, along the line of bifurcation of the left coronary artery into the anterior descending and left circumflex branches.

The surface ECG usually shows a *QRS morphology of right bundle branch block type (RBBB) with a right axis deviation.*

Fig. 5-A shows a typical case of left ventricular pacing. The pre-implantation tracing shows a second degree A-V block, Mobitz Type II. The post-implantation ECG and the vectocardiogram show an asynchronous pacemaker with the stimulating electrodes implanted over the left ventricle.

The electrical axis is deviated to the right; the QRS complexes are negative in L1 and aVL, and positive in V1 and aVF. These findings indicate an activation front directed from left to right and supero-inferior. They also localize the stimulation site high in the left ventricle. Notice that the spatial orientation of the mean vector of the stimulus-artifact (spike) is of little help in localizing the stimulation site. The QRS loop can be oriented to the right, anteriorly (or posteriorly) and inferiorly. Sometimes a terminal forces delay may be present and the ventricular activation forces assume a clockwise rotation.

The anterior or posterior propagation of the activation forces is related to the site of implantation of the electrodes. This may be on the antero-lateral or postero-lateral wall of the left ventricle. Similarly, the frontal plane orientation of the QRS loop is related to an inferior or superior position of the electrodes. In general, the vectocardiographic picture is similar to that of a complete right bundle branch block (RBBB) associated with a right ventricular hypertrophy. This justifies the posteriorly oriented terminal delay.

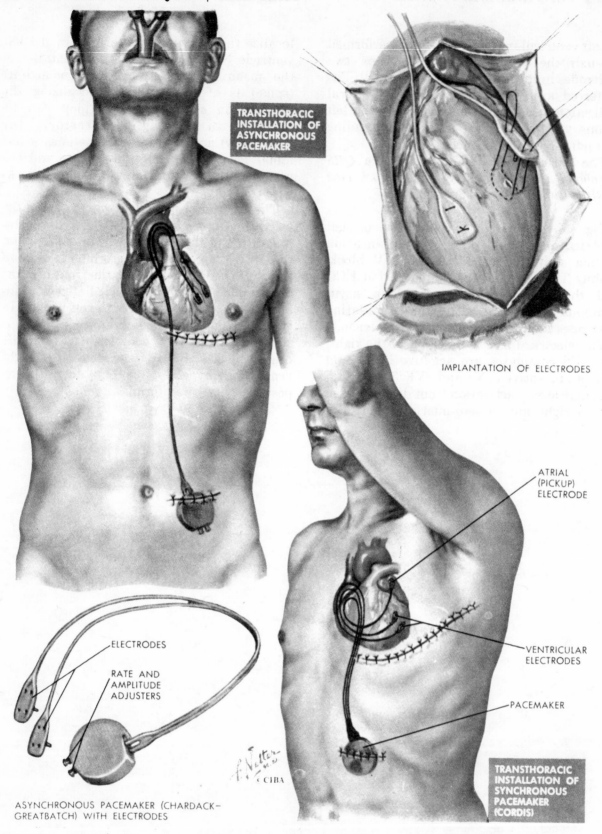

TRANSTHORACIC INSTALLATION OF ASYNCHRONOUS PACEMAKER

IMPLANTATION OF ELECTRODES

ELECTRODES

RATE AND AMPLITUDE ADJUSTERS

ASYNCHRONOUS PACEMAKER (CHARDACK–GREATBATCH) WITH ELECTRODES

ATRIAL (PICKUP) ELECTRODE

VENTRICULAR ELECTRODES

PACEMAKER

TRANSTHORACIC INSTALLATION OF SYNCHRONOUS PACEMAKER (CORDIS)

Fig. 6-A - Epicardial implantation of the electrodes through a transthoracic approach. See text.

The operative techniques for implantation of a permanent artificial pacemaker vary accordingly with the patient's age and the type of stimulator to be implanted. However, it is possible to distinguish two fundamental surgical approaches: a) epicardial implantation of the electrodes through a transthoracic route and, b) intracavitary insertion of the stimulating catheter through a venous route.

Thransthoracic Epicardial Implantation of Electrodes

This was the first technique used for direct stimulation of the heart in the therapy of complete A-V block (fig. 6-A). Except for the radio-frequency pacemaker, all other systems of artificial pacing have both the current generator and the stimulating electrodes implanted in the patient's body.

The number of electrodes to be sutured on the heart may vary from one to three depending on what type of pacemaker is selected for implantation. It is possible to find a fixed rate or a demand stimulator which uses only one electrode implanted on the heart while the second electrode (the indifferent electrode) is enclosed in the current generator. These are the *unipolar* systems where one pole is the cardiac electrode and the other is a metallic plate of the battery pack.

The *bipolar* type pacemaker, instead, requires the epicardiac implantation of two electrodes. The bipolar pacemakers vary from the "fixed rate" to several "demand" types.

In the case of a P-wave synchronous pacemaker, two or three electrodes are implanted. One of them (the *sensing* electrode of atrial potentials) is usually sutured on one of the atria. The *stimulating* electrode is sutured on the ventricular surface.

The ventricular electrode or electrodes are usually sutured in a cardiac area away from a main coronary artery. They may be installed on the lateral or postero-lateral wall or in the apical wall of the right or left ventricle. The electrode is located in relation to the type of thoractomy. This may be antero or postero-lateral, transdiaphragmatic or through a medial sternotomy. The pulse generator is usually implanted in a subcutaneous pocket in the axillary or abdominal wall depending upon the surgeon's preference.

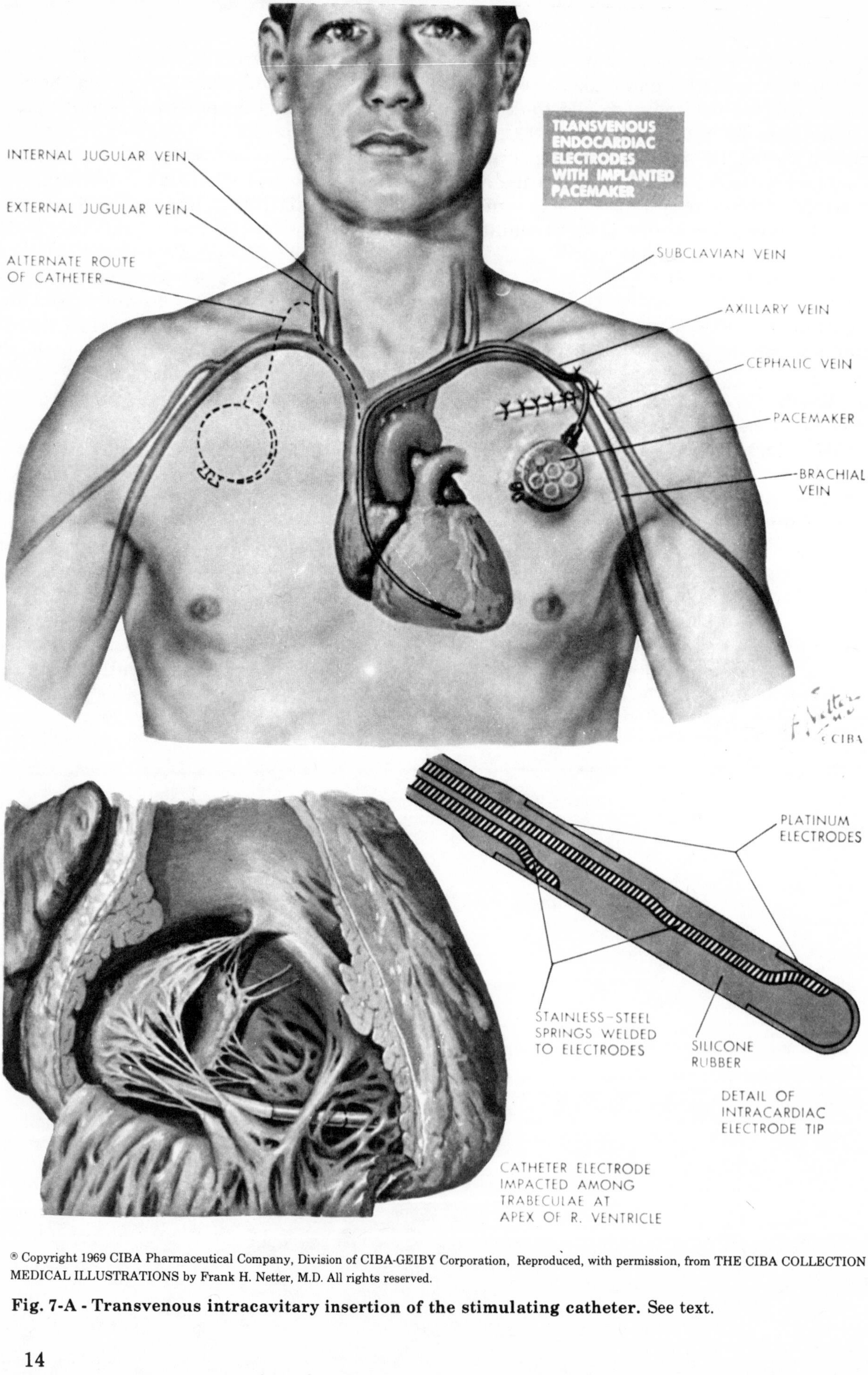

TRANSVENOUS
ENDOCARDIAC
ELECTRODES
WITH IMPLANTED
PACEMAKER

INTERNAL JUGULAR VEIN

EXTERNAL JUGULAR VEIN

ALTERNATE ROUTE
OF CATHETER

SUBCLAVIAN VEIN

AXILLARY VEIN

CEPHALIC VEIN

PACEMAKER

BRACHIAL
VEIN

PLATINUM
ELECTRODES

STAINLESS-STEEL
SPRINGS WELDED
TO ELECTRODES

SILICONE
RUBBER

DETAIL OF
INTRACARDIAC
ELECTRODE TIP

CATHETER ELECTRODE
IMPACTED AMONG
TRABECULAE AT
APEX OF R. VENTRICLE

Fig. 7-A - Transvenous intracavitary insertion of the stimulating catheter. See text.

OPERATIVE TECHNIQUES

Transvenous endocardial electrode

Once it was known that long periods of stable cardiac pacing were obtainable by placing a transvenous catheter into the apical trabeculae of the right ventricle, a new implantable generator-catheter stimulating system was introduced into clinical practice. This is the implantation technique most widely used today. The simplicity of this technique is based on the fact that the electrodes of a stimulating catheter are placed in contact with the right ventricular endocardium through a venous route (fig. 7-A). The main advantage of this technique is that it is relatively atraumatic because it does not require a thoractomy and a general anesthesia for the introduction of the electrodes.

The *generator* is essentially the same use in direct epicardial implantation. It is usually placed in a subcutaneous sac in the subclavicular or axillary area. The *catheter* has two platinum electrodes connected to stainless-steel springs which are immersed in silicone rubber and enclosed in a silastic tube.

The unipolar system has only one electrode at the tip of the catheter while the bipolar has a second ring electrode which is placed one or two centimeters from the tip. The catheter is usually introduced through one of the external or internal jugular veins or through a cephalic vein. It is then threaded under fluroscopic control into the right ventricular chamber until a stable position in the muscular trabeculae of the ventricular apex is obtained.

This implantation technique may be used with most stimulation systems, from the simplest "fixed rate" to the most sophisticated "demand" pacemakers. The exception is the P-wave synchronous pacemaker, which requires that an atrial sensing electrode be implanted on the atrial wall.

	Epicardial Implantation Of Electrodes	Endocardiac Insertion Of Electrodes
Thoractomy and general anesthesia necessary	Yes	No
Fluroscopy control necessary	No	Yes
Direct visualization of the electrodes implantation areas	Yes	No
Good electrodes contact	+	—
Operative mortality	+	—
Post-operative complications	+	—
Electrodes easy to reach in case of breakage	—	+
Preferred during open heart surgery complicated B; A-V block	+	—
Preferred in the treatment of A-V block of children	+	—
Preferred in the implantation of a P-wave synchronous pacemaker	+	—

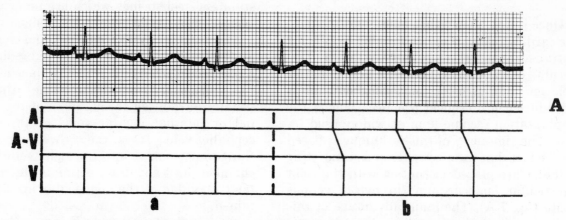

Fig. 8-A - Ladder diagram. A = atrial depolarization; A-V = conduction through the A-V junction; V = ventricular depolarization. Lines in section "a" of the diagram correspond to P waves and QRS complexes. In "b" they are connected by a diagonal line which indicates the A-V conduction.

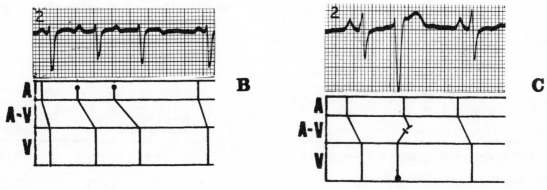

Fig. 8-B - Atrial extrasystoles.

Fig. 8-C - Ventricular extrasystole.

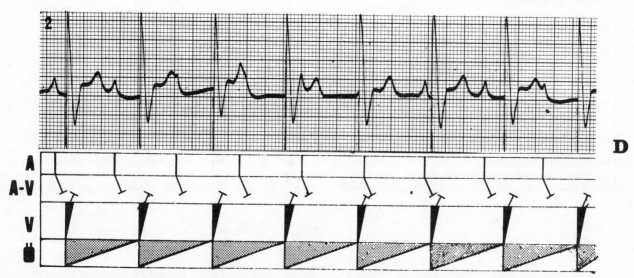

Fig. 8-D - Ladder diagram. Artificial pacemaker in the presence of a sinus rhythm with complete A-V block. The dotted area indicates the pacemaker recharging cycle.

This diagram, also called "Lewis lines," will be used to explain the mechanism of artificial pacemakers and the interaction between spontaneous and artificial rhythms. The classical format of a ladder diagram is presented in fig. 8-A. Each of the three spaces, A, A-V and V are separated by four horizontal lines which represent the conduction through the atrial and ventricular walls. These are diagrammed vertically below the ECG tracing. They must be accurately drawn so that line A coincides with the P-waves and line V with the QRS complex. During a normal sinus rhythm the atrial and ventricular depolarization is clearly shown on the ECG, while what occurs in the A-V junction is understood only in an indirect way.

Therefore, as a general rule, the P-waves and the QRS complexes (fig. 8-A...a) will be diagrammed first. When this is completed A's and V's will be connected and what occurs in the A-V junction will appear evident (diagonal lines). The direction in which the impulse travels will be obvious on the diagram when the atrial and ventricular activation lines are joined together (8-A...b). In the diagram a dot will be used to show the site of formation of ectopic impulses; a short bar at a right angle to the main line will indicate a block in impulse propagation.

Fig. 8-B presents a sinus rhythm interrupted by two atrial premature beats which show a progressive prolongation of the P^1-R interval (P^1 indicates an atrial depolarization wave of other than sinus origin).

The tracing of fig. 8-C shows a sinus rhythm with a ventricular premature beat (PVC). The impulse originating from the ventricles is blocked during the retrograde journey in the A-V junction. The same thing happens to the simultaneous sinus impulse which finds the A-V junction in a refractory state (for the concealed penetration of the PVC).

To represent the mechanism of action of an artificial pacemaker, a horizontal line will be added below the V line. The new space will represent the mechanism of action of the artificial pacemaker. The shaded area shows the recharging time of the pacemaker.

The *ventricular capture*, (which means ventricular depolarization due to the artificial impulse), will be represented by two slightly diverging lines and a darkened area. This indicates the aberrant and anomalous intraventricular conduction of the artificially induced activation front.

Fig. 8-D shows an artificial pacemaker of the asynchronous type, stimulating the ventricles at a fixed rate of 75/min. Each impulse is followed by a complete ventricular capture. A sinus rhythm co-exists with the artificial stimulation. This is indicated by the clearly visible presence of P-waves. None of the sinus impulses are capable of reaching the ventricles due to the presence of a complete A-V block. On the other hand, after depolarizing the ventricles, the pacemaker impulses are blocked while traveling in a retrograde fashion through the A-V junction.

REFERENCES

Castellanos, A., Jr., Lemberg, L., Salhaniek, L., and Berkovits, B.V.: *Pacemaker Vectorcardiography*, Amer. Heart J., 75:6, 1968.

Danielson, G.K., Shebatai, R., and Bryant, L.R.: *Failure of Endocardial Pacemaker Due to Late Myocardial Perforation*, J. Thorac. Cardiovasc. Surg., 54:42, 1967.

Dekker, E., Buller, J., and Shuilenbur, R.M.: *Aids to Electrical Diagnosis of Pacemaker Failure*, Amer. Heart J., 70:739, 1965.

Lister, J.W., Klotz, D.H., Jomain, S.L., Stuckey, J.H., and Hoffman, B.F.: *Effects of Pacemakers's Site on Cardiac Output and Ventricular Activation in Dogs with Complete Heart Block*, Amer. J. Cardiol., 14:494, 1964.

Mower, M.M., Aranaga, C. and Tabatznik, B.: *Unusual Patterns of Conduction Produced by Pacemaker Stimuli*, Amer. Heart J., 74:24, 1967.

Sodi Pallares, D., and Calder, R.M.: *New Bases of Electrocardiography*, St. Louis, The C. V. Mosby Co., 1956.

Barker, P.S., McLeod, A.G., and Alexander, J.: *The Excitatory Process Observed in the Exposed Human Heart*, Am. Heart J., 5:720, 1930.

Duchosal, P.W., and Sulzer, R.: *La Vectorcardiographie*, Basel, 1949, S. Karger AG.

Donzelot, E., Milanovich, J.B., and Kaufman, H.: *Etudes Practiques de Vectorgraphic*, Paris, 1950, L'Expansion Scientifique Française.

Massie, E., and Walsh, T.: *Clinical Vectorcardiography and Electrocardiography*, Chicago, 1960, Year Book Medical Publishers.

Barold, S. Serge, Narula, Onkar, S., Javier, Roger, P., Linhart, Joseph, W., Lister, John, W., and Samet, Philip: *Significance of Right Bundle-branch Block Patterns During Pervenous Ventricular Pacing*, Brit. Heart J., 1969.

Frank, E.: *An Accurate, Clinically Practical System of Spatial Vectorcardiography*, Circulation, 13:737, 1956.

Grant, R.P.: *Left Axis Deviation. An Electrocardiographic Pathologic Correlation Study*, Circulation, 14:233, 1956.

Siddons, H., and Sowton, E.: *Cardiac Pacemakers*, Springfield, Illinois, Charles C. Thomas, Publisher, 1967.

Furman, S., Escher, D.J.W., Solomon, N., and Schwedel, J.B.: *Implanted Transvenous Pacemakers*, Ann. Surg., 164:465, 1966.

Siddons, H., and Davies, J.G.: *A New Technique for Internal Cardiac Pacing*, Lancet, 2:1204, 1963.

Center, S., Castillo, A.A., and Keller, W.: *Permanent Pervenous Synchronous Pacing of the Heart*, Ann. Thorac. Surg., 4:218, 1967.

Weirich, W.L., Gott, V.L., and Lillehei, C.W.: *The Treatment of Complete Heart Block by the Combined Use of a Myocardial Electrode and an Artificial Pacemaker*, Surg. Forum, 8:360, 1957.

Chardack, W.M., Gage, A.A., and Greatbatch, W.: *A Transistorized Self-contained, Implantable Pacemaker for the Long Term Correction of Complete Heart Block*, Surgery, 48:643, 1960.

Hunter, S.W., Roth, N.A., Bernardez, D., and Noble, J.L.: *A Bipolar Myocardial Electrode for Complete Heart Block*, J. Lancet, 79:506, 1959.

Guilmet, D., Piwnica, A., and Pedeferri, G.: *Implantation d'un Stimulateur Cardiaque Interne par Sternotomie Mediane Verticale*, Ann. Chir. Thorac. Cardiov., 3:443, 1964.

Parsonnet, V., Gilbert, L., Zucker, I.R., and Assifi, I.: *Subcostal Transdiaphragmatic Insertion of Cardiac Pacemaker*, J. Thorac. Cardiov. Surg., 49:739, 1965.

Furman, S., Escher, D.J.W., Schwedel, J.B., and Hurwitt, E.S.: *Rechargeable Pacemaker for Direct Myocardial Implantation*, Arch. Surg., 91:796, 1965.

Silver, A.W., Root, G., Byron, F.X., and Sandberg, H.: *Externally Rechargeable Cardiac Pacemaker*, Ann. Thorac. Surg., 1:380, 1965.

Carlens, E., Johansson, L., Karlof, I., and Lagergren, H.: *New Method for Atrial-triggered Pacemaker Treatment without Thoracotomy*, J. Thorac. Cardiov. Surg., 50:229, 1965.

Greatbatch, W.: *Electrochemical Polarization of Physiological Electrodes*, Med. Res. Engin., 6:13, 1967.

Fisch, C.: *Pacemaker Electrocardiography. II*, J. Indian Med. Ass., 62:1028, 1969.

Kaiser, G.C., Barner, H.B., Willman, V.L., and Hanlon, C.R.: *Electrocardiographic Manifestation of Cardiac Pacing*, Missouri Med., 66:101, 1969.

Rosenbaum, M.B., and Lepeschkin, E.: *Bilateral Bundle Branch Block*, Amer. Heart J., 50:38, 1955.

Rosenbaum, M.B., Elizari, M.V., Lazzari, J.O., Nau, G.J., Levi, R.J., and Halpern, M.S.: *Intraventricular Trifascicular Blocks. Review of the Literature and Classification*, Amer. Heart J., 78:450, 1969.

Rosenbaum, M.B., Elizari, M.V., Lazzari, J.O., Nau, G.J., Levi, R.J., and Halpern, M.S.: *Intraventricular Trifascicular Blocks. The Syndrome of Right Bundle Branch Block with Intermittent Left Anterior and Posterior Hemiblock*, Amer. Heart J., 78:306, 1969.

Chou, T., and Helm, R.A.: *Clinical Vectorcardiography*, New York, Grune and Stratton, 1967.

Chapter II

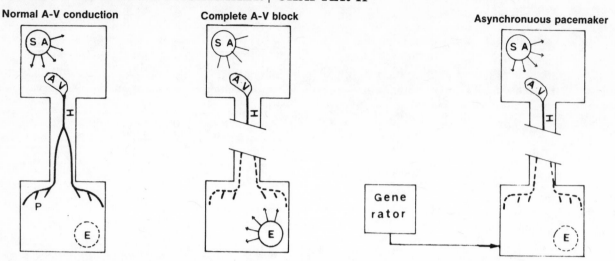

Fig. 9-A - **Asynchronous pacemaker in complete A-V block.** S-A = sino-atrial node; A-V = atrio-ventricular node; H = His bundle; P = Purkinje fibers; E = ectopic ventricular focus.

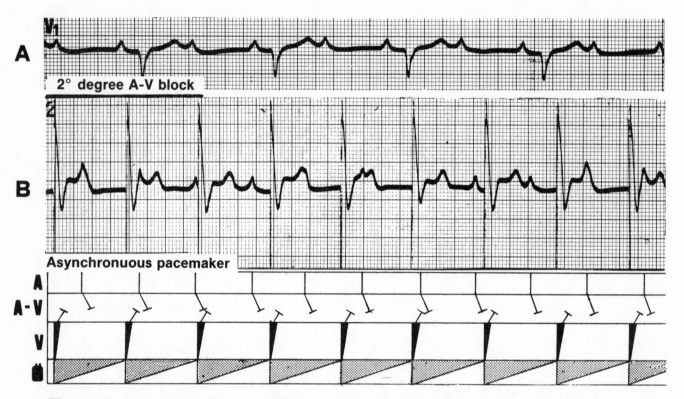

Fig. 9-B - **Asynchronous pacemaker.** "Fixed rate" ventricular pacing dissociated from a sinus rhythm.

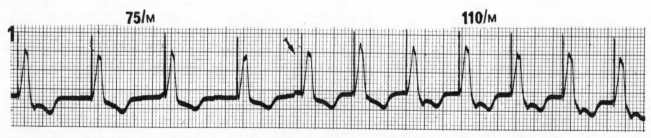

Fig. 9-C - **Asynchronous pacemaker.** Pacing is temporary and the rate is intentionally increased from 75/min. to 100/min.

THE ASYNCHRONOUS PACEMAKER

The asynchronous pacemaker was the first electrical prosthesis. It is still widely used, usually in the treatment of second and third degree A-V block, with bradycardic subsidiary pacemakers of either junctional or idioventricular origins.

The electronics of this artificial system is elementary (fig. 9-A). It consists of a simple current generator, without the complicated circuits, amplifiers and filters which make up the skeleton of the more complex "demand pacemaker" (see page 47).

An asynchronous pacemaker delivers impulses and stimulates the ventricles at a fixed, predetermined rate, usually between 55 and 80 beats per minute. It does not sense spontaneous cardiac potentials or other potentials of external origin.

Tracing A of fig. 9-B shows a patient with a second degree A-V block, Mobitz Type II, before artificial stimulation with an asynchronous pacemaker. Tracing B shows a "fixed rate" ventricular stimulation at 75/min., with *complete ventricular capture*. As it is shown by the P-P intervals, the atrial rhythm is still under sinus control. Its rate is 90/min. and is not very different from the pre-implantation rate. The sinus P waves and the artificially induced QRS complexes are independent and dissociated.

The rate of ventricular stimulation is constant, regular, preselected at the moment of implantation and is not altered by varying physiological demands. Therefore, this type of unit is also called a *"fixed rate pacemaker"*.

A certain confusion in terminology may arise when discussing asynchronous pacemakers. Some manufacturers supply asynchronous pacemakers whose "fixed rate" may, in particular clinical situations, be changed with a special external manipulation into a faster "fixed rate," to better comply with higher physiological requests. It is therefore useful to classify the Asychronous Pacemaker in two varieties:

a) *Fixed rate asynchronous pacemaker:* once implanted it is impossible to change the "fixed" stimulation rate of this unit into a faster one.

b) *Variable rate asynchronous pacemaker:* The stimulation rate of this unit may be increased following an increased cardiac output demand due to fever, exercise, increased metabolism, or hypotension. Depending on the manufacturer, the rate may be changed through one of the following external manipulations: 1) by inserting a percutaneous needle at a particular place of the generator. 2) by a coupling with an external magnetic switch placed on the skin overlying the generator. 3) by using a radio-frequency transmitter.

For example, cardiac pacing can be changed from a fixed rate of 60/min. to a different fixed rate of 80/min., and vice versa. It is obvious that this type of pacemaker, whatever the technique used for changing the rate, must be electronically more complex. It follows that the incidence of malfunction of a variable rate device is much higher than when using a fixed rate asynchronous pacemaker.

External asynchronous pacemakers which are used for temporary pacing are obviously all of the "variable rate" type. The rate is easily regulated with an external knob. This is shown in fig. 9-C where the temporary stimulation rate of an external pacemaker is intentionally increased from 75/min. to 100/min. (The transition is indicated by the arrow.)

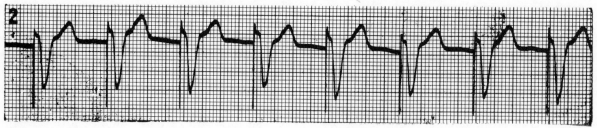

Fig. 10-A - Asynchronous pacemaker. Regular ventricular pacing and absence of atrial activity.

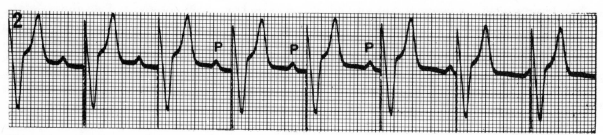

Fig. 10-B - Asynchronous pacemker. "A-P dissociation" (atrio-pacemaker). Sinus P-waves and pacemaker QRS's are independent and dissociated.

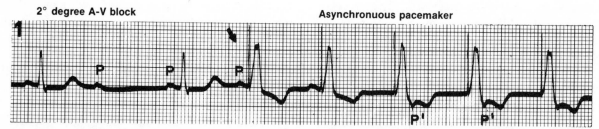

Fig. 10-C - Asynchronous pacemaker. Second degree A-V block. The artificial ventricular pacing shows a normal V-A (ventriculo-atrial) conduction. P^1 waves follow each pacemaker QRS.

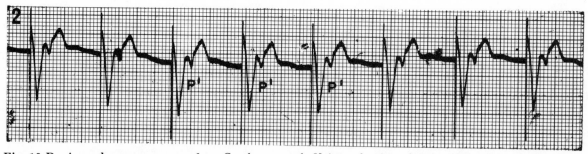

Fig. 10-D - Asynchronous pacemaker. Good retrograde V-A conduction of the artificial impulses with complete ventricular and atrial (P^1) activation.

Fig. 10-A belongs to a patient with an asynchronous pacemaker. From L2 alone it is difficult to determine whether the stimulation is of a unipolar or a bipolar type. It is possible, though, to recognize regular impulses with a rate of 75/min., each with good *ventricular capture*. Each artificial impulse is followed by a bizarre and anomalous QRS complex (QRS duration = 0.15 sec.).

Atrial activity (P or P1 waves) is not recognizable in this tracing. This indicates that, if present, the sinus rhythm must be very slow and that occasional P waves must be buried into the wide and bizarre QRS complexes.

Fig. 10-B shows a fixed rate pacing (rate = 73/min.) with a good and complete ventricular capture. Sinus P waves are easily recognized and their rhythm is independent and dissociated from the artificially induced rhythm. This situation is frequently encountered with the use of asynchronous pacemakers. When its rate is not too slow, the sinus rhythm may remain unchanged after the implant of a pacemaker. This may determine the so called *A-P dissociation* (atria-pacemaker dissociation) between the atrial depolarization (controlled by the S-A node) and that of the ventricles (controlled by the pacemaker).

Patients with abnormalities of the anterograde A-V conduction may have a normal retrograde ventriculo-atrial (V-A) conduction. This is usually found in all types of A-V block (first, second and third degree).

The tracing of fig. 10-C shows the beginning of a fixed rate ventricular pacing (75/min.), in a patient with a second degree A-V block Mobitz Type II. Sinus P waves are easily recognized in the first part of the tracing (rate equals 80/min.) while the ventricular rate (38/min.) is halved by the presence of a second degree A-V block. With the beginning of the artificial stimulation (arrow) the ventricular rate is almost doubled. Beginning with the third pacemaker induced QRS complex, it is possible to identify small and biphasic P1 waves. These indicate a retrograde penetration of the artificial impulse through the A-V junction and a retrograde activation of the atria (see page 156).

Therefore, the pacemaker stimuli "capture" both the ventricles and the atria, traveling backward through an A-V junction which shows a decreased forward conduction (second degree A-V block). The ventriculo-atrial (V-A) conduction time can be measured. It goes from the beginning of the pacemaker QRS to the beginning of the P1 waves. In this tracing it is within normal limits (0.16 sec.). Normal values fluctuate between 0.16 - 0.20 seconds. When it is prolonged it indicates a *retrograde V-A block*.

A "fixed rate" pacing (78/min.) is presented in fig. 10-D. Each QRS complex is followed by an obvious negative P1 wave. Also in this case the patient was treated for a complete A-V block. The retrograde V-A conduction time is normal and the atrial activation is under control of the artificial pacemaker.

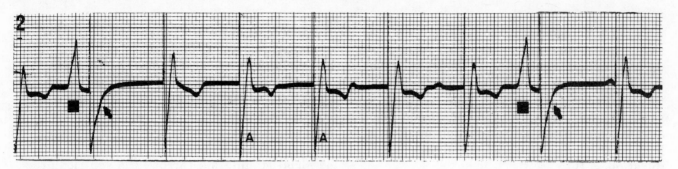

Fig. 11-A - Asynchronous pacemaker. Competition. The presence of ventricular extrasystoles (dark squares) does not disturb the regular pacemaker time-table. The impulses following the extrasystoles are not effective because they fall in the absolute ventricular refractory phase. Arrows indicate the "voltage-decay curves."

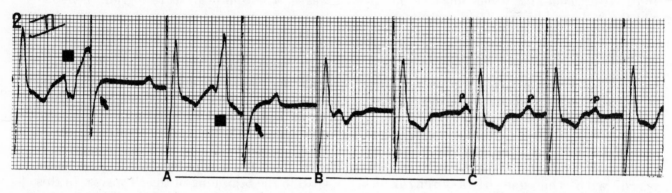

Fig. 11-B - Asynchronous pacemaker. Competition. Multifocal ventricular extrasystoles (dark squares) are followed by ineffective stimuli. Notice the voltage-decay curves (arrows) of the large amplitude unipolar impulses. The compensatory pause is complete (AB = BC).

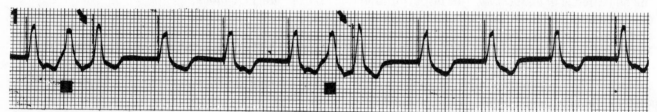

Fig. 11-C - Asynchronous pacemaker. Competition. Ventricular extrasystoles (dark squares) are interpolated and "sandwiched" between two artificial beats. The impulse which follows the extrasystole captures the ventricles during the excitability phase.

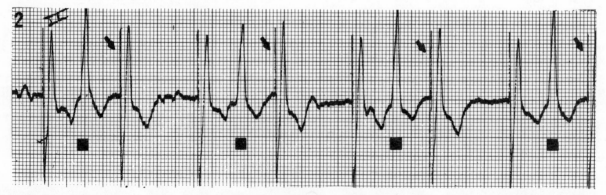

Fig. 11-D - Asynchronous pacemaker. Competition. The "interpolated bigeminy" is formed by two pacemaker beats and a ventricular extrasystole.

THE ASYNCHRONOUS PACEMAKER

The competition

The main disadvantage of an asynchronous pacemaker is its inability of sensing spontaneous cardiac potentials either of ventricular or of supra-ventricular origin. Spontaneous rhythms are not a rarity in patients with artificial pacemakers because:

a) many patients with Adam-Stokes seizures are in sinus rhythm at the moment of implantation of a pacemaker;

b) a sinus rhythm with a normal A-V conduction may reappear after some time in patients with A-V block who are being treated with artificial pacing;

c) any type of arrhythmia may arise during artificial stimulation (atrial or ventricular extrasystoles, atrial flutter or fibrillation, etc.).

These units do not have a *sensing mechanism,* of perception of cardiac potentials. Therefore they continue undisturbed to deliver impulses at a fixed rate, pre-selected at the moment of implantation, even in the presence of spontaneous QRS's. This creates the so-called *competition* between the artificial and the spontaneous pacemakers. The rhythms that follow are called *competitive rhythms*.

Fig. 11-A shows a fixed rate stimulation (73/min.) of an asynchronous pacemaker. Two ventricular extrasystoles are present (dark squares). These extrasystoles are not sensed by the artificial pacemaker which continues undisturbed to deliver stimuli according to its own time-table. Although they fall immediately after the extrasystoles (arrows) the impulses do not induce a ventricular response. Since they "land" during the absolute ventricular refractory period which follows the extrasystole, they are unable to "capture" the ventricles. It can be noted that the ineffective stimuli are followed by a prevalent negative deflection (arrows) quite different from the pacemaker QRS complexes. (Pacemaker automatic beats = A).

A base line deflection, induced by pacemaker stimuli which otherwise are not effective on the cardiac excitability, is typical of the unipolar stimulation. It is also present during a bipolar stimulation but the amplitude is so small as to be invisible on the ECG tracing. It may be either negative or positive, according to the lead being recorded and it represents a *voltage decay curve* which is an exponential curve of loss of voltage. It is also present when stimuli capture the ventricles and induces the noticeable QRS distortion which follows unipolar artificial impulses.

The decay curve artifact is particularly evident during unipolar pacing, because of the greater dipole between the stimulating and the indifferent electrodes, and it is mainly evident in those leads parallel to the decay curve vector. The decay curve must not be misinterpreted as a pacemaker QRS complex. A comparison between a decay curve (arrow) and a stimulus followed by "ventricular capture" is helpful in avoiding confusion.

Fig. 11-B shows another example of competition between the artificial impulses of an asynchronous pacemaker (rate 72/min.) and multifocal ventricular extrasystoles. The extrasystoles (dark squares) have opposite QRS morphologies. In both cases the following artificial impulse is not effective because it lands within the T wave of the extrasystoles, while the ventricles are still refractory. The voltage decay curves of the ineffective impulses (arrows) are very obvious. The pacing is of a unipolar type and the sinus rhythm (P-P intervals) is not disturbed by what happens into the ventricles (A-P dissociation).

In figures 11-A and 11-B, the *competitive rhythm* is determined by: a) the ventricular extrasystoles which prematurely interrupt the regular rhythm of the pacemaker and b) by the *complete compensatory pauses* (AB = BC) induced by the extrasystoles, since the impulses immediately following are not capable of capturing the ventricles (arrows).

When the artificial impulse "lands" far enough from the preceding extrasystole, it finds the ventricles in a normal excitability phase and therefore it may determine a propogated response. This is presented in fig.11-C where ventricular extrasystoles (dark squares) are "sandwiched" between two pacemaker QRS's. The artificial impulses following the extrasystoles (arrows) fall very late on the terminal portion of the extrasystolic T waves. They capture the ventricles which are repolarized and therefore are again excitable (see page 145).

An *interpolated bigeminy* is present in figure 11-D, where artificial stimuli (arrows) fall far enough from the preceding extrasystole (dark squares). Therefore, they land during the normal ventricular excitability phase. (The pacemaker QRS's preceding and following the extrasystoles are identical.)

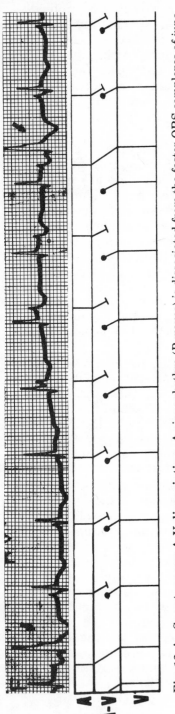

Fig. 12-A - Spontaneous A-V dissociation. A sinus rhythm (P waves) is dissociated from the faster QRS complexes of junctional origin. The arrows indicate the sinus impulses which cross the A-V junction and capture the ventricles (escape beats with ventricular capture; also called **escape capture beats.**)

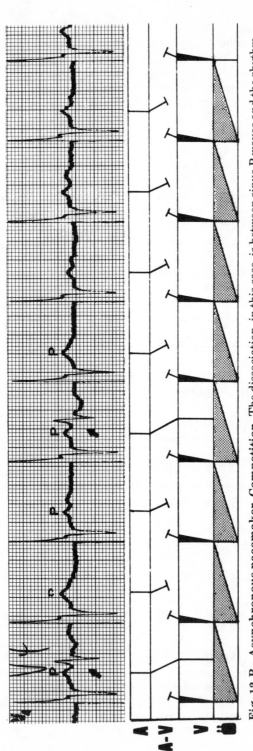

Fig. 12-B - Asynchronous pacemaker. Competition. The dissociation, in this case, is between sinus P waves and the rhythm induced by the pacemaker. Competitive beats are indicated by the arrows ("escape capture beats").

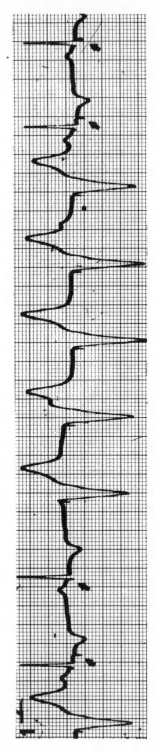

Fig. 12-C - Asynchronous pacemaker. Competition. The beats which "compete" with the pacemaker are of sinus origin and have a normal A-V conduction. Notice the small pacemaker spikes indicated by the arrows (bipolar stimulation). They fall during the ventricular refractory phase and, therefore, are not effective.

The competition

As mentioned previously, the presence of a sinus rhythm, independent and dissociated from that of an asynchronous pacemaker, is not a rarity. In such a situation a complete A-V block is usually present, and while the atria remain under sinus control, the ventricles beat through the artificial stimulator.

The most common cause of *competition* between a spontaneous rhythm and that of a pacemaker is the restoration of a normal A-V conduction in patients with A-V block at the moment of implantation. This situation is not rare and is present in almost 30% of patients treated with artificial pacing. Other causes of competition are represented by patients with sinus rhythm and normal A-V conduction, patients with intermittent A-V blocks at the moment of implantation of the asynchronous pacemaker, and patients exhibiting the so-called "super-normal conduction." (see page 159.)

When sinus impulses go through the A-V junction and reach the ventricles they "compete" with pacemaker beats. For a better understanding, it is useful to compare this iatrogenic phenomenon with a natural and extraordinary similar situation, the so-called "A-V dissociation with escape capture beats."

Figure 12-A shows a junctional rhythm dissociated from a slower sinus rhythm. When sinus P waves land far enough from the preceding and dissociated QRS complexes, they cross the A-V junction and capture the ventricles (arrows). These ventricular contractions of sinus origin, during an A-V dissociation, are called "escape beats with ventricular capture," or, briefly, "escape capture beats." Other P waves cannot cross the A-V junction because they find it refractory after the conduction of those junctional impulses which cause the A-V dissociation.

The examination of the tracing and of the diagram of fig. 12-B shows regular impulses from an asynchronous pacemaker with a rate of 73/min. Sinus P waves are also easily recognized. The sinus rhythm has a rate slightly slower (70/min.) than that of the artificial pacemaker. While the great majority of P waves are blocked, two of them are capable of crossing the A-V junction (arrows). This creates a situation altogether similar to the one illustrated in fig. 12-A, and, therefore, determines *escape beats with ventricular capture*, or "escape capture beats." The escape beats do not disturb the artificial pacemaker which continues to deliver regular impulses according to its own time-table. They are "sandwiched" between two pacemaker beats.

A similar situation is presented in fig. 12-C. In this tracing four sinus beats cross the A-V junction and reach the ventricles. The first QRS and the central sequence of the five wide and bizarre beats, are pacemaker induced. The pacemaker delivers impulses at a fixed rate. When they fall immediately after the sinus QRS, however, they are not effective because they find the ventricles in the absolute refractory period. The spikes are merely visible (arrows) because the stimulation is of a bipolar type.

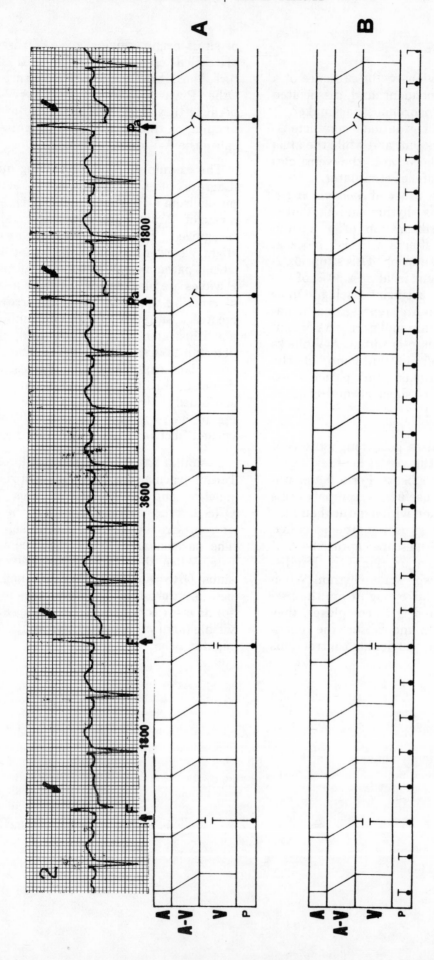

Fig. 13-A - Spontaneous ventricular parasystole. See text.

Iatrogenic pacemaker parasystole

Iatrogenic parasystoles are quite common in patients with asynchronous pacemakers. To illustrate this electrophysiologic situation it is useful to compare it with what happens spontaneously in a ventricular parasystole. One can then parallel the activity of a natural pacemaker with that of an artificial one and understand the definition of *iatrogenic pacemaker parasystole*.

"SPONTANEOUS VENTRICULAR PARASYSTOLE"

Ventricular parasystole is a strange phenomenon of electrical symbiosis where an ectopic focus, independent and protected, coexists and competes with a normal sinus rhythm. For this to happen it is necessary that one of the two pacemakers be immune to penetration from the other. The parasystolic focus, which operates side by side (para) to the primary cardiac pacemaker, is surrounded by a protective mechanism which makes it impenetrable from the invasion of sinus impulses.

In spontaneous ventricular parasystole, therefore, the ventricular ectopic focus delivers impulses in a regular and rhythmic fashion, undisturbed from sinus impulses. A classic example of ventricular parasystole is shown in the tracing of fig. 13-A.

The cardinal criteria for the diagnosis of this arrhythmia are:

a) the ventricular extrasystoles have *variable coupling intervals* (interval between the extrasystole and the preceding sinus beats);

b) the shortest *interectopic interval* (interval between two extrasystoles) must be a common denominator and therefore must easily divide the longer interectopic intervals;

c) presence of *fusion beats*. They are not essential for the diagnosis but, if present, they highly suggest the presence of a parasystolic focus.

In fig. 13-A, the parasystolic focus, with a rate of 36/min., coexists with impulses of sinus origin with a rate of 100/min. The coupling interval of the extrasystoles (interval with the preceding sinus beats) is variable. This suggests an independent mechanism, which means that the extrasystole does not have a cause-effect relation with the preceding sinus beat.

The mathematical relationship of the interectopic intervals is present with a common denominator of 1800 msec. The longest interectopic interval is twice (3600 msec.) the basic one. This suggests the presence of a protective mechanism or "entrance block" which prevents the interruption of the parasystolic rhythm. Fusion beats (F) are easily recognized. They are "hybrid" beats and their morphology is something in between that of sinus beats and that of the QRS of the parasystolic focus (Pa).

Therefore, the protective mechanism is the basic element of a spontaneous parasystole and is called "entrance block" or "protective block" (diagram A). The nature of this protective mechanism is not clear. The most common theory holds that an area of unidirectional block is present in the myocardial tissues surrounding the ectopic focus. This allows the exit of impulses from the ectopic focus but not its penetration from external sources (for ex. from impulses of sinus origin).

Others have recently suggested that parasystolic foci have an automaticity with a rate much higher than that recorded on the surface ECG. In other words, a parasystolic focus would conceal a potential ventricular tachycardia. The rapid depolarization and repolarization of the myocardial tissues surrounding the parasystolic focus would determine a physiologic refractory trench (entrance block) toward external stimuli, at the same time creating an "exit block." This explains the usually low parasystolic rates (30-60/min). For example, the automaticity of the parasystolic focus of fig. 13-A could be 180/min. This would determine a protective entrance mechanism. An exit block of 5:1, however, would produce a parasystolic rate of 36/min. (diagram B). This theory is interesting in that it is an electrophysiological attempt at explaining the entrance block. Furthermore, it agrees with the commonly acknowledged fact that ventricular parasystoles quite often degenerate in episodes of ventricular tachycardias.

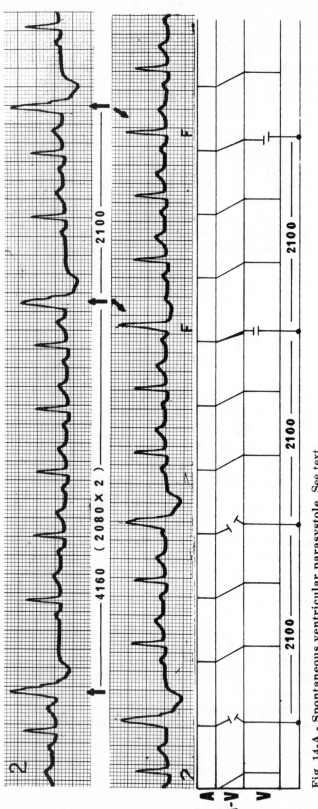

Fig. 14-A - Spontaneous ventricular parasystole. See text.

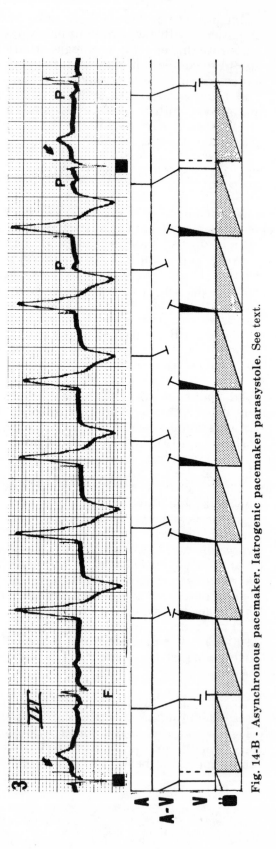

Fig. 14-B - Asynchronous pacemaker. Iatrogenic pacemaker parasystole. See text.

THE ASYNCHRONOUS PACEMAKER

Iatrogenic pacemaker parasystole

The tracings on the opposite page compare a spontaneous with an *iatrogenic ventricular parasystole*. The iatrogenic parasystole is due to an asynchronous pacemaker.

In fig. 14-A the sinus rhythm is punctuated by numerous ventricular extrasystoles which have variable coupling intervals with the preceding sinus beats. When the coupling interval becomes long enough and the extrasystoles fall immediately after the P wave, they show a morphology which is in between that of a sinus beat and that of a ventricular extrasystole. These are *ventricular fusion beats* (F).

The interectopic interval common denominator is 2100 msec. The longest interectopic interval (top tracing) is twice the basic interval. Therefore, all the criteria for the diagnosis of ventricular parasystole are present.

Fig. 14-B shows a central sequence of six pacemaker beats with complete ventricular capture. The stimulation rate is 75/min. Therefore, the interval between two QRS's is equal to 800 msec. The first and last QRS's are of sinus origin (dark squares). The pacemaker stimuli which follow the sinus QRS (arrows) do not determine a ventricular response. They fall into the absolute ventricular refractory period of the sinus beats which are conducted to the ventricles. The ineffective stimuli are outlined in the diagram.

Although they show a slightly different morphology, the second and the last QRS are both *ventricular fusion beats*. The ventricular depolarization is divided between the sinus impulse and the artificial stimulus, which falls immediately after the P wave (see diagram). The morphology of the fusion beats is the vectorial resultant of the amount of ventricular tissue depolarized from one or the other pacemaker. This explains the slight difference between the two fusion beats. The sinus rate can be easily determined by the last three P waves.

This tracing, therefore, satisfies all the requirements for the diagnosis of ventricular parasystole: a) interectopic interval common denominator; b) fusion beats, and c) a variable coupling interval of the pacemaker impulses with the preceding sinus beats. The peculiarity of this parasystolic focus is that it is not spontaneous, but it is induced by the human intervention with an artificial electrical source in the right ventricle (asynchronous pacemaker in the treatment of a complete A-V block). Therefore, the re-establishment of a sinus rhythm with a normal A-V conduction has created a new electrophysiologic situation called *iatrogenic ventricular parasystole*.

The iatrogenic parasystole, as the spontaneous one, is "protected" from the penetration of sinus impulses. The delivery of artificial impulses is undisturbed by the almost simultaneous sinus rhythm. The pacemaker follows quietly its own time-table which calls for an impulse every 800 msec. This occurs even when the ventricles are not excitable because they have been depolarized by the sinus impulse.

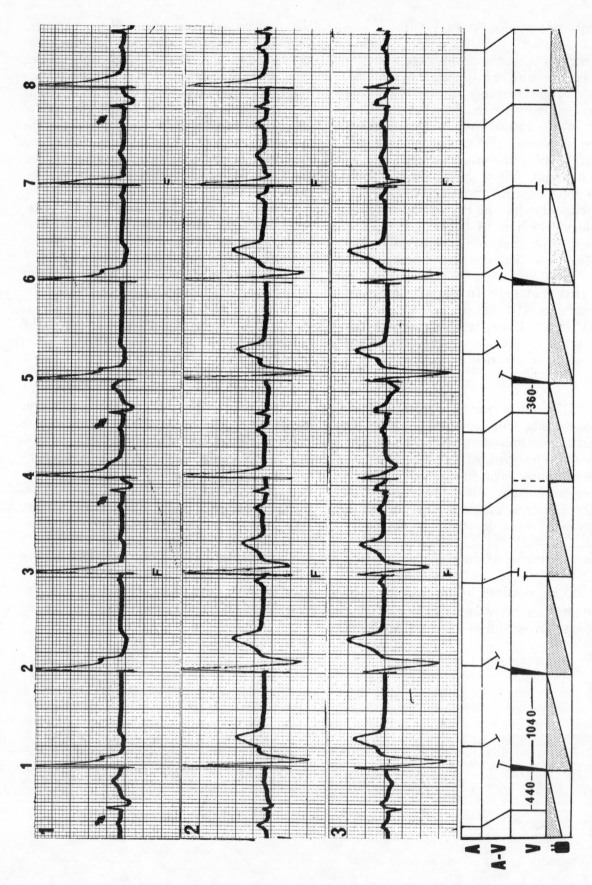

Fig. 15-A - Asynchronous pacemaker. Iatrogenic pacemaker parasystole.

THE ASYNCHRONOUS PACEMAKER

Iatrogenic pacemaker parasystole

The incidence of iatrogenic pacemaker parasystole is obviously related to the conduction capacity of the A-V junction. The higher the impairment of the A-V junction, the less the incidence of pacemaker parasystole. In complete A-V block this phenomenon cannot be present. In patients with sinus rhythm at the moment of implantation, and in those where a normal A-V conduction reappears sometime after pacing (even if a high degree of A-V block is present at the moment of implantation), the parasystole will commonly be observed.

Fig. 15-A shows another classic example of *iatrogenic parasystole* due to an *asynchronous pacemaker*. The three recorded leads are simultaneous. A fixed rate pacing is present with a rate of 58/min. (the interval between two stimuli equals 1040 msec). The artificial stimuli are numbered from 1 to 8. Furthermore, it is easy to recognize sinus beats which occasionally cross the A-V junction and activate the ventricles (top tracing arrows).

All the pacemaker impulses which fall beyond the absolute refractory period of the sinus beats depolarize the ventricles (first, second, fifth, and sixth impulse). The QRS morphology is the one typical of pacemaker beats with complete ventricular capture. The fourth and eighth impulses fall, instead, too close to the preceding QRS. Therefore, they do not elicit a propagated ventricular response (the non-effective stimuli are outlined in the diagram.) They only alter the isoelectric line because the pacing is unipolar. Here the voltage decay curve determines a deflection easily recorded on the surface ECG.

The examination of the *vector of the artifact-decay curve* of beat N.4 and N.8 (not of the spike! see page 25) shows that it is predominantly positive in all three leads. The vector on the frontal plain is equal to +70. Since this vector is directed from the generator to the intracardiac electrode, it is possible to determine the generator site. In this case the generator must be in the right pectoral area. (The examination of the axis of the decay curve on the frontal plane allows one to recognize the indifferent electrode site and, therefore, the location of the generator.)

The third and seventh stimuli determine QRS complexes with a morphology in between that of pacemaker beats with complete ventricular capture and that of sinus beats conducted to the ventricles. These are *ventricular fusion* beats (F). The ventricles are depolarized partly by the sinus impulse and partly by the almost simultaneous artificial impulse.

The different configuration of fusion beats is the vectorial resultant of the amount of ventricular myocardium activated by one or the other stimuli. In the first of the two fusion beats (N.3), ventricular activation is in great part, determined by the artificial impulse and only in a small part from the sinus impulse. In the other fusion beat (N.7), the situation is exactly the opposite (see diagram).

The *coupling interval,* which is the interval between a pacemaker beat and the preceding sinus QRS, is variable from 360 to 440 msec. and it suggests a complete independence of the two pacemakers.

The artificial pacemaker is "protected" from sinus impulses and it delivers impulses according to its own time-table, undisturbed from the sinus rhythm (interectopic interval of 1040 msec.).

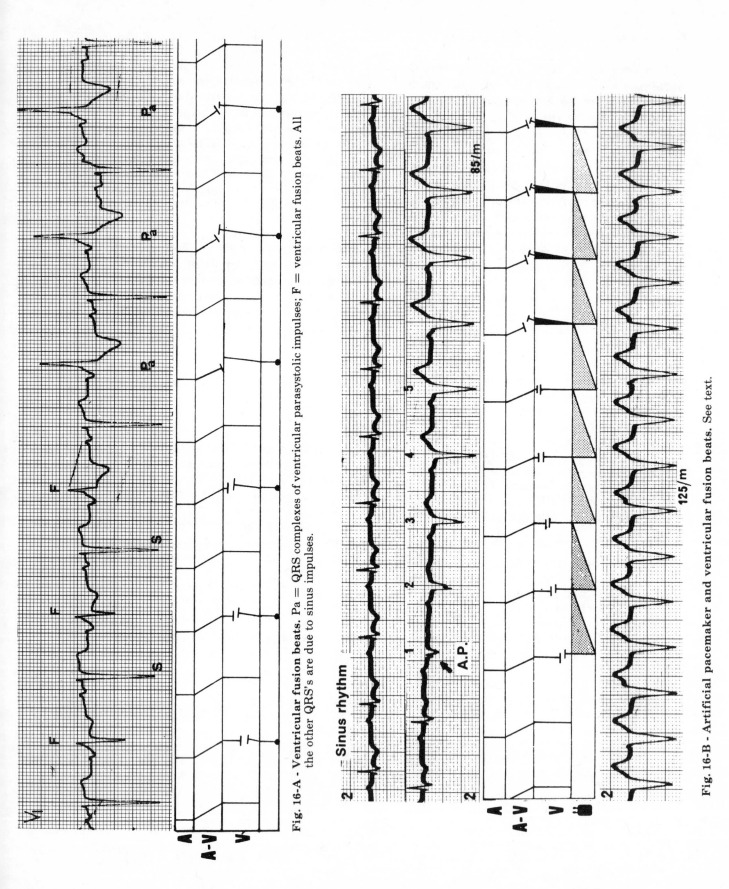

Fig. 16-A - Ventricular fusion beats. Pa = QRS complexes of ventricular parasystolic impulses; F = ventricular fusion beats. All the other QRS's are due to sinus impulses.

Fig. 16-B - Artificial pacemaker and ventricular fusion beats. See text.

Fusion Beats

Ventricular fusion beats (see pages 30-32) introduce another electrophysiologic situation which occurs with extraordinary similarity both spontaneously (ventricular parasystole) and in patients with asynchronous pacemakers. Fusion beats can be present practically with all types of pacemakers.

First of all, it is important to keep in mind that the morphology of a pacemaker QRS may change slightly in L3 in relation to respiratory cycles. This is a normal phenomenon and should not be interpreted as a pacemaker malfunction. Furthermore, when the impulse falls into the relative ventricular refractory period, (that is, on the descending branch of the preceding T wave), it may determine a QRS with a morphology slightly different than that of pacemaker beats with complete ventricular capture (determined from stimuli which fall in end-diastole).

Fig. 16-A illustrates a sinus rhythm in competition with a spontaneous ventricular parasystole. The resultant rhythm is an unusual form of ventricular bigeminy in which at least three *ventricular fusion beats* (F) are present. They are easily and clearly distinguished from sinus beats (S) and from parasystolic beats with ventricular capture (Pa). The QRS morphology of the three ventricular fusion beats is slightly different because the ventricular activation is shared by the sinus node and by the parasystolic focus,

and is quantitatively different. This is in relation to the gradual shortening of the coupling interval of the parasystolic impulses with the preceding sinus beats (note the fusion beats on the diagram).

A similar situation is presented in fig. 16-B in those beats which signal the beginning of an artificial ventricular stimulation (arrow in the second tracing). The first tracing shows a regular sinus rhythm before the insertion of a stimulating catheter. In the second tracing, starting from the third beat, a bipolar pacing is initiated with an external asynchronous pacemaker. The amplitude of the stimulus-artifact in this lead (L2) is so small as to be almost invisible and such that the artificial pacing simulates to perfection a ventricular tachycardia.

Before the QRS complexes of clear ventricular origin (beats N.6, etc.) there are five *ventricular fusion beats* whose morphology is in between that of sinus and that of pacemaker beats. It can also be noted that while the morphology of the first and second fusion beat is closer to that of sinus beats, the third, fourth and fifth fusion beats show an almost complete ventricular "capture" by the artificial focus (note the diagrammed presentation of fusion beats).

The bottom tracing confirms that the aberrant QRS's are in fact due to an artificial pacemaker. Here the stimulation rate is intentionally increased from 85 to 125/min. (external temporary pacemaker).

REFERENCES

Bluestone, R., Davies, G., Harris, A., Leatham, A., and Siddons, H.: *Long-term Endocardial Pacing for Heart Block*, Lancet, 2:307, 1965.

Burchell, H.B., Connolly, D.C., and Ellis, F.H., Jr.: *Indications for and Results of Implanting Cardiac Pacemakers*, Amer. J. Med., 37:764, 1964.

Chardack, W.M., Isbikawa, H., Fochler, F.J., Souther, S., and Gage, A.A.: *Pacing and Ventricular Fibrillation*, Ann. N. Y. Acad. Sci., 167:919, 1969.

Chardack, W.M.: *Heart Block Treated with an Implantable Pacemaker. Past Experience and Current Developments*, Progr. Cardiovasc. Dis., 6:507, 1964.

Chardack, W.M., Gage, A.A., and Greatbatch, W.: *A Transistorized Self-contained Implantable Pacemaker for the Long-term Correction of Complete Heart Block*, Surgery, 48:643, 1960.

Pick, A., and Langendorf, R.: *Approaches to the Diagnosis of Complex A-V Junctional Mechanisms, Mechanisms and Therapy of Cardiac Arrhythmias*, L. S. Dreifus and W. Likoff (ed.). New York: Grune & Stratton, p. 427, 1966.

Samet, P., Bernstein, W.H., Medow, A., and Nathan, D.A.: *Effect of Alterations in Ventricular Rate on Cardiac Output in Complete Heart Block*, Amer. J. Cardiol., 14:477, 1964.

Lister, J.W., Delman, A.J., Stein, E., Grunwald, R., and Robinson, G.: *The Dominant Pacemaker of the Human Heart, Antegrade and Retrograde Activation of the Heart*, Circulation, 35:22, 1967.

Schamroth, L.: *Principles Governing 2:1 A-V Block with Interference Dissociation*, Brit. Heart J., 31:780, 1969.

Castellanos, A., Jr., Mayer, J.W., and Lemberg, L.: *Intermittent Parasystole with Disturbance in Impulse Formation*, Acta Cardiol., 17:49, 1962.

Chardack, W.M., Gage, A.A., Federico, A.J., Schimert, G., and Greatbatch, W.: *Clinical Experience with an Implantable Pacemaker*, Ann. N. Y. Acad. Sci., 111:1075, 1964.

Chardack, W.M., Gage, A.A., Federico, A.J., Schimert, G., and Greatbatch, W.: *The Long-term Treatment of Heart Block*, Progr. Cardiovasc. Dis., 9:105, 1966.

Chardack, W.M., Gage, A.A., and Greatbatch, W.A.: *A Transistorized Self-contained Implantable Pacemaker for the Long-term Correction of Complete Heart Block*, Surgery, 48:643, 1960.

Furman, S., and Schwedel, J.B.: *An Intracardiac Pacemaker for Stokes-Adams Seizures*, New Eng. J. Med., 261:943, 1959.

Katz, L.N., and Pick, A.: *A Clinical Electrocardiography. Part. I. The Arrhythmias*, Philadelphia, Lea & Febiger, 1956.

Pick, A.: *Parasystole*, Circulation, 8:243, 1953.

Scherf, D.: *Zur Frage der Parasystolie*, Wien. Arch. Inn. Med., 8:155, 1924.

Sowton, E.: *Artificial Pacemaking and Sinus Rhythm*, Brit. Heart J., 27:311, 1965.

Zoll, P.M., Frank, H.A., and Linenthal, A.J.: *Four Years Experience with an Implanted Cardiac Pacemaker*, Ann. Surg., 160:351, 1964.

Zucker, I.R., Parsonnet, V., Gilbert, L., and Asa, M.M.: *Dipolar Electrode in Heart Block*, J.A.M.A., 184:549, 1963.

Portal, R.W., Davies, J.G., Leatham, A., and Siddons, A.H.M.: *Artificial Pacing for the Heart*, Lancet, 2:1369, 1962.

Lagergren, H., Johansson, L., and Edhag, O.: *One Hundred Cases of Treatment for Adams-Stokes Syndrome with Permanent Intravenous Pacemaker*, J. Thorac. Cardiov. Surg., 50:710, 1965.

Schwedel, J.B., and Escher, D.J.W.: *Transvenous Electrical Stimulation of the Heart. I.*, Ann. N. Y. Acad. Sci., 111:972, 1964.

Parsonnet, V., Zucker, I.R., Gilbert, L., and Myers, G.H.: *A Review of Intracardiac Pacing, with Specific Reference to the Use of a Dipolar Electrode*, Progr. Cardiov. Dis., 6:472, 1964.

Gordon, A.J.: *Catheter Pacing in Complete Heart Block: Techniques and Complications*, J.A.M.A., 193:1091, 1965.

Furman, S., Escher, D.J.W., Schwedel, J.B., and Solomon, N.: *Transvenous Pacing: A Seven Year Review*, Amer. Heart J., 71:408, 1966.

Tancredi, R.G., McCallister, B.D., and Manken, H.T.: *Temporary Transvenous Catheter-electrode Pacing of the Heart*, Circulation, 36:598, 1967.

Siddons, H., and Sowton, E.: *Cardiac Pacemakers*, Springfield, Ill., Thomas, 1967, chap. 5.

Thevenet, A., Hodges, P.C., and Lillehei, C.N.: *The Use of a Myocardial Electrode Inserted Percutaneously for Control of Complete Atrio-ventricular Block by an Artificial Pacemaker*, Dis. Chest., 34:621, 1958.

Bellet, S., Muller, O.F., De Leon, A.C., Sher, L.D., Lemmon, W.M., and Kilpatrick, D.G.: *The Use of an Internal Pacemaker in the Treatment of Cardiac Arrest and Slow Heart Rates*, Arch. Inter. Med., 105:361, 1960.

Solomon, N., and Escher, D.J.W.: *A Rapid Method for Pacemaker Catheter Electrode Insertion*, Amer. Heart J., 66:717, 1963.

Parsonnet, V., Zucker, R., Gilbert, L., and Asa, M.: *A Intracardiac Bipolar Electrode for Interim Treatment of Complete Heart Block*, Amer. J. Cardiol., 10:261, 1962.

Chapter III

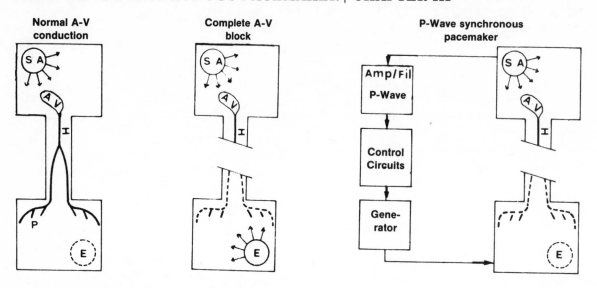

Fig. 17-A - P-wave synchronous pacemaker. The diagram illustrates the system atria-pacemaker-ventricles in the presence of a complete A-V block.

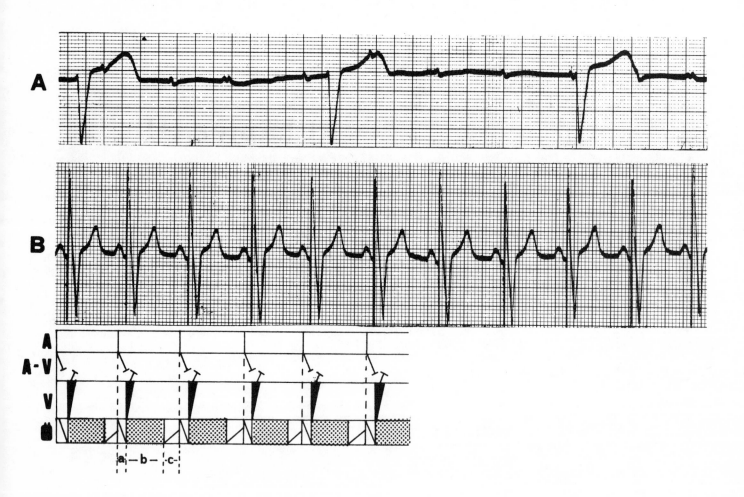

Fig. 17-B - P-wave synchronous pacemaker. The pacemaker restores a normal synchronism between atrial and ventricular contractions (B) also in the presence of a complete A-V block (A); a = A-P delay (atria-pacemaker); b = refractory period; c = recharging cycle.

This is the *only true A-V electrical prosthesis*. In patients with a complete A-V block this type of pacemaker re-establishes a rhythm and a cardiac function very close to normal. The cardiac rhythm produced by this "electronic A-V bridge" is very similar to a normal sinus rhythm. Even during electrical stimulation, the co-ordination between atrial and ventricular contractions is maintained within physilogical limits. Furthermore, within certain limits, this type of unit is the only one which usefully responds to physiological variation of the sinus rate. The P-wave synchronous pacemaker requires two electrodes. One must be attached to the atrial wall and the other electrode must be in contact with the ventricular musculature. (fig. 17-A). The atrial electrode is usually implanted on the epicardium and senses the atrial activation forces (sinus P waves, P¹ waves retrograde or secondary to atrial ectopic foci).

Since atrial potentials are usually of low voltage, the P *wave sensing* apparatus must be sufficiently sensitive, but unable to record electrical interference of other origin. In the great majority of cases, the sensitivity of the P wave-sensing system is kept around 0.90 - 1.1 mV. However, the signal received by the atrial electrode, which is the sensing electrode, is usually too weak to activate the circuit. Therefore, it must be magnified and this is obtained through the insertion of a filter-amplifier (fig. 17-A).

The ventricular electrode is the *stimulating electrode*. It is usually implanted on the right ventricular epicardium. After a time interval from sensing the P wave (similar to the physiologic P-R interval), this electrode delivers an impulse and activates the ventricles.

Therefore, the P wave guides the function of the pacemaker. A normal *A-P synchronism* (atrial-pacemaker) is maintained through the insertion of a circuit delay between the P-wave sensing system and the ventricular impulse emission circuit.

Tracing A of fig. 17-B shows a complete (third degree) A-V block. The atrial activity is independent from that of the ventricles. The sinus rate is 85/min., while that of the idio-ventricular ectopic focus is about 20/min.

Tracing B shows the same patient after the implantation of a P-wave synchronous pacemaker. The ventricular rate is now equal to the atrial rate. P waves precede each stimulus-artifact which induces a complete ventricular capture. The *P-stimulus interval* (P-S) is 0.16 seconds. The diagram illustrates the mechanism of the pacemaker. The P wave, which is blocked in the A-V junction, is sensed by the atrial electrode. After a time interval of 0.16 seconds, the atrial potentials activate the stimulating ventricular electrode and determine a ventricular depolarization (a = A-P delay; b = pacemaker refractory period; c = recharging cycle).

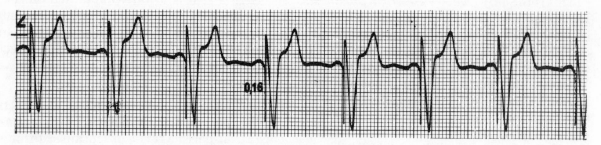

Fig. 18-A - P-wave synchronous pacemaker. The atria-pacemaker delay, represented by the P-S interval (P-stimulus), is equal to 0.16 sec. and is within normal limits.

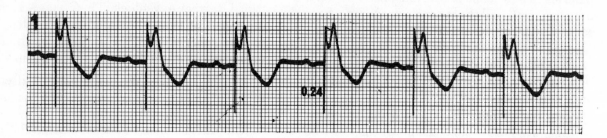

Fig. 18-B - P-wave synchronous pacemaker. Each P-stimulus interval is prolonged (0.24 sec.); therefore a first degree "A-P block" (atria-pacemaker) is present.

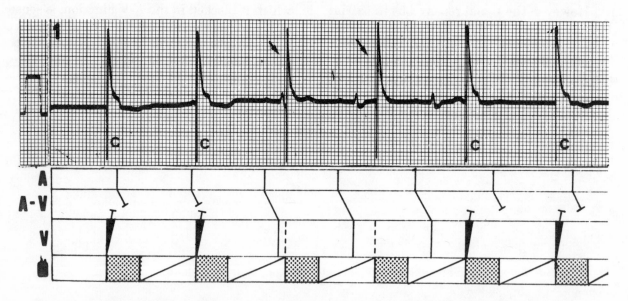

Fig. 18-C - P-wave synchronous pacemaker. The pacemaker is working in an automatic function and stimulates the ventricles at a fixed rate of 60/min. Notice the low voltage of the sinus P-waves and QRS complexes.

The A-P delay

Figure 18-A shows an artificial cardiac stimulation (69/min.) governed by the P wave. Sinus P waves precede each pacemaker QRS complex. Here, the P-S interval (P wave-stimulus) is 0.16 seconds. The artificially induced *A-P delay* (atrial-pacemaker) is a characteristic of only this type of pacemaker. It simulates to perfection the physiological A-V delay of a normal sinus rhythm.

The components of the A-P delay are determined by:

(1) the atrial electrode site. For example, if the electrode is placed over the right atrium a delay of 20 msec. may be present between the firing of the sinus impulse and its sensing by the atrial electrode;

(2) latency in the initiation of ventricular depolarization; this is due to propagation of the artificial impulse, through non-specific myocardial fibers which have a lower conduction velocity;

(3) the electronic delay of the P-wave synchronous pacemaker.

The first two factors are physiological and, together, they reach values of approximately 40 msec. The length of the electronic delay is usually preselected by the manufacturer and is about 120 msec. Therefore, a normal A-P delay or *P-S interval* (P wave-stimulus), for a P-wave synchronous pacemaker, should be about 160 msec. (This is the P-S interval of the Cordis Atricor). When the P-S interval is longer than 0.16 sec. a pacemaker malfunction must be suspected.

Figure 18-B shows a *first degree A-P block*. It belongs to a patient with a P-wave synchronous pacemaker which exhibits a battery exhaustion. The P-S interval (P stimulus) is equal to 0.24 seconds.

In the absence of a spontaneous atrial rhythm (sinus arrest, sino-atrial block) or in the presence of a very slow atrial rhythm (sinus bradycardia), the artificial pacemaker initiates a "fixed rate ventricular pacing" *(automatic pacing)* using a reserve electronic circuit. It usually stimulates with a rate of about 60/min. The same events would occur with a wire breakdown, involving the atrial sensing electrode, and in the presence of atrial potentials of very low voltage (ex. atrial fibrillation with small amplitude f waves), or in the presence of a sinus rhythm with P waves smaller than 1 mV.

The tracing of fig. 18-C belongs to a patient with a *P-wave synchronous pacemaker*. The stimulation is of a fixed rate type (60/min.). The first two and last two artificial impulses capture the ventricles (C). A sinus rhythm is present with a rate of 72/min. and with P waves and QRS complexes of low voltage. P waves are not sensed by the atrial electrode, and therefore, the A-P synchronism is missing. The artificial impulses which fall immediately after sinus QRS's (outlined in the diagram) are not able to capture the ventricles because they fall within the ventricular refractory period (arrows). They only determine voltage-decay artifacts (see page 25). Therefore, the P-wave synchronous pacemaker is working at a fixed rate of 60/min. and it is utilizing the safety reserve circuits. A similar behavior would be present in case of rupture of the atrial electrode.

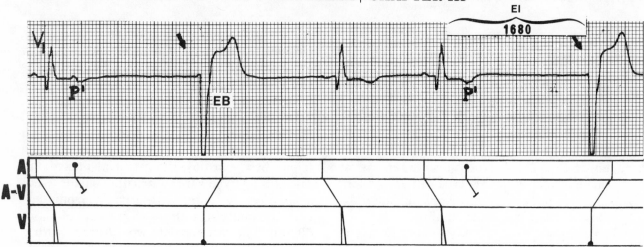

Fig. 19-A - Ventricular escape beats. The patient does not have a pacemaker; ventricular escape beats (EB) terminate the asystolic pauses following blocked atrial extrasystole (P¹). The escape interval is equal to 1680 msec.

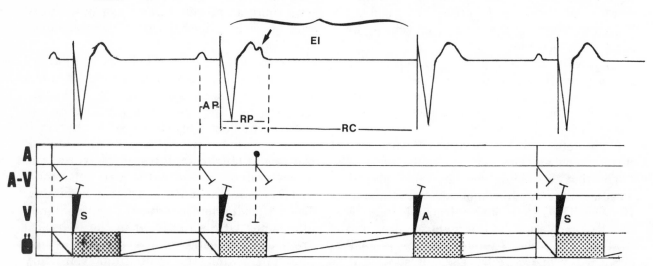

Fig. 19-B - P-wave synchronous pacemaker. The atrial extrasystole is not sensed by the pacemaker because it falls within the pacemaker refractory period. An automatic beat (A) appears at the end of the escape interval of 1 sec. AP = A-P delay; RP = refractory period; RC = automatic recharging cycle; EI = escape interval; S = synchronized beat; A = automatic beat.

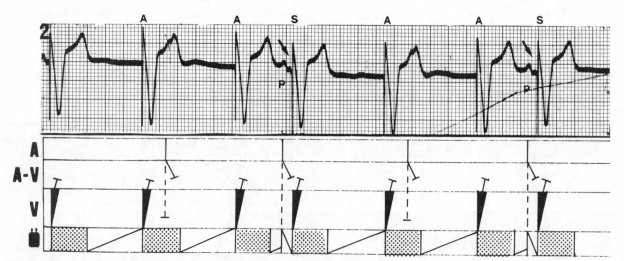

Fig. 19-C - P-wave synchronous pacemaker. Only the pacer beats indicated by the arrows are synchronous with P-waves. All the others are automatic pacemaker beats.

Escape interval and Automatic Pacing

To be usefully employed in clinical practice, this type of pacemaker must have a reserve stimulating circuit which will function when atrial potentials are not sensed. This safety device is what determines *automatic beats and automatic rhythms,* which are also called "pacemaker escape beats and escape rhythms". After a predetermined interval of time without perception of atrial activity (usually about one second), the pacemaker starts a "fixed rate" ventricular pacing through a reserve safety circuit.

This situation is very similar to what happens spontaneously during ventricular escape beats. Fig. 19-A shows a patient without an artificial pacemaker. Several sinus beats, conducted to the ventricles, are present together with two blocked atrial extrasystoles (P[1]) and two idioventricular beats (arrows). The PAC's temporarily supress the sinus pacemaker and are followed by a long and silent pause. The asystolic interval is terminated by beats of clear ventricular origin. *These are not extrasystoles* (premature beats) *but emergency beats* (idioventricular escape beats). They are not due to an increased ventricular excitability; they are spontaneous impulses of subsidiary centers which "escape" to the normal sinus control because of the long interval without cardiac activity. These beats are called *ventricular escape beats (ve)* and the interval of time which separates them from sinus QRS's is called *escape interval* (in this case EI = 1680 msec.).

Something extraordinarily similar happens when using P-wave synchronous pacemakers. Fig. 19-B begins with two sinus P-waves followed by impulses of a P-wave synchronous pacemaker and ventricular capture. Next is an atrial premature beat (arrow) which falls into the pacemaker refractory period. Therefore, it does not activate the stimulating circuit. This would occur also during a sinus arrest. The following pause ends with an *automatic or escape beat* (A) which is also pacemaker induced.

The interval between the automatic beat and the preceding P-wave synchronized beat is called *escape interval* (EI). This is formed by the refractory period of the pacemaker (RP)

and by the complete recharging cycle of the stimulating circuit (RC).

In one of the most commonly used P-wave synchronous pacemakers (Cordis Atricor), the escape interval is equal to one second. Therefore, if atrial activity is not present, the pacemaker fires at a "fixed rate" with impulses at one second interval (rate equals 60/min.).

Therefore the *automatic circuit* is a safety device. It guarantees an automatic ventricular pacing when: atrial activation waves are absent (for example: sinus arrest); when atrial impulses are of low voltage (for example: atrial fibrillation or P-wave amplitude <1mV), and in the presence of prolonged P-P intervals, (for example: atrial extrasystoles, temporary suppression of the S-A node, marked sinus bradycardia).

Fig. 19-C shows an irregular pacing. A superficial examination of the tracing may result in an interpretative error. It is clearly visible that the majority of impulses are regular (rate = 60/min.), except for the two impulses indicated by the arrows. These are obviously preceded by sinus P-waves.

Due to the presence of the two synchronized P-waves, it appears that the pacemaker is of the P-wave synchronous type. Here, the possibility of an intermittent synchronization, secondary to unit malfunction, can be ruled out. A sinus bradycardic rhythm is present (note the P-P interval) and some of the P-waves fall within the refractory period of the pacemaker (see diagram) and are effective on the synchronizing mechanism. Since the P waves are not sensed, they are followed by the delivery of pacemaker automatic impulses (indicated with A). Only when the P-waves fall far enough from the preceding stimulus, will they activate the stimulating circuit and will induce a premature firing within the automatic rhythm (synchronized beats = S). The entire sequence created by the interaction of spontaneous and artificial impulses is very similar to an A-V dissociation with escape beats (see page 27). It must be noticed that: a) the sinus impulse does not escape from the refractory period of the A-V junction (the P-waves are continuously blocked) but from the P-wave synchronous pacemaker and b) the ventricular capture is always determined by an artificial impulse.

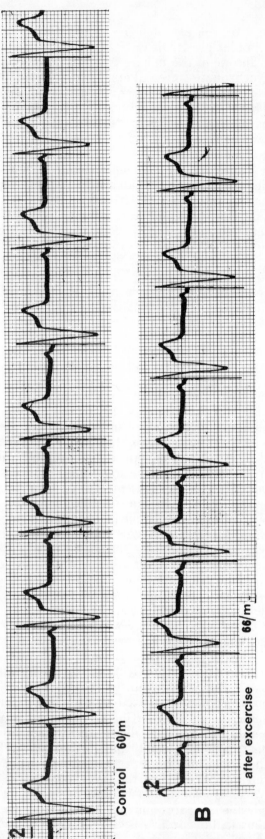

Control   60/m

after excercise   66/m

Fig. 20-A - P-wave synchronous pacemaker. Tracing A shows a pacemaker in automatic function and dissociated from a sinus rhythm. An increased sinus rate, obtained with exercise (B), triggers the mechanism of synchronization between the atrium and the pacemaker.

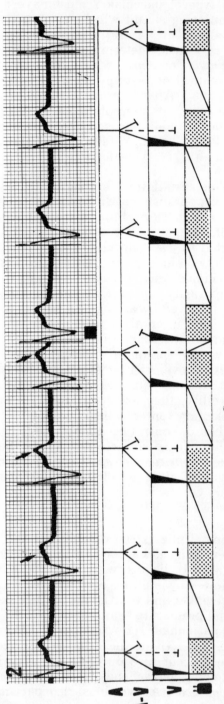

Fig. 20-B - P-wave synchronous pacemaker. See text.

THE P-WAVE SYNCHRONOUS PACEMAKER

The A-P Synchronism

Tracing A of fig. 20-A shows an artificial pacing with a fixed rate of 60/min., and with good ventricular capture. Several QRS complexes are preceded by a sinus P-wave which, however, does not have a constant time relation (variable P-S interval) with the ventricular complexes. Some of the P waves are too close to the QRS for a normal A-P (atria-pacemaker) synchronism, while others are not even recognizable, since they are buried within the pacemaker QRS's. The tracing, therefore, shows a fixed rate ventricular pacing dissociated from sinus activity. It is now necessary to establish whether the artificial stimulation is due to an asynchronous pacemaker (see page 21) or to a P-wave synchronous pacemaker working with an automatic reserve circuit. Tracing B was recorded after light exercise. It can be easily noticed that the pacing rate is increased (66/min.) and each QRS complex is now preceded by a P-wave with a constant P-S interval of 0.14 seconds. The slight increase of sinus rate, induced by exercise, has been enough to trigger the P wave-pacemaker synchronizing mechanism. These tracings clearly show how a slow sinus rate (in this case 60/min.) triggers the *automatic emergency pacing* which maintains the heart rate within more acceptable limits.

Fig. 20-B belongs also to a patient with a P-wave synchronous pacemaker. Among the regular automatic impulses, with a rate of 60/min. and with good ventricular capture, there suddenly appears an artificial impulse. This impulse is premature with respect to the pacemaker time-table but capable of depolarizing the ventricles (dark squares). A careful analysis of the tracing allows the identification of atrial activation waves (arrows). It is not easy to decipher the polarity of the P-waves and establish whether they are positive or negative. Two alternative explanations may be derived from this ECG tracing:

(a) there is a bradycardia (rate < 60/min.) with a slight sinus arrhythmia and the pacemaker is working at a fixed rate. When the P-wave falls outside the refractory period of the pacemaker it triggers the A-P synchronization.

(b) the automatic impulses of the P-wave synchronous pacemaker travels through the A-V junction in a retrograde fashion and depolarizes the atria, with a progressive V-A conduction delay (ventriculo-atrial). When the atrial activation is so delayed as to go beyond the refractory period of the pacemaker, the P[1] wave is sensed and the atrial-pacemaker synchronism is triggered. The entire sequence brings to mind that of a junctional or idioventricular rhythm with a retrograde V-A Wenckenbach and with an *echo beat* (reciprocal beat). This second explanation is diagrammed below the tracing.

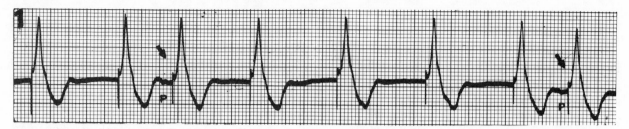

Fig. 21-A - P-wave synchronous pacemaker. Premature beats (arrows) are caused by markedly bradycardic sinus P waves which are normally synchronized with the pacemaker.

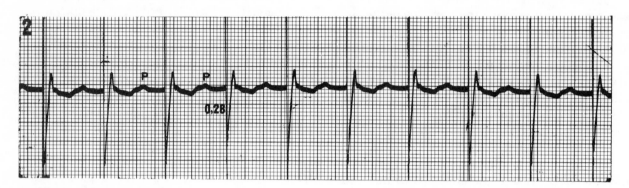

Fig. 21-B - P-wave synchronous pacemaker. A sinus tachycardia is synchronized with the pacemaker (ventricular response of 1:1). A first degree A-P block is present (P-S intervals = 0.28 sec.).

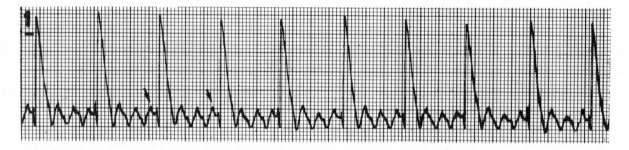

Fig. 21-C - P-wave synchronous pacemaker. The atrial flutter determines an A-P block (atrial-pacemaker) of 4:1. Arrows indicate synchronized F waves.

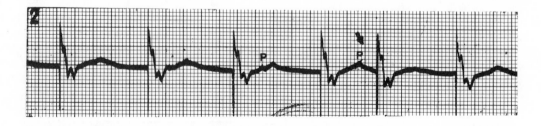

Fig. 21-D - P-waves synchronous pacemaker. Only one of the bradycardic P waves is synchronized with the pacemaker.

The refractory period

This type of stimulator is not only protected from absent or bradycardic atrial rhythm, but also from very fast atrial rates. Supraventricular tachycardias, atrial flutter and fibrillation (with high amplitude atrial waves) could, in fact, cause dangerous and rapid ventricular rates by utilizing the artificial A-V conduction pathway. One of the first objectives in the construction of this type of pacemaker has been the construction of a device capable of maintaining the stimulation rate within the so-called "physiological limits."

The maximum stimulation rate reached by an impulse generator is determined by the *refractory period*. This is an interval of time which follows the impulse delivery and during which the pacemaker is unable to sense a signal and, therefore, cannot deliver a new impulse. The refractory period may change from one manufacturer to another.

The next important objective has been to select a refractory period capable of protecting the circuits from internal or external electrical impulses. These include the pacemaker R waves, the re-entry of the stimulating impulse, and the presence of tall, peaked T waves which may pass through the filter-amplifier system, ventricular premature beats with short coupling intervals and, finally, external electrical signals. For example, the length of the refractory period of the Cordis Atricor is equal to 480 msec. The maximal pacing rate determined by a refractory period of 480 msec. is, therefore, equal to 125/min. The minimal pacing rate is determined by the *automatic interval* (see page 43) which, being equal to 1 second, allows for an automatic ventricular pacing of 60/min. Therefore, in the presence of an atrial rate higher than 125/min., the ventricular rate is halved by the presence of a *A-P block of 2:1,* similar to the physiological A-V block. Every other atrial impulse falls into the refractory period of the pacemaker. If the atrial rate is higher than 220/min. the *A-P block is of the 3:1 type.* When the atrial rate is lower than 60/min. the automatic mechanism is triggered.

Fig. 21-A shows the behavior of a P-wave synchronous pacemaker during a sinus bradycardia. The artificial pacemaker is synchronized with the P-waves only in two occasions (arrows); otherwise, it works at a fixed rate.

Fig. 21-B shows a sinus tachycardia (100/min.), with a ventricular response of 1:1, in a patient with a P-wave synchronous pacemaker. The P-S interval is prolonged (0.28 sec.) and indicates a *first degree A-P block,* due to pacemaker malfunction.

An atrial flutter is shown in fig. 21-C. In this case a *4:1 A-P block* is present because the atrial rate is particularly elevated. Similarly to what happens in the spontaneous A-V ratio of an atrial flutter, it is difficult to establish which of the F-waves, immediately preceding the pacemaker QRS, is the "synchronized F-wave". Since the A-P delay is fixed (see page 41), the synchronized F-wave which triggers the ventricular electrode is, in all likelihood, the one indicated by the arrow.

In a patient with a P-wave synchronous pacemaker, the finding of an occasional premature artificial impulse must bring to mind the presence of a bradycardic atrial rhythm (fig. 21-D). When P-waves are not easily identifiable and only occasionally synchronized with the pacemaker, the tracing sometimes may be erroneously interpreted as a pacemaker malfunction. In these cases, the technique of chest wall stimulation (CWS) identifies the normal sensing and synchronizing mechanisms of this type of stimulator (see page 189). CWS technique has been usefully adopted in the routine examination of patients with artificial pacemakers.

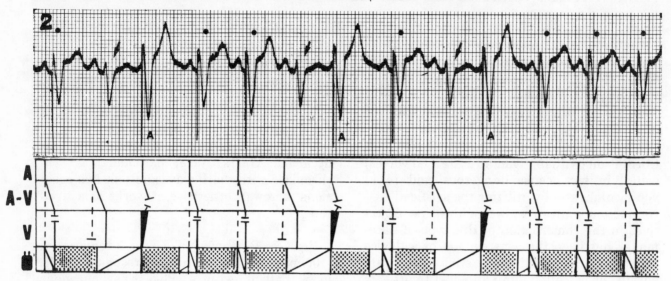

Fig. 22-A - P-wave synchronous pacemaker. The sinus beats indicated by the arrows are not sensed by the pacemaker. A = automatic beats; dots indicate ventricular fusion beats.

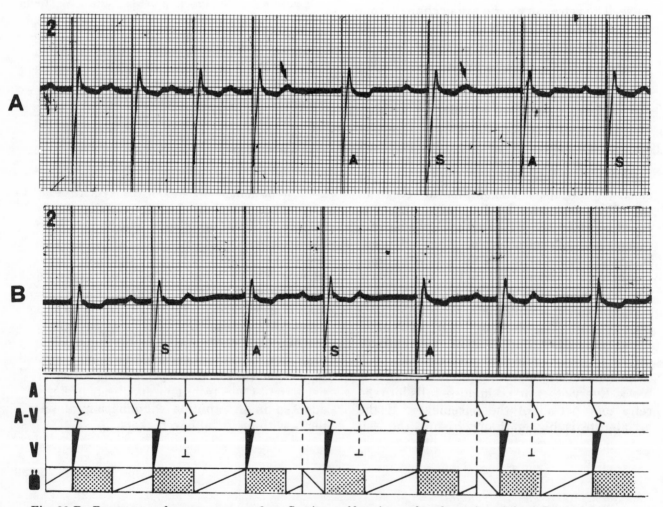

Fig. 22-B - P-wave synchronous pacemaker. Sensing malfunction and prolongation of the A-P interval.

The refractory period

The first sign of malfunction of a P-wave synchronous pacemaker is usually a loss of the sensing function and the perception of atrial signals. In this case the pacemaker is automatically switched into a fixed rate mode. However, attention must be paid not to diagnose a pacemaker malfunction every time P waves are not followed by a pacemaker stimulus.

In fig. 22-A, the patient with a P-wave synchronous pacemaker was admitted with a diagnosis of pacemaker malfunction. In this tracing three types of QRS's can be recognized: a) QRS of sinus origin, preceded by a P wave, and with a normal P-R interval (arrow); b) QRS complexes wide and bizarre, preceded by an artificial stimulus but not by a P wave (automatic beats = A); c) QRS complexes with a morphology in between that of a sinus beat and that of a pacemaker automatic beat. The latter are all preceded by a stimulus artifact and by a P wave with a constant P-S interval. They are *ventricular fusion beats* (dark dots).

The sinus rate is about 120/min. The rhythm is, therefore, a sinus tachycardia with a rapid atrial rate and with a 1:1 response from the pacemaker. A minimal variation of the P-P intervals is enough to determine an *A-P block* (atria-pacemaker block) and, at the same time, an *A-V block*. The not sensed P wave determines the 2:1 *A-P block* (atria-pacemaker), because it falls into the pacemaker refractory period. The following P-wave is buried within the pacemaker automatic QRS and is blocked in the A-V junction ("A-V block") because of the retrograde concealed penetration of the artificial impulse. The pacemaker impulses which follow the not sensed P waves are pacemaker *escape or automatic impulses* (beats A). The interval of time which separates them from the preceding impulse is equal to one second. This is the typical interval of an automatic mechanism. The QRS's of the automatic beats show complete ventricular capture.

The tracing shows, therefore, a *normal P-wave synchronous pacemaker behavior* in the presence of an atrial rhythm with a rate occasionally faster than 120/min. This determines the "intermittent A-P block" in which an occasional atrial wave is not able to trigger the synchronizing mechanism.

When the sinus rate is equal to 120/min., the ventricular depolarization is simultaneously induced by the sinus and by the artificial impulse. The resulting QRS'S are, therefore, *ventricular fusion beats* (F). This situation may be compared to a ventricular parasystole.

The first four beats of tracing A of fig. 22-B are due to regular pacemaker stimuli (rate = 90/min.) and are all preceded by sinus P-waves. The P-S interval, although constant, is markedly prolonged (0.28 sec.) and suggests a battery exhaustion (*1st degree A-P block*). The P-wave indicated by the arrow is not followed by an artificial impulse, but by a pause. After an interval of one second (escape interval), this pause ends with an automatic beat (A). The following QRS (indicated with S) is preceded by a P-wave with a prolonged P-S interval. It is then followed by another automatic beat (*second degree A-P block.*)

Tracing B and the diagram show a sequence of beats separated by intervals of different length which determine a "ventricular bigeminy". The rhythm is that of a malfunctioning P-wave synchronous pacemaker. It is due to alternate synchronized (S) and automatic beats (A). It is possible that the escape beats are caused by a very modest increase of the sinus rate (for example from 95/min. to 98/min.). During the bigeminy, one of the two P-waves is hidden within the QRS and falls within a period of time in which the pacemaker is refractory. Therefore, the unit is a *P-wave synchronous pacemaker with two obvious findings of malfunction:* a) marked increase of P-S interval (normal = 0.16 sec.); b) prolongation of the refractory period of the pacemaker and reduction of the upper limit of P-wave synchronization (normal up to 120/min., in this case about 100/min.).

P-wave synchronous pacemaker

Advantages

Absence of "competition" with spontaneous cardiac rhythm.

Rhythm and rate are governed by the S-A node.

Physiologic response to nervous control.

Improved hemodynamic conditions because of A-V synchronism.

Disadvantages

More complicated electronic circuits.

Necessity of an atrial electrode through thoracotomy.

Upper limit of ventricular rate equals 120/min.

Marked sensitivity of the sensing circuit and possiblity of recording external signals.

REFERENCES

Carlens, E., Johansson, L., Karlof, I., and Lagergren, U.: *New Method for Atrial-triggered Pacemaker Treatment without Thoracotomy*, J. Thorac. Cardiovasc. Surg., 50:229, 1965.

Castellanos, A., Jr., Lemberg, L., Rodriguez-Tocker, L., and Berkovits, B.V.: *Atrial Synchronized Pacemaker Arrhythmias: Revisited*, Amer. Heart J., 76:199, 1968.

Linden, R.J., and Mitchell, J.N.: *Relation Between Left Ventricular Diastolic Pressure and Myocardial Segment Length and Observation of the Contribution of Atrial Systole*, Circ. Res., 8:1092, 1960.

Skinner, S.K., Mitchell, J.H., Wallace, A.G., and Sarnoff, S.J.: *Hemodynamic Effects of Altering the Timing of Atrial Systole*, Amer. J. Physiol., 205:499, 1963.

Bonnabeau, Jr., R.C., et al.: *Observations of Sudden Death During Pacemaker Stimulation in Complete Atrioventricular Block, Leading to Development of P-wave Pacemaker without Atrial Leads*, Trans. Amer. Soc. Artif. Intern. Organs, 9:158, 1963.

Nathan, D.A., Center, S., Samet, P., and Wu, C.Y.: *The Application of an Implantable Synchronous Pacer for the Correction of Stokes-Adams Attacks*, Ann. N.Y. Acad. Sci., 111:1093, 1964.

Elmquist, R., et al.: *Artificial Pacemaker for Treatment of Adams-Stokes Syndrome and Slow Heart Rate*, Amer. Heart J., 65:731, 1963.

Samet, P., Jacobs, W., Bernstein, W.M., and Shane, R.: *Hemodynamics Sequelae of Idioventricular Pacemaking in Complete Heart Block*, Amer. J. Cardiol., 11:594, 1963.

Castellanos, Agustin, Jr., and Lemberg, Louis: « *Electrophysiology of Pacing and Cardioversion* », Appleton-Century-Crofts, New York, 1969.

Dittmar, H.A., Friese, G., and Holder, E.: *Erfahrungen uber die langfristige elektrische Reizung des menschlichen, Herzens*. Z. Kreislaufforsch, 51:66, 1962.

Center, S., Nathan, D.A., Wu, C.Y., and Duque, D.: *Two Years of Clinical Experience with the Synchronous Pacer*, J. Thorac. Cardiov. Surg., 48:513, 1964.

Samet, P., Bernstein, W.M., Nathan, D.A., and Lopez, A.: *Atrial Contribution to Cardiac Output in Complete Heart Block*, Amer. J. Card., 16:1, 1965.

Siddons, H., and Sowton, E.: « *Cardiac Pacemakers* », Charles C. Thomas, Illinois, 1967.

Nathan, D.A., Samet, P., Center, S., and Wu, C.Y.: *Long Term Correction of Complete Heart Block. Clinical and Physiologic Studies of a New Type of Implantable Synchronous Pacer*, Prog. Cardiov. Dis., 6:538, 1964.

Mitchell, J.H., Gilmore, J.P., and Sarnoff, S.J.: *The Transport Function of the Left Atrium*, Amer. J. Cardiol., 9:237, 1962.

Braunwald, E., and Frahm, C.J.: *Studies on Starling's Law of the Heart. Observations on the Hemodynamic Functions of the Left Atrium in Man*, Circulation, 24:633, 1961.

Greenwood, R.J., and Finkelstein, D.: « *Sinoatrial Heart Block* », Charles C. Thomas, Publisher, Springfield, Ill., 1964.

Dack, S.: *Pacemaker Therapy in Heart Block and Stokes-Adams Syndrome*, J.A.M.A., 10:142, 1965.

Lemberg, L., Castellanos, A., and Berkovits, E.E.: *Pacemaking on Demand in A-V Block*, J.A.M.A., 191:106, 1965.

Najmi, M., Segal, B.L., Likoff, W., and Dreifus, L.S.: *Atrial Pacemaker Block; a New Electrocardiographic Syndrome Associated with Implanted Synchronous Pacemakers*, Dis. Chest, 48:1, 1965.

Nathan, D.A., Center, S., Wu, C.Y., and Keller, W.: *An Implantable Synchronous Pacemaker for the Long Term Correction of Complete Heart Block*, Amer. J. Cardiol., 11:362, 1963.

Center, S., Nathan, D.A., Wu, C.Y., Samet, S., and Keller, W.: *The Implantable Synchronous Pacer in the Treatment of Complete Heart Block*, J. Thorac. Cardiov. urg., 46:744, 1963.

Carlens, E., Johansson, L., Karlof, I., and Lagergren, U.: *New Method for Atrial-triggered Pacemaker Treatment without Thoracotomy*, J. Thorac. Cardiovasc. Surg., 50:229, 1965.

Freidberg, C.K., Donoso, E., and Stein, W.G.: *Nonsurgical Acquired Heart Block*, Ann. N.Y. Acad. Sci., 3:835, 1964.

Adams, C.W.: *Retrograde Atrial Conduction with Complete Heart Block Following Implantation of an Internal Ventricular Pacemaker*, Dis. Chest, 43:544, 1963.

Furman, Seymour, and Escher, Doris, J.W.: « *Principles and Techniques of Cardiac Pacing* », Harper & Row, New York, 1970.

Lev, M.: *The Normal Anatomy of the Conduction System in Man and Its Pathology in Atrioventricular Block*, Ann. N.Y. Acad. Sci., 3:817, 1964.

Dreifus, L.S., Likoff, W., and Moyer, J.H.: « *Mechanisms and Therapy of Cardiac Arrhythmias* », Grune and Stratton, New York and London, 1966.

Winternitz, M., and Langendorf, R.: *Auriculoventricular Block with Ventriculoauricular Response*, Amer. Heart J., 27:301, 1944.

Nathan, D.A., Center, S., Wu, C.Y., and Keller, W.: *An Implantable Synchronous Pacemaker for the Long Term Correction of Complete Heart Block*, Circulation, 23:682, 1963.

Chardack, W., and Greatbatch, W.: *Failure Rate Report. Chardack: Greatbatch Implantable Pacemakers*. Circulated Communication, November, 1964.

Braunwald, N.S., and Morrow, A.G.: *Accelerated Fatigue Testing of Pacemaker Electrodes. A Comparison of Available Electrodes with an Elgiloy Wire Coil*, Surgery, 58:846, 1965.

Castellanos, A., Jr., Lemberg, L., Rodriguez-Tocker, L., and Berkovits, B.V.: *Atrial Synchronized Pacemaker Arrhythmias: Revisited*, Amer. Heart J., 76:199, 1968.

Castellanos, A., Jr., Lemberg, L.: *Arrhythmias Appearing After the Implantation of Synchronized Pacemaker*, Brit. Heart J., 21:747, 1964.

Chalnot, P., Faivre, G., Frisch, R., and Cherrier, F.: *Utilization d'un nouveau stimulateur implantable; le pacemaker synchrone de Nathan*, Ann. Med. (Nancy), 3:295, 1964.

Chapter IV

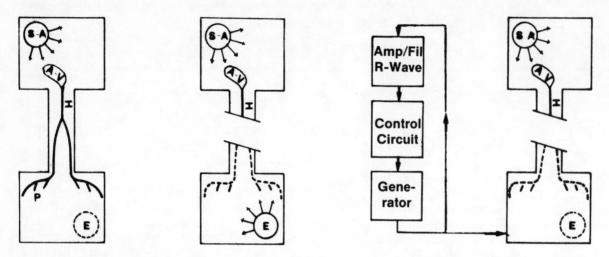

Fig. 23-A - QRS-synchronous "demand" pacemaker. The diagram illustrates the function of the pacemaker in a complete A-V block.

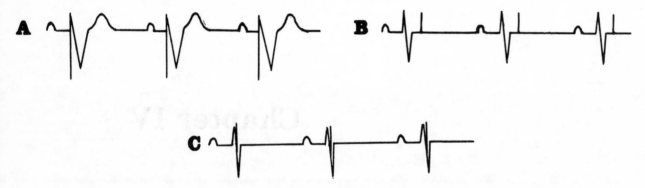

Fig. 23-B - A = P-wave synchronous pacemaker; **B** = first model of QRS-synchronous **"demand" pacemaker.** A stimulus is delivered 0.16 secs. after spontaneous ventricular potentials; **C** = Recent model of a ventricular-triggered pacemaker. The impulse is delivered 20 msec. after the sensing of ventricular potentials.

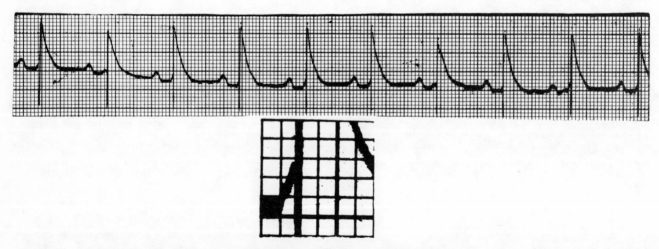

Fig. 23-C - QRS-synchronous "demand" pacemaker and sinus rhythm. The impulse is delivered by the pacemaker 20 msecs. after the beginning of spontaneous ventricular depolarization and is not effective because it falls within the ventricular refractory period.

THE "DEMAND" PACEMAKER

This type of artificial stimulator was essentially created to avoid some of the inconveniences of the asynchronous pacemaker and of the P-wave synchronous pacemaker. The motivations behind the production of new types of stimulators which would not interfere with spontaneous cardiac rhythms have been: a) the widespread clinical use of cardiac pacing, not anymore limited only to complete A-V blocks and Adams-Stokes seizures, and b) the evidence of restoration of a sinus rhythm, with a normal A-V conduction, sometime after artificial pacing. This situation occurs in a good percentage of patients with a complete A-V block at the time of implantation.

The absence of "competition" between the pacemaker and a spontaneous cardiac rhythm is, therefore, the essential characteristic of a *"demand pacemaker"*. Furthermore, the use of this type of stimulator has shown that the intracavitary stimulation may be preferred even using electronically more complex units. Only the P-wave synchronous pacemaker requires a thoracotomy to maintain a constant and stable atrial-pacemaker synchronism.

The "demand pacemakers" are essentially divided into two types: a) *QRS-synchronous "demand" pacemaker* or *ventricular-triggered* pacemaker.

b) *QRS-inhibited "demand" pacemaker* or *ventricular-inhibited pacemaker*.

A. THE QRS-SYNCHRONOUS "DEMAND" PACEMAKER

This type of stimulator appeared as a variant of a P-wave synchronous pacemaker. The great majority of stimulators available require that only one electrode be in contact with the ventricular wall. This works at the same time as a *sensing apparatus* (to sense the intracardiac potentials) and as a *stimulating electrode* (fig. 23-A).

The first "demand" models were nothing else than P-wave synchronous pacemakers. Instead of sensing atrial potentials, these units were adapted to be synchronized with ventricular potentials and to deliver an impulse after an interval of time of 0.14 - 0.16 seconds, after sensing the spontaneous QRS. Since the P-S interval (P-stimulus) of a P-wave synchronous pacemaker is similar to the physiologic P-R interval, the artificial impulse depolarizes the ventricles and it maintains the atrio-ventricular synchronism (A fig. 23-B). Instead, the impulse of a QRS-synchronous pacemaker is synchronized with ventricular potentials and falls within the refractory period of the ventricular excitability.

Therefore it is ineffective (B fig. 23-B).

In recent models, which are now universally adopted, the QRS-stimulus synchronism has been markedly shortened to values of about 20 msec. Therefore, the *stimulus falls within the QRS complex 20 msec. after the beginning of spontaneous ventricular depolarization* (C fig. 23-B) and *finds the ventricles refractory*. Thus, it is *ineffective*.

This type of pacemaker also has an *automatic reserve mechanism.* In case of the absence of spontaneous cardiac activity the safety mechanism starts working at a "fixed rate", after a predetermined interval of time *(escape interval or automatic interval)*. The QRS-synchronous pacemaker, therefore, guarantees a basic, fixed ventricular rate and is neutralized by the reappearance of a sinus rhythm. In this case it delivers impulses into the ventricular refractory period following each spontaneous QRS. In this way the possibility of stimulating the ventricles during the period of ventricular excitability is eliminated. At the same time, at any given moment, it is possible to recognize the activity of the pacemaker by the continuous presence of the stimulus-artifacts on the surface EKG. They appear either as ineffective spikes overimposed on a spontaneous QRS or as automatic impulses with "ventricular capture".

Not being synchronous with atrial activity, this type of pacemaker does not respond to changes in sinus rates. The name "ventricular-triggered" means that the pacemaker is synchronized with the QRS complex and that it continuously delivers impulses, either in the presence, or in the absence of spontaneous cardiac potentials.

Fig. 23-C shows how the impulse of a QRS-synchronous pacemaker alters the QRS morphology of a sinus rhythm with normal A-V conduction. Each QRS complex shows a pacemaker spike falling 20 msec. from the beginning of the ventricular depolarization. The stimulus does not capture the ventricles which are already into the absolute refractory phase.

In a way, the distorted morphology of the spontaneous QRS may simulate the ECG changes caused by a current of injury. Attention must be paid not to diagnose the presence of coronary artery or pericardial disease (see voltage-decay curve page 25).

The enlarged detail of fig. 23-C shows a spontaneous QRS with a synchronized pacemaker spike. The "QRS-spike interval" is characteristic of a QRS-synchronous pacemaker in the presence of spontaneous cardiac activity. The spike is delivered 20 msec. after the beginning of the ventricular depolarization.

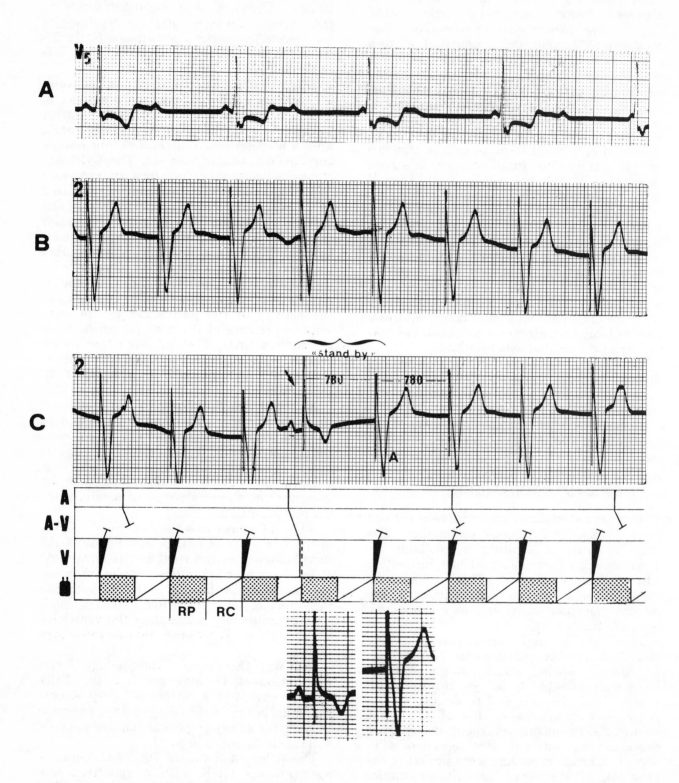

Fig. 24-A - QRS-synchronous "demand" pacemaker. See text.

THE QRS-SYNCHRONOUS "DEMAND" PACEMAKER

Escape interval

The QRS-synchronous "demand" pacemaker continuously delivers impulses either in the absence or in the presence of spontaneous ventricular potentials. In the first case, it captures the ventricles and stimulates in automatic fashion, at a "fixed rate"; in the other case, the impulse is not effective. The spike, which falls immediately after the beginning of a spontaneous QRS, eliminates the possibility of competition with supraventricular or idioventricular beats, and, at the same time, gives information about the presence and the normal function of the pacemaker.

This type of stimulator captures the ventricle only when *requested* (on "demand"). This happens when, after a certain interval of time, spontaneous cardiac activity is not present. The interval of time during which the pacemaker "stands-by" is called *stand-by or escape interval*.

Tracing A of fig. 24-A belongs to a patient with a complete A-V block before the implantation of a pacemaker. Sometime later, the cardiac rhythm is totally under control of a pacemaker. Tracing B shows artificial impulses with good ventricular capture at the "fixed rate" of 75/min. This tracing would be identical to that of a patient with an asynchronous pacemaker. The examination of tracing C indicates the true nature of the stimulator which is a QRS-synchronous "demand" pacemaker.

The beat indicated by the arrow is a sinus beat conducted to the ventricles. In this case an artificial impulse is fired 20 msec. after the beginning of the QRS complex and is followed by a 780 msec. pause without ventricular activity. This ends with a pacemaker impulse with complete ventricular capture (A).

The interval of time which separates the ineffective spike, buried within the spontaneous QRS, from the following "automatic" impulse with ventricular capture is called *escape interval*. During this interval the pacemaker is "stand-by". Therefore, if a continuous spontaneous activity is not present, the pacemaker "demand" function is requested and it fires at a fixed, automatic rate.

The automatic beats which terminate the asystolic pause (A) behave like true ventricular escape beats. The stand-by interval is equal to the one separating two pacemaker automatic beats. After the sinus beat which is conducted to the ventricles, there is no spontaneous activity. Therefore, after a pause of 780 msec. the pacemaker starts an automatic pacing with a rate of 75/min. and with complete ventricular capture. In the underlying diagram the synchronized impulse of the ventricular-triggered pacemaker is easily identified among the automatic impulses. The shaded area represents the refractory period of the pacemaker (RP) which follows each impulse delivery and is followed by a recharging cycle (RC). It can be seen that all of the recharging cycles, except one, are complete. This means that they terminate the automatic delivery time and that only one is interrupted by a premature delivery of the stimulus. This cycle is the one synchronized with the sinus beat.

In the enlarged detail below the diagram there are shown an automatic beat and a spontaneous beat synchronized with the pacemaker. It can be seen that the stimulus-artifact of the automatic beat is sharply delineated on the isolectric line. In the spontaneous beat, however, the impulse is delivered 20 msec. after the beginning of the QRS complex.

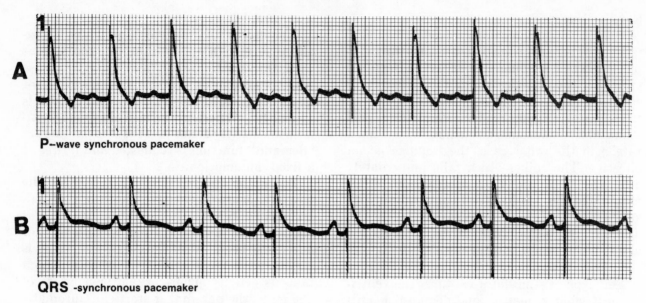

Fig. 25-A - QRS-synchronous pacemaker. When a sinus rhythm is present, a QRS-synchronous pacemaker (B) may have remarkable similarities to a P-wave synchronous pacemaker (A).

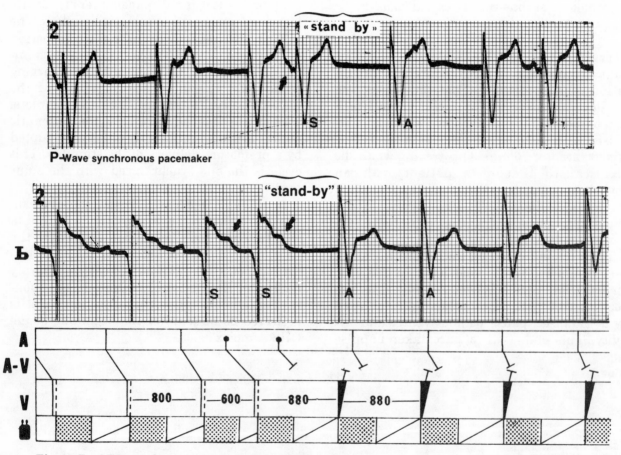

Fig. 25-B - QRS-synchronous pacemaker. Marked morphological differences are present between an automatic and a synchronized beat; QRS-synchronous pacemaker (B) and P-wave synchronous pacemaker (A).

THE QRS-SYNCHRONOUS "DEMAND" PACEMAKER

Escape beats

Tracing A of fig. 25-A shows an artificial stimulation at a rate of 72/min. Each spike is preceded by a P-wave and by a constant P-S interval (P-stimulus) of 0.18 sec. Each spike is sharply delineated on the isolectric line of the P-R interval. Therefore, since the pacemaker is a P-wave synchronous type, the ventricles are activated by artificial impulses synchronized with atrial depolarization waves.

Tracing B shows a situation which appears very similar to the preceding one. The artificial impulses at the beginning of each bizarre, aberrant, wide QRS complex are all preceded by P-waves and by constant P-S intervals. Again in this case, the presence of a P-wave synchronous pacemaker may be diagnosed. A closer examination of the ventricular complexes shows a positive initial deflection immediately preceding each pacemaker spike. This indicates the presence of a spontaneous ventricular depolarization which triggers a pacemaker of the QRS-synchronized type. Delivered 20 msec. after the beginning of the ventricular depolarization, the artificial impulse alters the QRS morphology, but is not effective because it falls within the ventricular refractory period. The rhythm is, therefore, of sinus origin with a normal A-V conduction in a patient with a QRS-synchronous "demand" pacemaker.

Another useful element in the differential diagnosis between a P-wave synchronous pacemaker and a QRS-synchronous "demand" pacemaker is offered by the careful morphological analysis of the *escape or automatic beats*. Both types of stimulators have a reserve mechanism which triggers an "emergency circuit", when spontaneous cardiac activity is not present, and induces a fixed rate stimulation. The automatic pacing begins after an interval of time (stand-by interval) which is predetermined by the different manufacturers.

Tracing A of fig. 25-B shows a P-wave synchronous pacemaker in the presence of a sinus bradycardia (see page 43). Only two of the artificial impulses are synchronized with a P-wave and have a P-S interval of 0.16 secs. (arrows). All the other spikes are delivered automatically at "fixed rate" (A). The P-wave synchronized impulses determine two ventricular contractions, slightly premature within the slower and more regular automatic rhythm. It should be noted that the morphology of the QRS which is synchronized with the atrium (S) is identical to that of the fixed rate automatic beats (A). This is because both the automatic impulses and the P-wave synchronized impulses "capture" and depolarize the ventricle.

Tracing B shows a similar situation in the presence of a *QRS-synchronous pacemaker*. The first three beats are of sinus origins and are conducted to the ventricles with a first degree A-V block (notice the prolonged P-R interval). Each sinus QRS is altered by an artificial impulse; this indicates a good synchronization with a "demand" pacemaker of the QRS-synchronous type. Two atrial extrasystoles follow (P[1] waves indicated by the arrows). The first one is conducted to the ventricle with a longer P-R interval, while the second is blocked within the A-V junction. The pause which follows the blocked atrial extrasystole is terminated, after a stand-by interval of 880 msec., by a pacemaker escape beat which initiates an automatic, fixed rate, pacing (69/min.). Notice how the morphology of the automatic escape beats (A) is totally different from that of sinus beats conducted to the ventricles and *synchronized* with the pacer (S). The morphology of the sinus QRS is altered by the pacemaker spike, while the *automatic QRS* is bizarre, wide and typical of a pacemaker beat.

The diagram below the tracing shows some of the R-R intervals of the spontaneous and the automatic beats. It should be noted that the duration of the *stand-by interval* (interval between the last spontaneous QRS and first automatic one) is equal to the duration of the *pacemaker automatic cycles* (880 msec.).

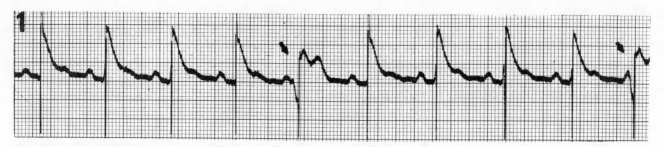

Fig. 26-A - QRS-synchronous pacemaker. Sinus QRS's and ventricular extrasystoles (arrows) show a spike 20 msecs. after the beginning of spontaneous ventricular depolarization.

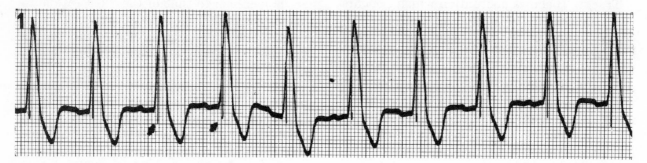

Fig. 26-B - QRS-synchronous pacemaker. A sinus rhythm is present with a complete left bundle branch block. Arrows indicate demand pacemaker spikes.

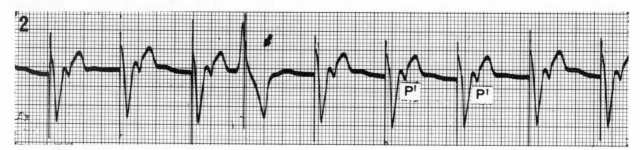

Fig. 26-C - QRS-synchronous pacemaker. The rhythm is controlled by the pacemaker in automatic function. A retrograde conduction to the atria is present (P¹). A single ventricular extrasystole (arrow) reveals the type of pacemaker in use.

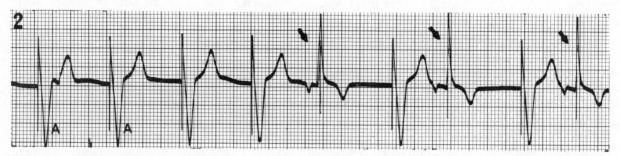

Fig. 26-D - QRS-synchronous pacemaker. The first four QRS's are automatic pacemaker beats. The following bigeminal rhythm is formed by a spontaneous QRS, synchronized with the pacemaker (arrow), and by an automatic pacemaker beat.

THE QRS-SYNCHRONOUS "DEMAND" PACEMAKER

Sensing function and automatic pacing

Fig. 26-A shows artificial impulses, with a rate of about 80/min., followed by aberrant, bizarre QRS complexes and preceded by P-waves with a constant P-stimulus interval (P-S interval). A superficial examination of the tracing suggests a pacing due to a P-wave synchronous pacemaker. However, two elements identify the type of pacemaker; a) the spike is not sharply demarcated on the isolectric line of the P-R interval but appears 20 msec. after the beginning of the spontaneous Q-wave (see page 53); b) the beats indicated by the arrows are ventricular extrasystoles which also clearly show pacemaker spikes within the QRS complexes.

Therefore, a sinus rhythm is present in a patient with a *QRS-synchronous pacemaker*. The artificial impulses are not effective because they all fall within the ventricular refractory period which follow both the sinus beat and the ventricular extrasystoles. The pacemaker shows, therefore, a *good sensing function* toward spontaneous ventricular potentials either of sinus or ectopic origin.

The tracing in fig. 26-B shows a patient with a sinus rhythm, a left bundle branch block, and a QRS-synchronous "demand" pacemaker. All the beats conducted to the ventricles show a pacemaker spike falling immediately after the spontaneous ventricular depolarization. At this point it is necessary to note that the aberration of the QRS morphology, induced by the stimulus-artifact (spike), may be confused with the QRS widen-ing due to an intraventricular conduction defect. Indeed, sometimes it is very difficult to determine whether an aberrant QRS complex is due to a bundle branch block, or is induced by the voltage decay curve of a unipolar stimulus.

When the cardiac rhythm is totally induced by artificial impulses, it may be difficult to recognize the type of "demand" pacemaker working. It may be useful, in such a case, to wait for the appearance of a spontaneous beat, either of a supraventricular or of a ventricular origin.

In the case of fig. 26-C, a fixed rate stimulation of 75/min., with a clear retrograde atrial activation (P[1]), is interrupted by a single ventricular extrasystole (arrow). Clearly showing a spike, the PVC suggests that the artificial stimulation is performed with a *ventricular-triggered "demand" pacemaker*.

Figure 26-D depicts a similar situation where the first four beats (A) are determined by automatic impulses of a pacemaker with complete ventricular capture. Here, the arrows indicate spontaneous beats which alternate with automatic pacemaker beats and determine sequences of a bigeminal type. The spontaneous QRS's clearly show the pacemaker spikes, immediately after the beginning of the ventricular depolarization. Thus, the pacemaker *is synchronized with the QRS* and, since it fires within the ventricular refractory period, it does not capture the ventricles.

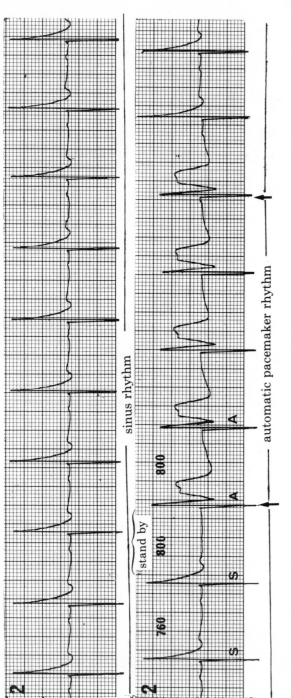

Fig. 27-A — QRS-synchronous pacemaker. The upper tracing shows a sinus rhythm perfectly synchronized with the pacemaker. A short automatic sequence is present in the lower tracing (beat A).

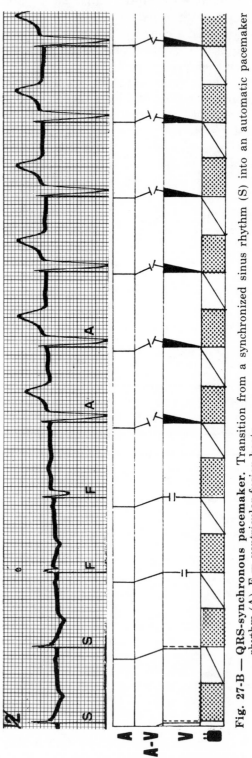

Fig. 27-B — QRS-synchronous pacemaker. Transition from a synchronized sinus rhythm (S) into an automatic pacemaker rhythm (A). F = ventricular fusion beats.

QRS-SYNCHRONOUS "DEMAND" PACEMAKER

Sensing Function and Automatic Pacing.

The tracings of fig. 27-A show a classical example of the stand-by, "demand" function of a ventricular-triggered pacemaker. They show the transition from a sinus rhythm (upper tracing) into an automatic pacemaker rhythm (lower tracing). The sinus beats conducted to the ventricles clearly show the pacemaker spike inscribed 20 msec. after the beginning of the spontaneous ventricular depolarization. The spikes are not effective on the myocardium and they only distort the QRS morphology of the sinus beats. Being continuously delivered and synchronized with the QRS's, the artificial impulses indicate a good pacemaker *sensing function*. After each synchronized impulse the pacemaker "stands-by" and waits. It will fire and capture the ventricles only when requested. This is what happens after the second sinus beat of the lower tracing. The asystolic pause, probably determined by a slowing of the sinus rate or by a sinus arrest, is ended by a sequence of five automatic pacemaker beats (A). The QRS morphology of the automatic beats is sharply different from that of sinus beats synchronized with the pacemaker (S). After the brief "fixed rate" sequence, the rhythm is again under sinus control. This is shown by the last two sinus QRS's which are synchronized with the pacemaker.

The tracings show the two typical functions of the QRS-synchronous pacemaker: a) *the sensing function* and synchronization with spontaneous cardiac potentials; and, b) *the pacing function*.

The time interval between the first synchronized sinus QRS and the first automatic beat is the *escape or stand-by interval*. In this case it is equal to 800 msec. and it must be equal to the R-R intervals of the automatic paced beats. The escape interval will never be shorter than the R-R interval of spontaneous, synchronized beats.

The transition from a spontaneous into an automatic rhythm of a QRS-synchronous pacemaker is not always so abrupt as in the case of fig. 27-A. It usually develops through one or several fusion beats, where the ventricular depolarization is shared between the spontaneous and the artificial impulses. Therefore, the morphology of fusion beats will be something in between that of spontaneous beats and pacemaker QRS's.

The first two beats of fig. 27-B are of sinus origin, normally conducted to the ventricles and synchronized with the pacemaker (S). The ventricular depolarization is entirely due to the artificial impulse; the pacemaker spike is not effective and only deforms the QRS morphology (as indicated by the dotted line on the diagram).

From the fifth beat and on the ventricular activation is entirely determined by the pacemaker which fires at a "fixed rate" (A). In fact, the QRS morphology is markedly different and resembles that of ventricular extrasystoles. The configuration of the third and fourth QRS complexes (F) is in between that of beats S and A. Because of a sinus arrhythmia, the third and fourth sinus impulses are slightly slower than the first two and appear just when the pacemaker delivers an escape, automatic beat (its automatic pacing function was "demanded" by the ventricular silence). Thus the ventricular depolarization is temporarily shared by two impulses, the sinus and the artificial one. The resulting beats are *ventricular fusion beats*.

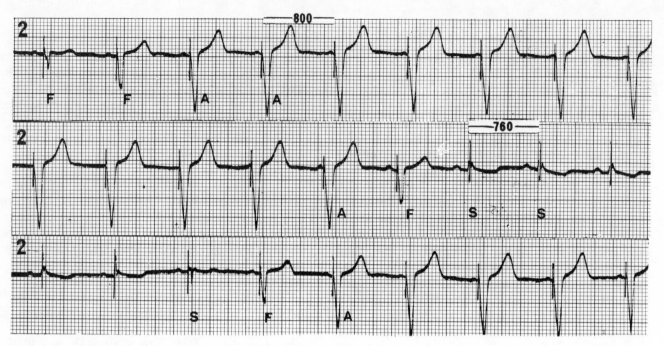

Fig. 28-A - QRS-synchronous pacemaker. "Concertina effect" - S = synchronized sinus beats; F = ventricular fusion beats; A = pacemaker automatic beat.

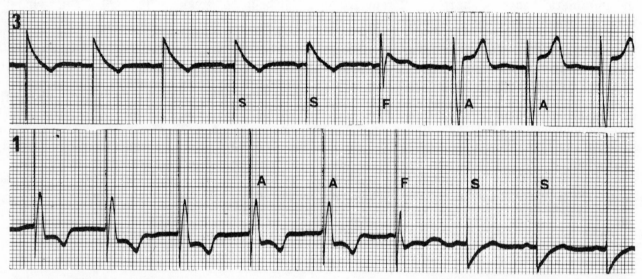

Fig. 28-B - QRS-synchronous pacemaker. Transition from a sinus rhythm into a pacemaker automatic rhythm (L3) and vice-versa (L1).

THE QRS-SYNCHRONOUS "DEMAND" PACEMAKER

Sensing function and automatic pacing

Tracings of fig. 28-A re continuous and clearly record the normal behavior of a QRS-triggered pacemaaker. The two sequences show a quiet transition of a sinus rhythm, normally conducted to the ventricles and synchronized with a QRS-synchronous pacemaker (S), into an automatic pacemaker (A) rhythm. These sequences are punctuated by several fusion beats (F), and they are often called *"concertina effect,"* since they recall the motion of an accordion bellow.

The automatic recharging cycle of the pacemaker is 800 msec., and, therefore, it determines a pacing rate of 75/min. When the S-A node cycles are shorter than 800 msec., the pacemaker is not effective. This means that it does not capture the ventricles and it fires within the sinus QRS. When the S-A cycle is of a longer duration, the ventricular rhythm is totally controlled by the pacemaker (automatic beat with complete ventricular capture). *Ventricular fusion beats* appear during the transition between sinus and pacemaker beats. Here the sinus rate is almost identical to the automatic rate of the pacemaker.

Similar sequences are presented in fig. 28-B, where the control of the cardiac rhythm is shared between the S-A node and an artificial pacemaker. Sinus beats, conducted to the ventricles and synchronized with a pacemaker (S), are replaced by automatic beats, with a different QRS morphology (A in the upper tracing) and vice versa (lower tracing). Fusion beats (F) counterpoint the rhythm and signal the transition between sinus and automatic QRS complexes.

It is worthwhile to remember that, sometimes, it is difficult to recognize the initial portion of a synchronized QRS (which precedes the stimulus-artifact by 20 msec.). This may depend on the particular electrocardiographic lead being recorded. In fig. 28-B the sinus beats conducted to the ventricles (S) are better visualized in L3 than in L1, and clearly show the initial portion of the Q waves which precede the pacemaker spike.

Great care must be paid in examining the initial part of the QRS complex. This is because it may be difficult to separate a synchronized from an automatic beat (see page 52). The 20 msec. interval is necessary to permit the accumulation of enough spontaneous ventricular potentials to be sensed by the pacemaker. They, in turn, will trigger an impulse into the ventricular refractory period.

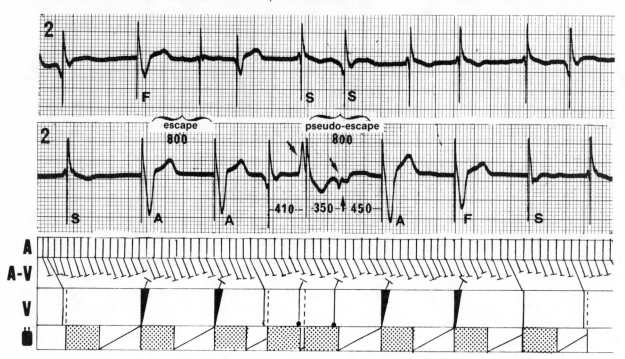

Fig. 29-A - QRS-synchronous pacemaker. The second ventricular extrasystole (second arrows) is not sensed by the pacemaker. The following automatic beat terminates a "pseudo-escape interval". The true escape interval follows an asystolic pause of 800 msec.

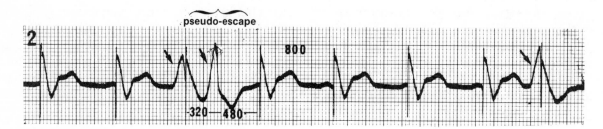

Fig. 29-B - QRS-synchronous pacemaker. The second ventricular extrasystole is not sensed because it falls within the pacemaker refractory period (400 msec.). The pacemaker works normally.

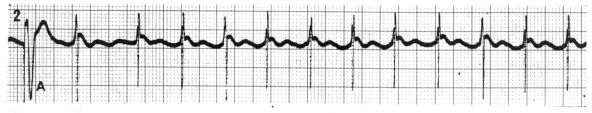

Fig. 29-C - QRS-synchronous pacemaker. The atrial flutter has a fast ventricular response (140/min.) and is normally synchronized with the pacemaker.

Refractory period

This type of stimulator, like the P-wave synchronous pacemaker, is protected from rapid cardiac rates by the insertion of a *refractory period*. This is a period in which the pacemaker does not sense intracavitary spontaneous potentials and does not synchronize with them.

The presence of a refractory period means that, when the R-R interval of a spontaneous beat is very short, the pacemaker does not deliver QRS-synchronized impulses. The great majority of ventricular-triggered pacemakers have a refractory period which is in between 400 and 500 msec. (see page 207). Therefore a spontaneous beat which falls within the *pacemaker refractory period* will not be sensed.

Tracings of fig. 29-A show an irregular ventricular rhythm of an atrial fibrillation in a patient with a QRS-synchronous pacemaker. Three types of QRS's are present: 1) supraventricular beats conducted to the ventricles and synchronized with the pacemaker (S); 2) pacemaker automatic beats (A); 3) fusion beats (F).

The cardiac cycles and, therefore, the R-R intervals are irregular. The pacemaker behavior follows the different penetration of atrial impulses through the A-V junction. When the R-R interval is short (400-460-480 msec. etc.) the pacemaker impulse is synchronized with the conducted QRS and it falls right within the ventricular complex. When the A-V conduction slows down, longer R-R intervals appear (>800 msec.), and the pacemaker "escapes" and initiates an automatic pacing with a rate of 75/min. (beats A). Therefore, the *escape interval* of the pacemaker in question is equal to 800 msec.

When the cardiac cycle is shorter than 400 msec. the situation is different. Notice the two extrasystoles indicated by the arrows in the lower tracing. The first beat closes a cardiac cycle of 410 msec. Thus it is *sensed* and *synchronized* by the pacemaker. The second is slightly more premature (350 msec.) and falls within the *pacemaker refractory period*. This is not sensed and, for the pacemaker, it is like being in the presence of a long asystolic pause (which starts from the preceding stimulus). After an escape interval of 800 msec., the pacemaker delivers an *automatic impulse* (A). The behavior of the pacemaker is normal. However, the automatic beat which follows the not sensed extrasystole is not a true escape beat. Furthermore, the interval of time between the synchronized PVC and the automatic beat is not a true escape interval.

We have defined as an *escape beat* a subsidiary, emergency beat (see pages 43 and 57) and, as such, it must always appear after a long cardiac pause. In this case, the *escape beat* appears after an asystolic pause of 800 msec., while the interval between the automatic pacemaker beat and the not sensed extrasystole is much shorter (450 msec.). The interval of 800 msec. (350 + 450 msec.) is called *"pseudo-escape interval."*

Similar situation is the one of fig. 29-B. The third and fourth QRS are ventricular extrasystoles. While the first PVC is sensed and synchronized with the pacemaker, the second PVC falls too prematurely (320 msec. from the preceding beat), and, therefore, into the refractory period of the pacemaker. It is not sensed and causes a *pseudo-escape, automatic beat*. Also in this case, the automatic cycles are equal to 800 msec. and the stimulation rate is equal to 75/min.

A *refractory period* of 400 or 500 msec. does not permit pacemaker synchronizations with rates faster than 125/min. or 150/min. The Cordis Ectocor, for example, originally had a a refractory period of 500 msec. This has later been shortened to 400 msec. to allow for a synchronization with faster cardiac rates. With such a refractory period, spontaneous cardiac rates up to 150/min. can be synchronized with the pacemaker. This is shown in fig. 29-C where an atrial flutter is present, with a 2:1 A-V block and a ventricular rate of 140/min. Except for the first QRS, which is a pacemaker beat with ventricular capture, all other spontaneous QRS's are synchronized with the pacemaker. Here the spikes are clearly visible within the ventricular complexes.

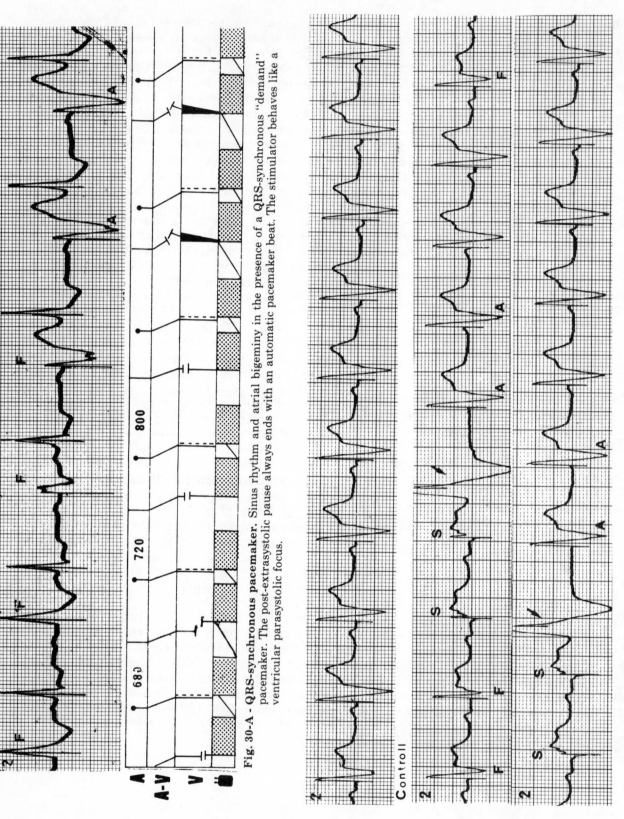

Fig. 30-A - **QRS-synchronous pacemaker.** Sinus rhythm and atrial bigeminy in the presence of a QRS-synchronous "demand" pacemaker. The post-extrasystolic pause always ends with an automatic pacemaker beat. The stimulator behaves like a ventricular parasystolic focus.

Fig. 30-B - **QRS-synchronous pacemaker.** Tracing A may simulate an asynchronous or a P-wave synchronous pacemaker. Tracing B reveals the true nature of the stimulator.

THE QRS-SYNCHRONOUS "DEMAND" PACEMAKER

Iatrogenic pacemaker parasystole

Fig. 30-A shows a sinus rhythm with an atrial bigeminy in a patient with a ventricular-triggered pacemaker. By just glancing at the tracing it is easy to spot pacemaker spikes, within spontaneous QRS complexes of supraventricular origin, and to recognize the type of stimulation (QRS-triggered pacemaker).

Atrial extrasystoles alternate with sinus beats. They are easily recognized because the P^1-wave morphology (dots in the diagram) is different from that of sinus P-waves (which are notched and of longer duration). The QRS complexes indicated by A are pacemaker automatic beats with complete ventricular capture. All the other complexes are ventricular fusion beats (F) with a morphology gradually approaching that of automatic pacemaker beats.

It should be noted that, while fusion and automatic pacemaker beats always appear at the end of a constant time interval (800 msec.) from the preceding atrial extrasystole (escape interval), the sinus impulse following the PAC appears with an always increasing delay (680-720-800 msec.). The different morphology of the fusion beats (first, third, fifth, and seventh QRS), is due to the progressive delay of the sinus impulses which depolarize an always smaller area of ventricular myocardium. Meanwhile, that which is activated by the automatic pacemaker impulses becomes increasing larger, until a complete ventricular capture (A). This tracing recalls the features of a spontaneous ventricular parasystole. As is commonly found with the use of asychronous pacemakers (see page 32), the ventricular-triggered pacemakers may also induce a form of iatrogenic ventricular parasystole. Opposite to what happens with the asynchronous pacemaker, *the artificial parasystolic focus,* created by a QRS-synchronous pacemaker, is not protected from the influence of sinus impulses. While the asynchronous pacemaker delivers impulses at a fixed rate, undisturbed by ventricular potentials of sinus origin (see the "entrance block" of a natural parasystole), the QRS-synchronous "demand" pacemaker is easily and intentionally influenced by spontaneous ventricular potentials. In fact, they determine the delivery of a pacemaker impulse in a moment of the cardiac cycle which is electrophysiologically inert, thus avoiding "competition" with the spontaneous beats.

Tracing A of fig. 30-B is of a patient with a QRS-synchronous pacemaker. The ventricular stimulation in this case is of a "fixed rate" type (73/min.). This may suggest the presence of an asynchronous type of pacemaker. Each QRS is preceded by a P-wave with a constant P-S interval (P-stimulus). This factor would be indicative of a P-wave synchronous pacemaker.

Tracings B, recorded only a few minutes later, allows a precise identification of the type of pacemaker. The sinus QRS complexes are synchronized with the pacemaker (S) and the ventricular extrasystoles indicated by the arrows (note the pacemaker spike synchronized also with the extrasystole) are followed by long sequences of automatic beats (A). Several fusion beats (F) are also present.

This tracing shows that: a) occasionally, long tracings are necessary to spot spontaneous beats and recognize the type of pacemaker in use; b) the presence of fixed rate stimuli does not necessarily mean "asynchronous pacemaker"; c) P waves, constantly preceding pacemaker beats, do not necessarily indicate the presence of a P-wave synchronous pacemaker and, d) the QRS-synchronous pacemaker parasystole is not protected from the influence of sinus beats. In fact, the sinus impulses do not allow the pacemaker to capture the ventricles.

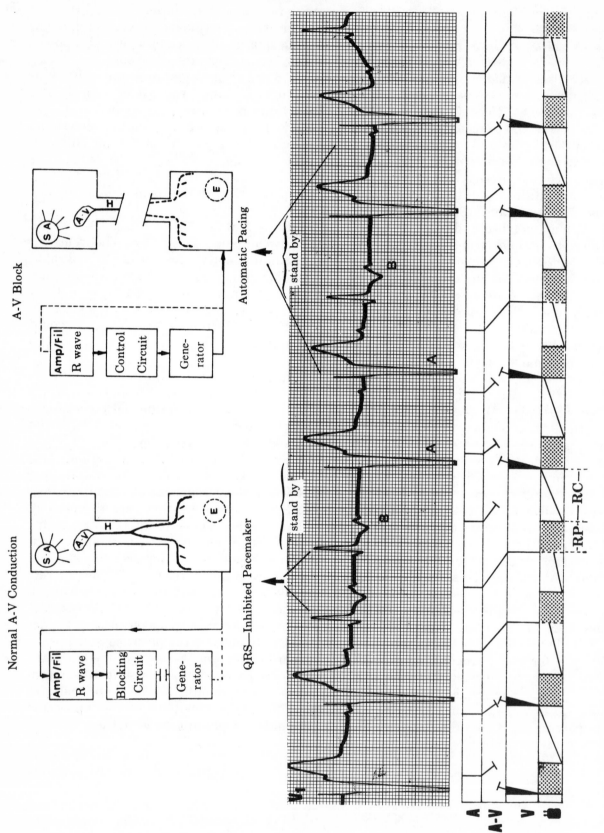

Fig. 31-A - QRS-inhibited "demand" pacemaker. Symbiosis and interaction between a sinus rhythm, with a second degree A-V block, and the non-competitive rhythm of an artificial stimulator. Dashes in the diagram indicate spontaneous impulses inhibiting the pacemaker. (R-P = pacemaker refractory period; RC = recharging cycle).

B. THE QRS-INHIBITED "DEMAND" PACEMAKER

Sensing function and automatic pacing

Also called *QRS-blocking* or *ventricular-inhibited*, this type of pacemaker is the one highly preferred in clinical practice, when it is necessary to avoid competition between a spontaneous rhythm and that of the artificial pacemaker. This is especially true in cases of intermittent A-V block. Similarly to the QRS-synchronous pacemaker, the ventricular-inhibited pacemaker has an *automatic mechanism* which stimulates the ventricles at a fixed rate, preselected at the moment of implantation, when spontaneous cardiac activity is not present. Thus, artificial pacing is performed *only when necessary,* not continuously but at "demand". *In the presence of spontaneous ventricular potentials, the delivery of a pacemaker impulse is "blocked" by a specialized inhibiting circuit and the pacemaker spike does not appear on the surface electrocardiogram.*

The presence of the *blocking circuit* is a unique feature of a QRS-inhibited pacemaker and it substantially differentiates this unit from a QRS-synchronous 'demand" pacemaker (see page 53). After a determined interval of time from the preceding ventricular contraction *(escape or stand-by interval),* if cardiac activity is not present, the ventricular-inhibited pacemaker will stimulate the heart at a fixed rate. On the other hand, the pacemaker is automatically suppressed when the R-R interval of spontaneous beats become shorter than the automatic pacing interval.

The tracing and diagram of fig. 31-A clearly show the mechanism of a QRS-inhibited pacemaker. A sinus rhythm is present and it controls the ventricles through sequences of second degree A-V block. After the first two beats, which are pacemaker automatic beats (rate = 60/min.), sinus impulses cross the A-V junction, with some delay, and activate the ventricles with a sequence of a 3:2 A-V Wenckebach. Notice that the first of the conducted P-waves has a P-R interval of 0.32 sec. and that a right bundle branch block is also present. The third P-wave of the Wenckebach period is blocked within the A-V junction (B) and the following asystolic pause is terminated by two pacemaker automatic beats (A). The rhythm continues with another short sequence of sinus beats, with a 2:1 A-V block, followed by an asystolic pause and by automatic pacemaker beats.

The pacemaker is, therefore, a *QRS-inhibited "demand" type* which is quiescent when sinus beats are conducted to the ventricles. The pacemaker delivers impulses only when the spontaneous cardiac rate falls below the intrinsic automatic rate of the pacemaker (which, in this case, is 60/min.).

The QRS-inhibited pacemaker has a *sensing mechanism* which responds to cardiac potentials picked up by the ventricular electrode. When activated, this circuit blocks the delivery of impulses from the generator for an interval of time whose length is determined at the moment of implantation. This interval is the *escape or stand-by interval,* which also determines the desired automatic pacing rate. In some of the models the escape interval can be changed through a percutaneous insertion of a needle-screw into the generator pack. Thus, slower or faster pacing rates can be obtained after implantation.

If spontaneous ventricular potentials, either of sinus or ectopic origin, do not appear at the expiration of the escape interval, the pacemaker continues to deliver automatic impulses. If, instead, a spontaneous ventricular contraction is present, the pacemaker is suppressed and the escape interval is reset.

In the case presented in fig. 31-A the automatic rate ("fixed rate"), preselected at the moment of implantation of the pacemaker, is equal to 60/min. (the interval between two automatic beats = 1 sec.). Each sinus impulse conducted to the ventricles suppresses the pacemaker for one second. This means that each spontaneous QRS, occurring before the end of the one second interval, blocks the generator delivering mechanism and starts a new recharging cycle of one second. If, at the end of the escape interval spontaneous ventricular potentials are still absent, the pacemaker delivers an impulse and continues to stimulate the ventricles with a fixed rate of 60/min. (impulses at one second interval); the automatic pacing continues until reappearance of spontaneous cardiac activity. Thus, the automatic interval is nothing else than an escape interval during which the pacemaker is "alert", "stand-by" and, ready to sense spontaneous ventricular potentials, or, in their absence, to stimulate the ventricles.

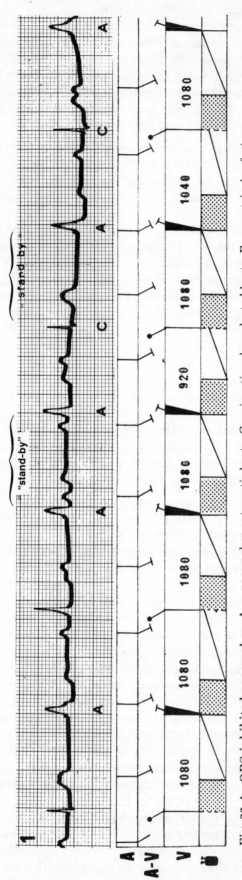

Fig. 32-A - QRS-inhibited pacemaker. A = pacemaker automatic beats; C = junctional conducted beats; F = ventricular fusion beat.

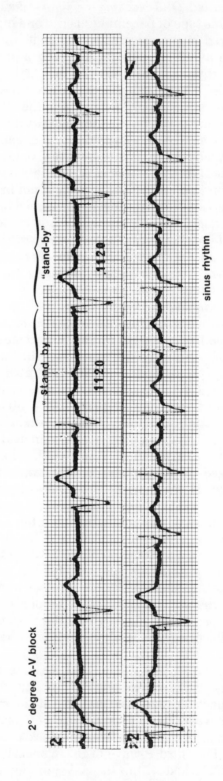

Fig. 32-B - QRS-inhibited pacemaker. A second degree A-V block triggers the "demand" pacemaker (top tracing); the reappearance of a normal A-V conduction and of a sinus rhythm suppress the artificial pacemaker.

THE QRS-INHIBITED "DEMAND" PACEMAKER

Sensing function and automatic pacing

Fig. 32-A shows a patient with a complete A-V block and a junctional rhythm (beats "C") in symbiosis to that of an artificial pacemaker (beats "A"). The stimulator is a QRS-inhibited "demand" type and the pacemaker spikes are not present within the spontaneous QRS's. The "fixed rate" stimulation is equal to 55/min. and the *escape interval* (automatic or "stand-by" interval) is equal to 1080 msec. The rate of sinus P-waves, which are blocked within the A-V junction and independent from the ventricular rhythm, is equal to 85/min.

Ventricular contractions are alternatively determined by pacemaker and by junctional impulses conducted to the ventricles. Beat F is a *ventricular fusion beat;* this is due partially by a junctional impulse and partially by an almost simultaneous artificial impulse. Here the junctional impulse is fired right at the end of the pacemaker stand-by interval of 1080 msec. The shaded area of the diagram indicates the *pacemaker refractory period* during which the pacemaker is unable to sense spontaneous ventricular potentials and to trigger the blocking circuit.

The refractory period has been intentionally inserted to avoid that the pacemaker senses: a) the electrical potentials created by its own impulses; b) the stimulus induced myocardial potentials. Both could cause a premature pacer inhibition. Therefore, the stimulus delivered by the pacer is, at the same time, blocking the pacer sensing mechanism for a certain interval of time. In the QRS-in-hibited "demand" pacemakers of several manufacturers, this time interval ranges between 200 and 400 msec. (see page 203).

The diagonal lines of the diagram indicate the impulse *recharging cycle*. The length of a recharging cycle is obviously different when included between two automatic beats then when between an automatic beat and a spontaneous one. The latter is always shorter than an automatic cycle. The escape interval between two automatic beats (A-A interval) and that between a spontaneous and an automatic beat (C-A interval) is always the same. In both circumstances, the escape interval includes a complete pacemaker recharging cycle.

Tracings of fig. 32-B show the reappearance of a sinus rhythm, with a normal A-V conduction (lower tracing), in a patient with a second degree A-V block Mobitz type II. Here the blocked P-waves are indicated with a dark dot. The upper tracing shows the interaction between sinus impulses, conducted to the ventricles (C), and pacemaker automatic impulses following blocked P-waves (A). The artificial stimulation rate is quite slow (53/min.) and the pacemaker behavior is that typical of a *QRS-inhibited "demand" type*. The conducted QRS's do not show a stimulus-artifact. Spikes appear and capture the ventricles only after asystolic pauses of 1120 msec.

With the reappearance of the sinus rhythm and a normal A-V conduction (lower tracing), the pacemaker is suppressed and remains silent throughout the sinus sequences (the sinus rate of 90/min. is faster than the pacemaker automatic rate).

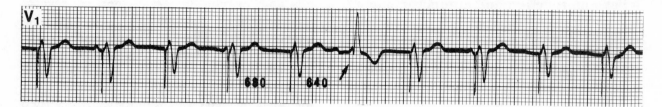

Fig. 33-A - QRS-inhibited pacemaker. The stimulation is almost entirely automatic except for the sinus beat normally conducted to the ventricle (arrow).

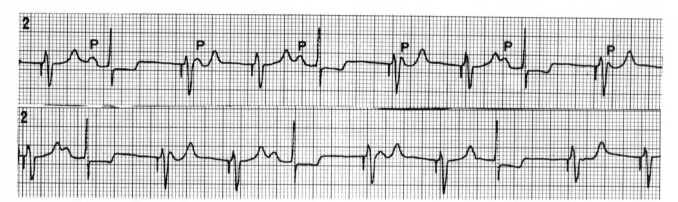

Fig. 33-B - QRS-inhibited pacemaker. The ventricular trigeminy results from the symbiosis of a bradycardic sinus rhythm (note the P-P intervals) and the automatic rhythm of a "demand" QRS-inhibited pacemaker. Every other sinus P wave is not conducted to the ventricles.

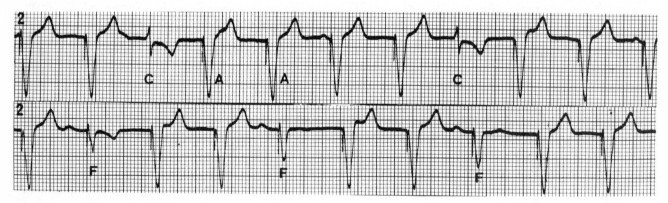

Fig. 33-C - QRS-inhibited pacemaker. C = sinus beat conducted to the ventricle; A = pacemaker automatic beats; F = ventricular fusion beats.

THE QRS-INHIBITED "DEMAND" PACEMAKER

Sensing function and automatic pacing

It is now a well known fact that a sinus rhythm, with a normal A-V conduction, may reappear in approximately 20-30% of patients with advanced degrees of A-V block and treated with artificial pacing. The electrical potential of sinus beats which are conducted to the ventricles do not compete with the activity of a QRS-inhibited permanent pacemaker. In fact, the R-wave potentials are first sensed by the pacemaker, then selectively amplified and, finally, transmitted to a blocking circuit which inhibits the delivery of pacemaker impulses.

Fig. 33-A shows a regular pacing (88/min.), with good ventricular capture, interrupted only once by a sinus beat conducted to the ventricles. The spontaneous beat is slightly more premature (640 msec.) than the automatic cardiac cycles (680 msec.).

The generator firing schedule is preselected at the moment of implantation and, in this case, one impulse each 680/msec. The impulse delivery is interrupted by early sinus beats. The sensed R-wave terminates the recharging cycle and starts a new one. The duration of the *recharging cycle* may be determined by the stimulus interval (in this case = 680/msec.) minus the pacemaker refractory period (see page 203). The majority of QRS-inhibited pacemakers have automatic pacing rates between 50 and 100 impulses/min., while the refractory period ranges between 200-400 msec.

Tracings of fig. 33-B show the interaction between a bradycardic sinus rhythm (the sinus P-waves are indicated in the upper tracing) and that of a *ventricular inhibited "demand"* pacemaker. Every other P-wave is blocked within the A-V junction and is partially buried in the pacemaker QRS. It is difficult to establish whether P-waves are blocked by the concealed retrograde V-A conduction of the pacemaker beats, or if a second degree A-V block is present. Thus the rhythm is a "ventricular trigemy type", where the two regular beats are those of the pacemaker and the premature beat is a sinus beat conducted to the ventricles.

Fig. 33-C is also from a patient with a *QRS-inhibited "demand" pacemaker*. It is possible to recognize pacemaker automatic beats with complete ventricular capture (A), sinus beats conducted to the ventricles with a first degree A-V block (C) and beats with a morphology between A and C. The latter are *ventricular fusion beats* (F) where the ventricular depolarization is partially due to sinus and partially to pacemaker impulses (see page 83). Once again, the pacemaker mechanism is clearly revealed by the sinus beats without pacemaker spikes. This indicates a QRS-inhibited "demand" system in action.

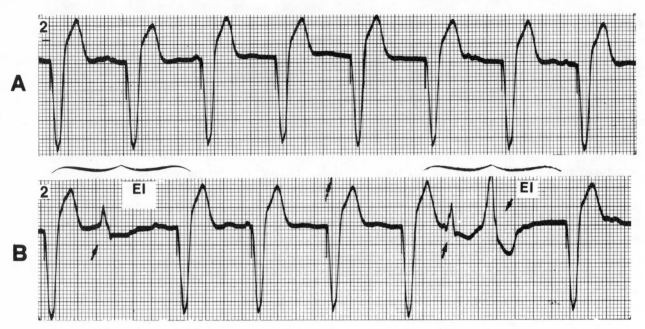

Fig. 34-A - QRS-inhibited pacemaker. Tracing A shows a cardiac rhythm entirely under control of an artificial pacemaker. Tracing B shows multifocal ventricular extrasystoles which suppress the "demand" QRS-blocking pacemaker.

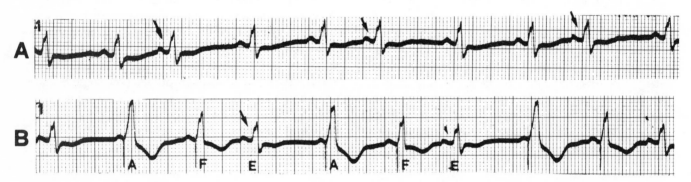

Fig. 34-B - QRS-inhibited pacemaker. Tracing A shows an atrial trigeminy. The "triplets" in tracing B are formed by an automatic pacemaker beat (A), a fusion beat (F), and an atrial extrasystole (E).

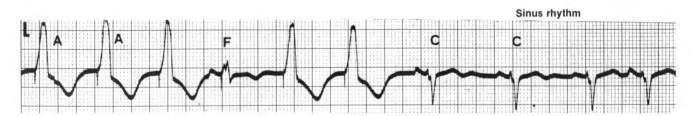

Fig. 34-C - QRS-inhibited pacemaker. The automatic pacemaker rhythm is suppressed by the reappearance of a sinus rhythm; F = ventricular fusion beat.

THE QRS-INHIBITED "DEMAND" PACEMAKER

Sensing function and automatic pacing

This type of pacemaker senses spontaneous ventricular potentials and is temporarily "inhibited". This means that it does not deliver impulses unless there are asystolic pauses longer than the escape automatic interval. It follows that "inhibitory ventricular potentials" and will not necessarily be only those of sinus beats. The QRS-blocking pacemaker may also be suppressed by ventricular and atrial extrasystoles, by ventricular complexes of atrial flutter and fibrillation, and by ventricular potentials of other origins, as long as they fall outside its refractory period and are sensed by the pacemaker (see page 203).

Fig. 34-A shows two tracings from the same patient. Tracing A shows a regular pacing with a rate of 73/min. and complete ventricular capture. Tracing B shows two intervals of different length (large parenthesis) induced by the presence of multifocal and repetitive ventricular extrasystoles (arrows); the PVC's are sensed and temporarily inhibit the pacemaker. In the second sequence, the interval between the two pacemaker impulses is slightly longer because the recharging cycle is interrupted twice by the extrasystoles. It follows that, while the interval between two successive automatic stimuli may be different (depending upon the number of spontaneous QRS's which are being sensed) the *escape interval* (interval between a pacemaker automatic impulse and the preceding ventricular contraction) is always the same.

It should be noted that, in the presence of spontaneous ventricular beats with wide and aberrant QRS's (for example ventricular extrasystoles), the escape interval cannot be exactly measured. This is because it may be difficult to know at which point, from the beginning of the widened QRS, the pacemaker senses the ventricular potentials and then is suppressed.

Tracing A of fig. 34-B shows a sinus rhythm with an atrial trigeminy. Each beat indicated by the arrow is an atrial premature beat. After the implantation of a *QRS-blocking pacemaker*, (tracing B) a trigeminal rhythm is still present. The "triplets" are formed by: a) a pacemaker automatic beat (A), which ends the pause following the atrial extrasystoles (arrow); b) a ventricular fusion beat (F), due to the fusion of a sinus and an artificial impulse and, c) the atrial extrasystole which inhibits the pacemaker (E).

The tracing of fig. 34-C starts with a brief automatic sequence of a QRS-inhibited pacemaker (beats A). The emergence of a sinus rhythm, with a normal A-V conduction (final sequence of the tracing), suppresses the "demand" pacemaker. In this case, again, a ventricular fusion beat (F) is present and is due to an occasional sinus impulse which crosses the A-V junction and fuses with a simultaneous artificial impulse.

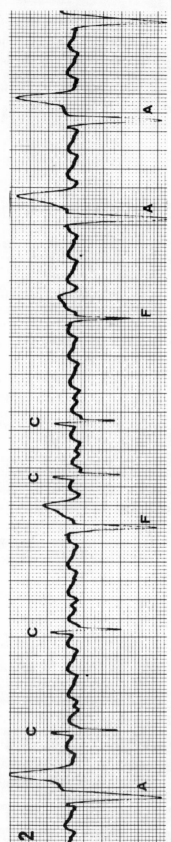

Fig. 35-A - QRS-inhibited pacemaker and atrial flutter. A = pacemaker automatic beats; C = beats conducted to the ventricle; F = ventricular fusion beat.

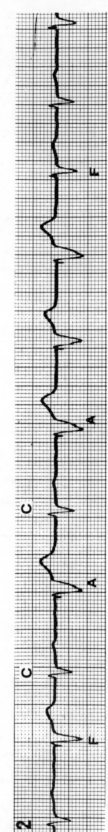

Fig. 35-B - QRS-inhibited pacemaker and atrial fibrillation. See text.

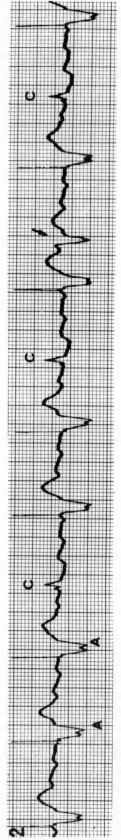

Fig. 35-C - QRS -inhibited pacemaker and atrial flutter. See text.

THE QRS-INHIBITED "DEMAND" PACEMAKER

Sensing function and automatic pacing

The ventricular potentials of an atrial flutter or fibrillation are sensed by a QRS-blocking pacemaker in the same way as potentials of sinus or extrasystolic origin. This is shown in the tracing of the opposite page.

Fig. 35-A shows an atrial flutter with a variable A-V ratio. The irregular ventricular response is due to: 1) impulses conducted to the ventricles from the atria (C); 2) pacemaker automatic beats (A), which appear after the long ventricular asystolic pauses due to an increase of the A-V block; 3) fusion beats (F) between atrial and pacemaker impulses. The *QRS-inhibited pacemaker* protects the ventricles from prolonged asystolic intervals, which are often present in an atrial flutter with a high degree of A-V block. On the other hand, it does not compete with spontaneous ventricular beats.

A similar behavior is present in a patient with atrial fibrillation and a high degree of A-V block (fig. 35-B). Again the ventricular com-plexes of the atrial fibrillation (conducted beat = C) can be separated from those of pacemaker beats (A). A ventricular fusion beat (F) is occasionally present and has a morphology between that of artificial and spontaneous QRS's.

The performance of the "demand" pacemaker during an atrial fibrillation is requested only by the absence of cardiac activity. This is usually secondary to a reduced conduction of the atrial impulses through the A-V junction.

A QRS-inhibited "demand" pacemaker may be suppressed either by supraventricular or by idioventricular potentials. Fig. 35-C presents an atrial flutter with occasional transmission of atrial impulses to the ventricles (conducted beats = C). The spontaneous QRS's are sensed by the "demand" pacemaker which temporarily blocks the delivery of automatic impulses (beat A). The single ventricular extrasystole, indicated by the arrow, is also able to block the pacemaker's impulse delivery and to start a new recharging cycle.

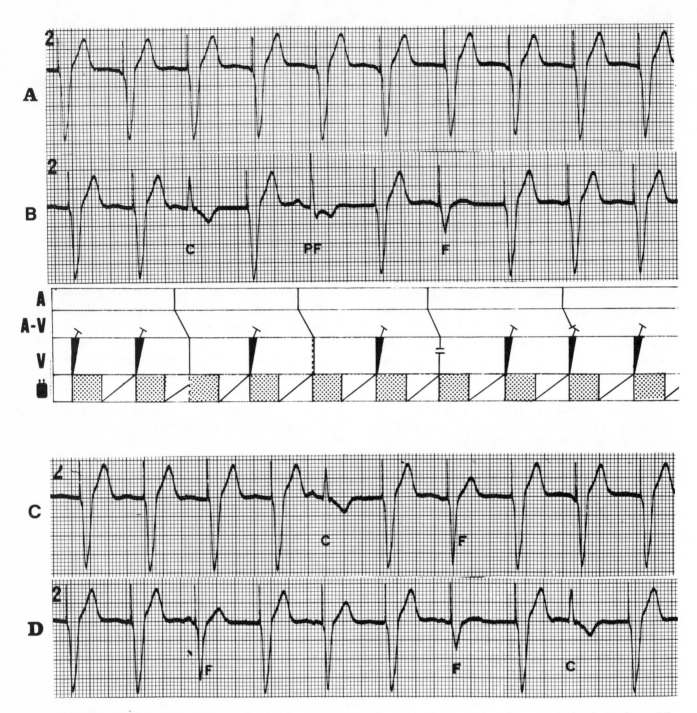

Fig. 36-A - QRS-inhibited pacemaker. C = sinus beats conducted to the ventricles; F = ventricular fusion beat; PF = pseudo-fusion beats.

THE QRS-INHIBITED "DEMAND" PACEMAKER

Fusion and pseudofusion beats

The presence of spontaneous cardiac activity may suppress a ventricular-triggered pacemaker for hours, days, weeks or even months. The stimulator fires only when "demanded" by asystolic pauses longer than the intrinsic automatic cycles of the pacemaker. On the other hand, this unit may stimulate the ventricles at a fixed rate for days, months, and simulate the presence of an asynchronous pacemaker.

When facing a rhythm like that of tracing A of fig. 36-A it is difficult to know whether the ventricular pacing is caused by a QRS-synchronous or QRS-inhibited "demand" type pacemaker, or by an asynchronous pacemaker. However, the occasional presence of spontaneous beats, of sinus or ectopic origin, may be helpful in the differential diagnosis.

Tracing B shows three beats of sharply different configuration when compared to pacemaker automatic beats. The first is a sinus beat with normal ventricular conduction (C); the third is a ventricular fusion beat (F) due to the almost simultaneous propagation of the sinus and of the pacemaker impulse. The second beat, however, is a sinus beat conducted to the ventricles, and shows a pacemaker spike immediately after the beginning of the ventricular activation. Thus, the sinus beat exhibits the so called "pseudo-fusion" (PF) with the pacemaker impulse.

Spontaneous beats altered by ineffective spikes are not a rare finding when in the presence of a QRS-inhibited pacemaker. This is a particular situation where the spontaneous ventricular depolarization begins just at the end of the pacemaker escape interval; the pacemaker, therefore, delivers an automatic impulse since it has not sensed the spontaneous ventricular potentials. The spike does not capture the ventricular myocardium which is entirely depolarized by the sinus impulse. Thus, the resulting beat is a *pseudo-fusion beat*. It is not a true fusion beat where the ventricles are partially depolarized by the S-A node and partially by the pacemaker impulse. Also it is not a pacemaker *automatic beat* with a complete ventricular capture by the artificial impulse. It is, instead, a normal sinus beat conducted to the ventricles which shows a pacemaker spike inscribed on it. This is called *"pseudo-fusion"* because it simulates a true fusion, but it is only a recording phenomenon of the pacemaker spike simultaneous with the sinus QRS on the surface EKG. Pseudo-fusion beats are often misinterpreted by the beginner as pacemaker malfunction and may delay the exact identification of the type of pacing. For example, in this case, they may suggest the presence of a QRS-synchronous pacemaker or they may be misdiagnosed as pacemaker malfunction.

Tracing C and D belong to the same patient. They show additional sinus beats conducted to the ventricles (C) and true fusion beats (F).

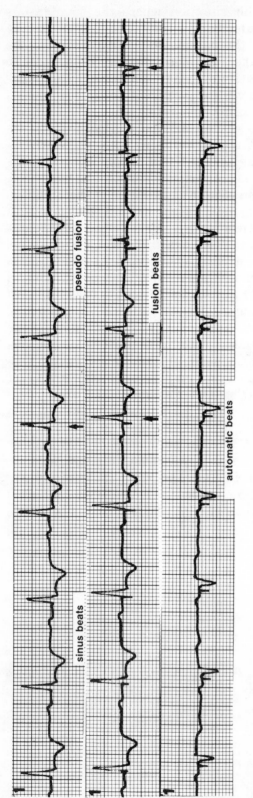

Fig. 37-A - QRS-inhibited pacemaker. The transition from the sinus rhythm (upper tracing) to the pacemaker automatic rhythm (third tracing) goes through numerous pseudo-fusion and ventricular fusion beats (middle tracing).

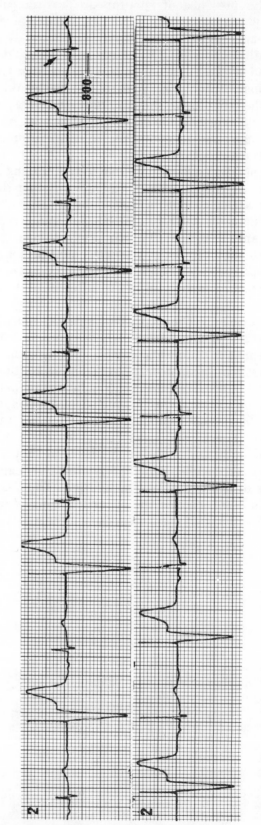

Fig. 37-B - QRS-inhibited pacemaker. The ventricular bigeminy is due to alternating pacemaker automatic beats and sinus beats. Notice the pseudo-fusion beats in the lower tracing.

THE QRS-INHIBITED "DEMAND" PACEMAKER

Fusion and pseudofusion beats

At this point it is necessary to clarify the following terminology:

a) *ventricular fusion beat* (true fusion); it appears when the activation of the ventricular chambers is shared by the simultaneous propagation of impulses coming from two different foci. Therefore, the QRS morphology of a fusion beat is the vectorial summation of the different amounts of myocardium activated by one or the other pacemaker.

b) *pseudofusion beat;* it is present anytime a spontaneous QRS and a pacemaker spike are simultaneously recorded and overimposed on the surface electrocardiogram. The pacemaker impulse falls into the absolute ventricular refractory period and it is inscribed on a spontaneous QRS. A pseudofusion beat calls to mind the simultaneous ECG recording of a P wave and a QRS complex during A-V dissociation, ventricular extrasystoles and ventricular tachycardia.

The duration of the pacemaker escape interval is preselected at the moment of implantation and triggers the automatic pacing mechanism. Therefore, when spontaneous ventricular potentials are formed just at the end of the escape interval, they may not be able to inhibit the pacemaker which has already reached the critical time of impulse delivery. This causes the simultaneous surface EKG recording of a stimulus-artifact and a spontaneous QRS and the so-called *pseudofusion beat*. The ventricular depolarization is determined entirely by the sinus impulse and the spike is totally ineffective.

When the sinus impulse reaches the ventricles only a few milliseconds after the critical impulse-emission time, the pacemaker and the S-A node share the ventricular depolarization and, then, *true ventricular fusion beats* are recorded on the surface EKG. If the sinus impulse is delayed further over the critical emission time, the artificial pacemaker captures the entire ventricular myocardium *(automatic beats)*.

Fig. 37-A is a continuous recording of the transition from a sinus rhythm into a ventricular rhythm of a *QRS-inhibited pacemaker*. The delivery rates of the S-A node and of the artificial pacemaker are very similar. However, at a certain point a slight and constant delay of the S-A node time-table enables the emergence of the QRS-blocking "demand" pacemaker (arrow on the upper tracing). Therefore, the first four beats are of sinus origin and are conducted to the ventricles (a slight prolongation of the P-R interval is present). From the fifth to the fourteenth beat the morphology of the QRS is essentially the same. Here, however, the spikes can be seen inscribed in the ventricular complexes and inducing a slight QRS deformity. These impulses do not capture the ventricles; they "fuse" with a sinus QRS on the surface ECG and, therefore, are *pseudofusion beats*.

Due to a slight but progressive delay of the S-A node emission rate, the pacemaker spikes fall always more prematurely with respect to the ventricular depolarization of sinus origin. Note that while the fifth QRS has a pacemaker spike inscribed on the peak of the R wave, the fourteenth QRS "begins" with a spike. From the fifteenth complex (first arrow of the second tracing) to the eighteenth (second arrow) the QRS morphology begins to change and exhibits four different configuration. From the twentieth beat and on (the entire lower tracing), the ventricular rhythm is totally under control of the pacemaker firing at a fixed rate. While the QRS's of the bottom tracing are *automatic beats,* those from the fifteenth through the eighteenth complexes are *true ventricular fusion beats*. The different morphology of the fusion beats indicates that the amount of ventricular myocardium depolarized by the sinus impulse decreases while that activated by the almost simultaneous artificial impulse is increasing progressively, until it reaches a point where the pacemaker captures the entire ventricular myocardium.

Thus this sequence illustrates the transition from a sinus rhythm to an automatic rhythm of a QRS-inhibited pacemaker, going through several pseudo-fusion and true fusion beats. In this case, the first four sinus beats without spikes indicate the presence of a QRS-inhibited type "demand" pacemaker.

Tracings of fig. 37-B show an unusual type of ventricular bigeminy. The "couplets" are made of a sinus and a QRS-inhibited "demand" pacemaker beat.

The first five sinus QRS's, which alternate with pacemaker automatic beats, do not show a stimulus-artifact and thereby indicate the type of pacing in action (QRS-blocking). Beginning with the beat indicated by the arrow, the sinus QRS's show a spike at the top of the R wave. These are *pseudofusion beats* and they alternate with *automatic pacemaker beats* with complete ventricular capture.

The continuous presence of the pacemaker spike, either during the recording of spontaneous QRS's or at the beginning of paced beats, allow the measurement of the pacemaker automatic cycle. In this case it is equal to 800 msec. (escape interval); therefore, the automatic pacing rate is 75/m although the interval between two automatic QRS's in the upper tracing would suggest a stimulation rate of 32/m.

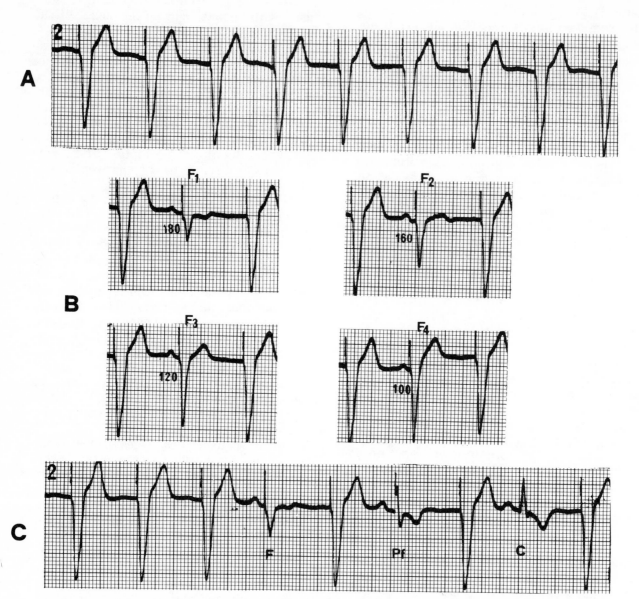

Fig. 38-A - QRS-inhibited pacemaker. Tracing A shows a fixed rate ventricular pacing. Four ventricular fusion beats (F1 .... F4) are present in tracing B. Tracing C shows automatic pacemaker beats (A), a ventricular fusion beat (F), a pseudo-fusion beat (Pf) and a sinus beat conducted to the ventricles (C).

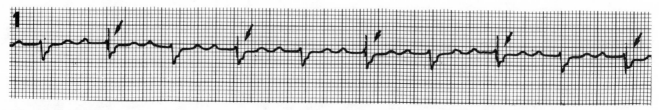

Fig. 38-B - QRS-inhibited pacemaker. Every other QRS shows a pseudo-fusion with a pacemaker spike.

THE QRS-INHIBITED "DEMAND" PACEMAKER

Fusion and pseudofusion beats

Tracing A of fig. 38-A shows a regular artificial pacing at a rate of 85/min. Each impulse is followed by a QRS indicating a good ventricular capture by the pacemaker. From this tracing alone it is difficult to establish what type of pacemaker is working. A similar tracing would be present in a patient with: a) an asynchronous pacemaker; b) a P-wave synchronous pacemaker working in automatic function (fixed rate pacing) or, c) a QRS-synchronous or QRS-inhibited "demand" pacemakers also working in their automatic functions.

Tracing C solves the dilemma by recording: 1) *pacemaker automatic beats* (A); 2) *one fusion beat* (F); 3) *a sinus beat with pseudo-fusion* (Pf); and, 4) *a sinus beat normally conducted to the ventricles* (C). The sinus QRS which does not show a pacemaker spike indicates the presence of a ventricular-inhibited "demand" pacemaker.

The tracings of section B analyze four ventricular fusion beats of different morphology (F1-F4) caused by the simultaneous ventricular propagation of the sinus and pacemaker impulses. First of all, it may be noticed that the QRS duration of fusion beats is always shorter than that of automatic pacemaker beats. The time interval between the sinus P-wave and the pacemaker spike (P-S interval) is slightly different and decreases from F1 to F4. The longer the P-S interval, the greater the amount of ventricular myocardium activated by the sinus impulse. Here the QRS morphology of F1, with P-S equals 180 msec., is closer to that of the sinus beat in the bottom tracing. With a decreasing P-S interval, due to a slowing of the sinus rate, (160-120-100 msec.), the ventricles are progressively captured more by the artificial impulse then by the sinus impulse and the morphology of the fusion beats F2, F3 and F4 is closer to that of pacemaker automatic beats (A).

Fig. 38-B shows a sinus rhythm with a 1st degree A-V block and a right bundle branch block. Only every other QRS has a spike falling into the initial portion of the ventricular complex. The tracing could lead one to the following misinterpretation: sensing malfunction of either a QRS-synchronous or of a QRS-blocking pacemaker. The right diagnosis is, instead, a normally functioning *QRS-inhibited pacemaker* and presence of *pseudo-fusion beats* (see page 81).

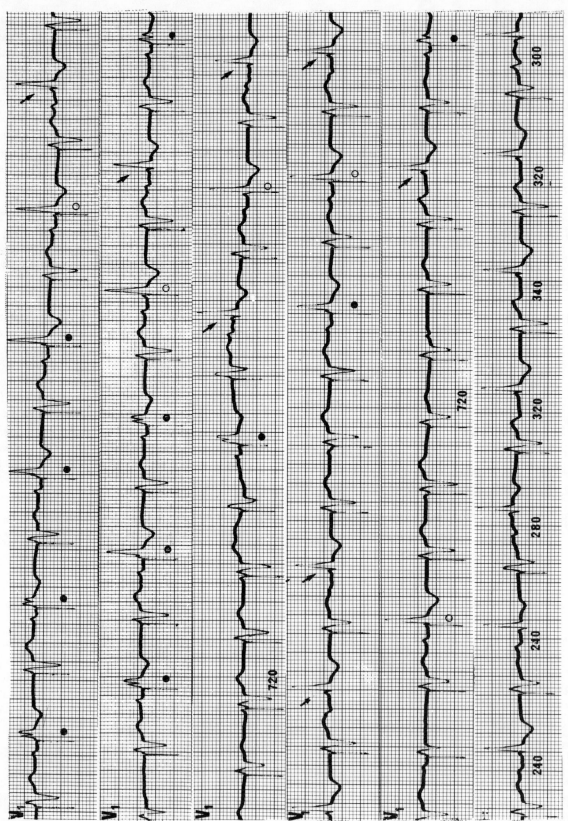

Fig. 39-A - QRS-inhibited pacemaker. The arrows indicate the beats conducted to the ventricles; the clear circles are pseudo-fusion beats; dark circles indicate ventricular fusion beats.

Fusion and pseudofusion beats

Fig. 39-A is a beautiful synthesis of the normal behavior of a *ventricular-inhibited pacemaker*. It illustrates the interaction between a spontaneous and an artificial cardiac rhythm.

A bradycardic sinus rhythm is easily recognized (P-P interval), alternating with that of an artificial pacemaker. P-waves occasionally go through the A-V junction and activate the ventricles. The QRS complexes indicated by arrows are sinus beats conducted to the ventricles with a right bundle branch block. Sinus impulses depolarize the ventricles when P-waves fall close enough to the preceding pacemaker spike and before the expiration of the pacemaker automatic interval (720 msec.).

The sinus impulses which are delivered slightly later because of sinus arrhythmia are not sensed by the pacemaker. Following its own characteristics, the unit delivers an automatic impulse at the end of the stand-by interval. The ineffective spikes are recorded on the surface ECG simultaneously with the sinus beats and determine the so-called pseudo-fusion beats (indicated by a clear circle). At other times, the artificial and sinus impulses share the ventricular depolarization. The resulting complexes are ventricular fusion beats (indicated by a dark circle), with a QRS morphology that is in between that of sinus and pacemaker beats.

When sinus impulses fall too early after a captured pacemaker beat, they are blocked within the A-V junction and induce the "escape" of *pacemaker automatic beats* with complete ventricular capture. At this point the automatic interval may be exactly measured and is 720 msec.; the automatic pacing rate is therefore, 85/min.

The presence of a sinus arrhythmia illustrates another interesting finding, that is the variability of the P-R intervals of the sinus beats conducted to the ventricles. (The P-R intervals are indicated in msec. on the bottom tracing.) The more premature the P-wave from the preceding pacemaker beat, the longer the P-R interval. The decreased conduction velocity in the A-V junction is also due in part to a concealed retrograde conduction of the artificial impulse through the A-V junction (see page 156).

REFERENCES

Ectocor Synchronous Standby Pacer, 3d ed. Miami, Cordis Corporation, 1968.

McHenry, Malcolm, M., Nelson, Charles, G., Hopkins, Donald, M., and Smeloff, Edward, A.: *Permanently Implanted Transvenous Pacemakers*, Circulation, 38, 1968.

Neville, J., Miller, K., Keller, W., and Abildskov, J.A.: *An Implantable Demand Pacemaker*, Clin. Res., 14:256, 1966.

Sowton, E.: *Ventricular-triggered Pacemakers: Clinical Experiences*, Brit. Heart J., 30:363, 1960.

Castellanos, A., Jr., Gage, A.A., Federico, A.J., Schimert, G., and Greatbatch, W.: *Clinical Experience with an Implantable Pacemaker*, Ann. N.Y. Acad. Sci., 111:1075, 1964.

Escher, D.J.W.: *The Present Status of Clinical Cardiac Pacing*, Amer. Heart J., 74:126, 1965.

Furman, S., and Escher, D.J.W.: *Ventricular Synchronized Demand Pacing*, Amer. Heart J., 76:445, 1968.

Furman, S., Escher, D.J.W., Schwedel, J.B., and Solomon, N.: *Transvenous Pacing*, Amer. Heart J., 71:408, 1966.

Furman, S., Escher, D.J.W., and Solomon, N.: *Standby Pacing for Multiple Cardiac Arrhythmias*, Ann. Thorac. Surg., 3:327, 1967.

Sowton, E.: *Artificial Pacemaking and Sinus Rhythm*, Brit. Heart J., 27:311, 1965.

Furman, S., Escher, D.J.W., Schwedel, J.B., and Solomon, N.: *Transvenous Pacing: A Seven Year Review*, Amer. Heart J., 71:408, 1966.

Overbeck, W., and Buchner, C.: *Indikation und operative Technik bei der Implantation kunstlicker Schrittmacher*, Langenbeck. Arch. Klin. Chir., 313: 582, 1965.

Jensen, N.K., Schmidt, R., Garamella, J.J., Lynch, M.F., and Peterson, C.A.: *Intracavitary Cardiac Pacing*, J.A.M.A., 195:916, 1966.

Zoll, P.M., Frank, H.A., and Linenthal, A.J.: *Four-year Experience with an Implanted Cardiac Pacemaker*, Ann. Surg., 160:351, 1964.

Furman, Seymour, and Escher, Doris, J.W.: « *Principles and Techniques of Cardiac Pacing* », Harper & Row, New York, 1970.

Hoffman, B.F., and Cranefield, P.F.: « *Electrophysiology of the Heart* », McGraw-Hill, New York, 1960.

Katz, L.N., and Pick, A.: « *Clinical Electrocardiography: I. The Arrhythmias* », Lea and Febiger, Philadelphia, 1956.

Dreifus, L.S., Likoff, W., and Moyer, J.H.: « *Mechanisms and Therapy of Cardiac Arrhythmias* », Grune and Stratton, New York and London, 1966.

Greenwood, R.J., and Finkelstein, D.: « *Sinoatrial Heart Block* », Charles C. Thomas, Publisher, Springfield, Ill., 1964.

Siddons, H., and Sowton, E.: « *Cardiac Pacemakers* », Charles C. Thomas, Illinois, 1967.

Hurst, J.W., and Logue, R.B.: « *The Heart* », New York, McGraw-Hill Co., 1970.

Thalen, H.J. Th., Van Den Berg, J.W., Homan Van Der Heide, J.N., and Nieveen, J.: « *The Artificial Cardiac Pacemaker* », Netherlands, Charles C. Thomas, 1969.

Chardack, W.M.: « *Discussion* », *in Cardiac Pacing and Cardioversion*, Philadelphia, Charles Press, 1967, p. 27.

Escher, D.J.W.: *The Present Status of Clinical Cardiac Pacing*, Amer. Heart J., 74:126, 1967.

Nathan, D.A., Center, S., Wu, C.Y., and Keller, W.: *An Implantable Synchronous Pacemaker for the Long-term Correction of Complete Heart Block*, Amer. J. Cardiol., 11:362, 1963.

Castellanos, A., Jr., Lemberg, L., and Berkovits, B.V.: *The Use of the Demand Pacemaker in Auriculoventricular Conduction Disturbances*, J. Cardiov. Surg., 7:92, 1966.

Parsonnet, V., Zucker, I.R., Gilbert, L., and Myers, G.H.: *Clinical Use of an Implantable Standby Pacemaker*, J.A.M.A., 196:784, 1966.

Goetz, R.H., Dormandy, J.A., and Berkovits, B.: *Pacing on Demand in Treatment of Atrioventricular Conduction Disturbances of the Heart*, Lancet, 2:599, 1966.

Furman, S., Escherm, D.J.W., Solomon, N., and Krauthamer, M.: *Electrocardiographic Manifestation of Standby Pacing*, J. Thorac. Cardiov. Surg., 54:723, 1967.

Zuckerman, W., Zaroff, L.I., Berkovits, B.V., Matoff, J.M., and Harken, D.E.: *Clinical Experiences with a New Implantable Demand Pacemaker*, Amer. J. Cardiol., 20:232, 1967.

Lemberg, L., Castellanos, A., Jr., and Berkovits, B.V.: *Pacemaking on Demand in A-V Block*, J.A.M.A., 191:12, 1965.

Nathan, D., Center, S., Wu, C.Y., and Keller, W.: *An Implantable Synchronous Pacemaker for the Long-term correction of Complete Heart Block*, Amer. J. Cardiol., 27:862, 1963.

Parsonnet, V., Zucker, I.R., Gilbert, L., and Asa, M.M.: *The Development of an Intracardiac Dipolar Catheter Electrode for the Treatment of Complete Heart Block*, Surg. Forum, 13:179, 1962.

Parsonnet, V., Zucker, I.R., Gilbert, L., and Myers, G.H.: *A Review of Intracardiac Pacing with Specific Reference to the Use of a Dipolar Electrode*, Progr. Cardiov. Dis., 6:472, 1964.

Parsonnet, V., Zucker, I.R., Gilbert, L., and Myers, G.H.: *Clinical Use of an Implantable Demand Pacemaker*, J.A.M.A., 196:104, 1966.

Pick, A.: *Parasystole*, Circulation, 8:243, 1953.

Sowton, E.: *Artificial Pacemaking and Sinus Rhythm*, Brit. Heart J., 27:311, 1965.

Sowton, E.: *Cardiac Pacemakers and Pacing*, Med. Concep. Cardiovasc. Dis., 36:31, 1967.

Zuckerman, W., Zaroff, L.I., Berkovits, B.V., Matloff, J.M., and Harken, D.E.: *Clinical Experiences with a New Implantable Demand Pacemaker*, Amer. J. Cardiol., 21:232, 1967.

Furman, S.: *Fundamentals of Cardiac Pacing*, Amer. Heart J., 73:261, 1967.

Neville, J.F., Millar, K., Keller, W., and Abildskov, J.A.: *An Implantable Demand Pacemaker*, Clin. Res., 14:256, 1966.

Furman, S., and Escher, D.J.W.: *Ventricular Synchronous and Demand Pacing*, Amer. Heart J., 76:445, 1968.

« *A Symposium Cardiac Pacing and Cardioversion* », The Charles Press, Philadelphia, 1967.

De Carvalho, A.P., De Mello, W.C., and Hoffman, B.F.: « *The Specialized Tissues of the Heart* », Amsterdam, Elsevier Publishing Co., 1961.

Marshall, R.J., and Shepherd, J.T.: « *Cardiac Function in Health and Disease* », Philadelphia, W.B. Saunders Co., 1968.

Castellanos, Augustin, Jr., and Lemberg, Louis: « *Electrophysiology of Pacing and Cardioversion* », Appleton-Century-Crofts, New York, 1969.

Cosby, Richard, S., and Bilitch, Michael: « *Heart Block* », McGraw-Hill, 1972.

Chapter V

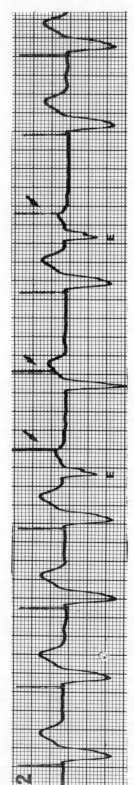

Fig. 40-A - Asynchronous pacemaker malfunction. The ineffective impulses indicated by the arrows, do not indicate a pacemaker malfunction. In fact, they fall within the ventricular refractory period following the extrasystoles (E).

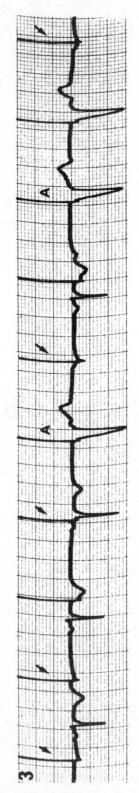

Fig. 40-B - Asynchronous pacemaker malfunction. The spikes indicated by the arrows, although they fall in diastole and therefore within a normal cardiac excitability phase, are not followed by a depolarization. The sporadic nature of the ventricular capture (A) allows to diagnose a pacemaker malfunction.

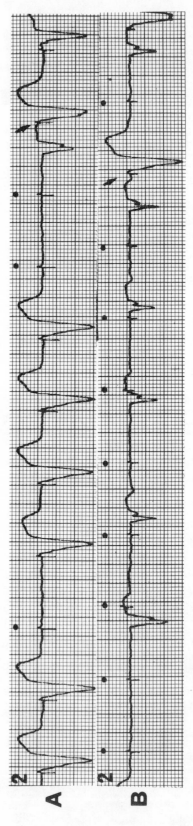

Fig. 40-C - Asynchronous pacemaker malfunction. The tracings are recorded with an interval of a few hours. Dots indicate ineffective pacemaker impulses while the arrows point to spikes which capture the ventricles during the supernormal excitability phase.

PACEMAKER MALFUNCTIONS

In recent years the number of patients treated with permanent cardiac pacemakers has markedly increased. This has enabled researchers to accumulate a remarkable amount of data on malfunctions of the different pacing systems, from the simple asynchronous units to the more sophisticated "demand" pacemakers. For example, it has been established that when it involves the generator-myocardial connecting system; a pacemaker malfunction may be related to the different implantation technique (epicardic or intracavitary); otherwise, malfunctions may be present with both approaches when they involve the generator pack and the electrode-myocardial junction.

The most common causes of pacemaker malfunction are: a) changes of resistance and of cardiac excitability threshold; b) fracture or dislocation of the electrode tip; c) fracture or dislocation of the cable connecting the generator to the myocardium; d) malfunction of the generator electronic components and, e) premature battery exhaustion.

A common ECG finding of *pacemaker malfunction* is the presence of artificial impulses with absent or sporadic "ventricular capture." The radiographic and fluoroscopic examination, the electronic analysis of the impulse rate, amplitude and duration, and the measurement of cardiac excitability threshold usually allow investigators to pinpoint the exact cause of pacemaker malfunctions.

Before considering more complex examinations, it is often quite easy to recognize early signs of pacemaker malfunction from the simple analysis of a surface ECG. Also, one must avoid misdiagnosing a pacemaker malfunction when the rhythm of a normally functioning pacemaker interacts with a spontaneous cardiac rhythm.

The ECG strip when associated with simple, non invasive techniques (see page 169), is the *single most valuable examination* in the diagnosis of pacemaker malfunction.

ASYNCHRONOUS PACEMAKER MALFUNCTION

One of the most common mistakes in the ECG evaluation of an asynchronous pacemaker behavior is to interpret the presence of spikes which are not followed by a ventricular depolarization as pacemaker malfunction. While this is a typical finding of malfunction of a "demand" pacemaker, it is commonly found when in the presence of normally functioning pacemakers of the asynchronous type. It must be noted that an asynchronous pacemaker does not sense spontaneous cardiac potentials, and that impulse delivery is on a continuous basis, according to the pacemaker "fixed" time schedule. Therefore, when spontaneous cardiac activity is present, pacemaker impulses may fall within different phases of the spontaneous cardiac cycles. Those which fall during ventricular diastole, and within the excitability phase, depolarize the ventricles. All others, although recorded on the surface ECG are not effective on the heart muscle.

In fig. 40-A, for example, the spikes indicated by the arrows do not "capture" the ventricles since they fall into the absolute ventricular refractory phase of the preceding spontaneous beats (two ventricular premature and one escape beats). Otherwise, the asynchronous pacemaker works normally at a fixed rate of 72/min. and with a good ventricular response.

The presence of *pacemaker spikes which do not depolarize the ventricles when falling in diastole* (that is after the preceding T wave) is substantial evidence of *pacemaker malfunction*. The artificial impulses in fig. 40-B are delivered with a constant regularity but are not always followed by a ventricular response (as in beats indicated by A). One must not be deceived by the presence of sinus QRS's, because ventricular depolarization should also be expected from the spikes which are indicated by the arrows. These obviously fall in areas of normal cardiac excitability. The diagnosis is that of a sinus rhythm with a second degree A-V block, Mobitz type II, and a malfunctioning asynchronous pacemaker. A dislocation of the stimulating electrode tip within the right ventricular chamber was at the base of the pacemaker malfunction.

Tracings A and B of fig. 40-C also belong to a patient with a malfunctioning asynchronous pacemaker, and are recorded a few hours apart. Tracing A shows three ineffective artificial impulses (see dots) within an otherwise regular artificial rhythm. The patient was admitted for a generator change 28 months after implantation. Tracing B shows the reappearance of a spontaneous cardiac activity and more ineffective pacemaker impulses (see dots). Here it may be noted that only two spikes (indicated by the arrows) are capable of depolarizing the ventricles. As will be seen in later discussion, these impulses capture the ventricles because they fall into the supernormal phase of ventricular excitability (see page 149).

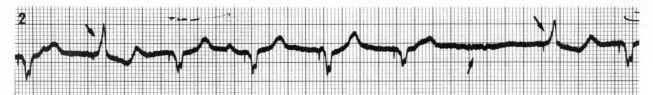

Fig. 41-A - Asychronous pacemaker malfunction. The bottom arrow indicates an impulse not followed by a ventricular response. The different QRS morphologies (top arrows) are due to changing ventricular activation areas.

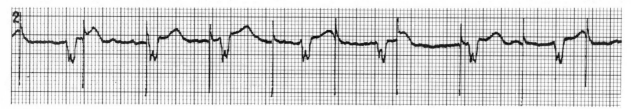

Fig. 41-B - Asynchronous pacemaker malfunction. All the artificial impulses are ineffective and independent from the irregular ventricular rhythm.

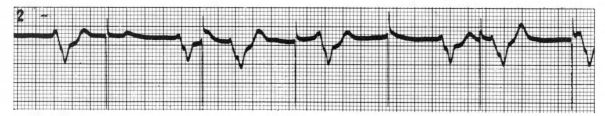

Fig. 41-C - Asynchronous pacemaker malfunction. Chaotic ventricular action in the presence of a totally ineffective artificial pacing.

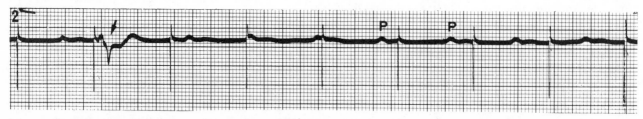

Fig. 41-D - Asynchronous pacemaker malfunction. Ventricular asystole is present within a sinus rhythm completely blocked in the A-V junction. All but one pacemaker spikes are totally ineffective (arrow).

Ineffective cardiac pacing is not always symptomatically signaled by the patient with a permanent pacemaker. This may be due either to the presence of a spontaneous rhythm or to the sporadic nature of the ineffective pacing. The necessity for a periodic control of patients with permanent pacemakers, and the usefulness of an early diagnosis of pacer malfunction, will appear obvious from the cases presented in fig. 41-A through D.

Fig. 41-A is recorded from an asymptomatic patient with an asynchronous pacemaker which was implanted through an intracavitary route. The tracing shows a 75/min. pacing rate, not followed in one occasion (middle arrow) by a ventricular response. Two unusual QRS complexes which are preceded by an artificial impulse may also be recognized (first and last arrows); they show a QRS morphology sharply different from the others. In this patient the tip of the catheter, not well wedged into the trabeculae of the right ventricular apex, was floating to and fro within the pulmonary outflow tract. The loss of ventricular capture was only occasional, occurring when the catheter tip would cross the semilunar valves. The QRS morphology was related to the changing stimulation site, from the apex to the right ventricular septal wall (see page 8). In such a case the fluoroscopic

examination, associated with a surface ECG, may be useful in clearing the diagnosis. The catheter must always be relocated in the optimal ventricular pacing site. At other times, the sudden rhythm changes, associated with a pacemaker malfunction, may be noticed by patients, and they can even induce episodes of Adams-Stokes.

Fig. 41-B presents an irregular ventricular rhythm, associated with a totally ineffective artificial pacing, due to electronic component failure. Atrial activity is not recognizable (probably because of atrial fibrillation), and not one of the pacemaker spikes (90/min.) induces a ventricular response.

The idio-ventricular rhythm, emerging during a pacemaker malfunction, may occasionally degenerate into ventricular tachycardia and or fibrillation. It may also slow down in prolonged asystolic pauses. Fig. 41-C shows an irregular, chaotic cardiac action in a comatose patient with a malfunctioning asynchronous pacemaker. The QRS complexes are slow, irregular, widened and bizarre, and are typical of an agonal rhythm.

In fig. 41-D ventricular activity is almost totally absent. Sinus activity is present (75/min.) but all P waves are blocked within the A-V junction. A regular artificial stimulation from a malfunctioning pacemaker is not followed by a ventricular capture, except in one instance (QRS indicated by the arrow).

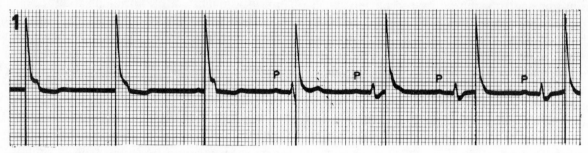

Fig. 42-A - P-wave synchronous pacemaker. The pacemaker is in automatic function because of low voltage P waves. Only the first three impulses capture the ventricles.

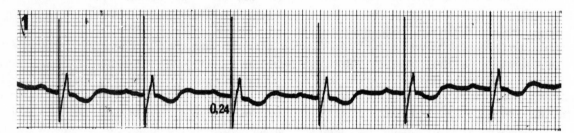

Fig. 42-B - P-wave synchronous pacemaker malfunction. First degree A-P block (atrial-pacemaker). The P-S interval (P-spike) is equal to 0.24 sec.

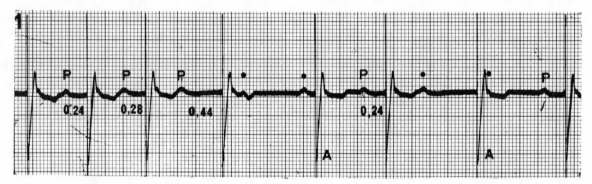

Fig. 42-C - P-wave synchronous pacemaker malfunction. Second degree A-P block. The P waves synchronized beats show a progressively longer P-S interval. The P waves which are not synchronized and blocked within the A-V junction are indicated by a dot. A = automatic pacemaker beats.

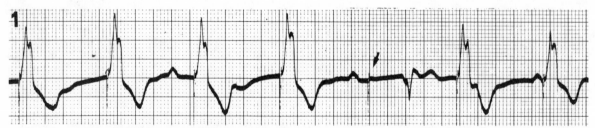

Fig. 42-D - P-wave synchronous pacemaker malfunction. There is no A-P synchronism and the automatic pacing is occasionally ineffective (arrow).

P-WAVE SYNCHRONOUS PACEMAKER MALFUNCTION

A P-wave synchronous pacemaker malfunction may be recognized by abnormalities of: a) synchronization with atrial signals, b) A-V ratio and, c) ventricular pacing. The patient presented in fig. 42-A has already been encountered (see page 40). In this patient, a P-wave synchronous pacemaker does not sense the low voltage sinus P waves and it works with the automatic reserve mechanism. Only the first three impulses capture the ventricles, while the others fall into the ventricular refractory phase of sinus QRS's. Such pacemaker behavior may be induced by fibrotic changes around the electrode implanted on the atrial wall, by exhaustion of the generator batteries, or by instability of the atrial catheter, in those instances where the stimulation is performed with transvenous catheters.

Thus, the loss of P-wave synchronization and the presence of automatic ventricular pacing are the first signs of a P-wave synchronous pacemaker malfunction. The autonomy of the automatic reserve circuit may last several months.

A common sign of malfunction is also represented by an excessive prolongation of the A-P delay (atrial-pacemaker). This is usually secondary to battery exhaustion or alterations of the generator electronic components.

Fig. 42-B shows a *first degree A-P block (atrial-pacemaker)* in a patient with a P-wave synchronous pacemaker. The P-S interval (P-stimulus) is equal to 0.24 sec. (normal = 0.16 sec.), but the ventricular rhythm is still guided by the P waves, regularly preceding each QRS complex.

A second degree A-P block is presented in fig. 42-C. The blocked P waves, which are not synchronized with the pacemaker, are indicated by black dots, while "A" indicates automatic escape beats. Note here that the P-S interval of the first four synchronized beats is progressively prolonged. In this patient the synchronizing mechanism is altered, while the automatic pacing system is still working well. In similar circumstances the generator must be changed within a short time.

After the loss of the P-wave synchronism, the pacemaker may stimulate with intermittent ventricular capture. This is presented in fig. 42-D, where the regular pacing of a P-wave synchronous pacemaker is, at one point, not followed by a ventricular response (arrow).

Chest wall stimulation (CWS) is very useful in evaluating a P-wave synchronous pacemaker which is working in an automatic fashion. This technique permits one to test the pacemaker synchronizing capacity by using low voltage stimuli on the thoracic wall, which are interpreted by the pacemaker as atrial signals (see page 189).

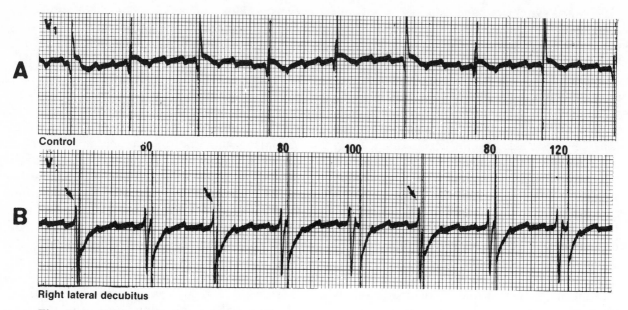

Fig. 43-A - QRS-synchronous pacemaker malfunction. The sensing malfunction is revealed in tracing B recorded in a right lateral decubitus.

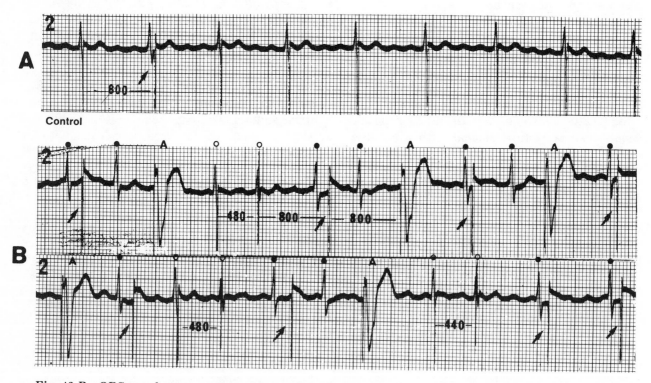

Fig. 43-B - QRS-synchronous pacemaker malfunction. See text.

QRS-SYNCHRONOUS PACEMAKER MALFUNCTION

A QRS-synchronous pacemaker malfunction may involve the sensing and stimulating mechanisms, separately or simultaneously. In the presence of: a) increased cardiac excitability threshold; b) dislocations of the intracavitary catheter tip and c) battery exhaustion is usually the capacity of sensing spontaneous cardiac signals the first to disappear. This is presented in fig. 43-A. The tracings were obtained from a patient with a ventricular synchronized pacemaker, inserted to improve the ventricular rate of an atrial flutter with a high degree of A-V block. Tracing A, recorded with the patient supine, clearly shows the presence of F waves (350/min.), conducted to the ventricles with a 4:1 ratio. The spontaneous QRS's are deformed by high amplitude stimulus-artifacts (unipolar stimulation), falling 20 msec. from the beginning of the Q wave and thus within the ventricular refractory period. The pacemaker, therefore, shows a normal synchronizing mechanism with spontaneous ventricular potentials. In this case, no statements can be made about the pacemaker stimulating capacity, in the event of a high degree of A-V block and the disappearance of spontaneous ventricular beats.

Tracing B was recorded with the patient in a right lateral decubitus. Stimulus-artifacts are still present but, except for those indicated by the arrows, they are not synchronized with spontaneous QRS's and are delivered in an automatic fashion (with a 75/min. rate). In this case the automatic pacing rate is very close to the spontaneous ventricular rate (the atrial flutter also has a ventricular rate of about 75/min.). This may suggest that the spikes are still synchronized with spontaneous QRS's. Instead, they are almost totally dissociated with the QRS's and fall at different intervals from the beginning of spontaneous ventricular depolarization (60-120 msec.). The impulses do not capture the ventricles because they fall within the ventricular refractory period of spontaneous QRS's. This indicates that the *sensing and synchronizing mechanisms are abnormal* because of dislocation of the catheter tip.

It is usually difficult to evaluate the underlying pacing capacity of a malfunctioning ventricular-synchronized pacemaker. This is especially true when a tracing shows signs only of an abnormal sensing mechanism. In fact, the presence of synchronized or of non-synchronized pacemaker spikes does not guarantee a pacing with a good ventricular capture, when needed. In such a case, it may be useful to assay the presence and the efficacy of pacemaker impulses on the ventricular myocardium through the technique of chest wall stimulation (see page 183).

Fig. 43-B shows an atrial flutter with an A-V ratio of 4:1 and a good ventricular rate (tracing A) in a patient with a QRS-triggered pacemaker. All the QRS's are normally synchronized with the demand pacer, except for the beat indicated by the arrow. The spike, in fact, is too far from the beginning of the QRS. This also suggests that the artificial impulse is delivered in an automatic fashion by the pacemaker, because of a missed perception of the ventricular signal at the end of the intrinsic escape interval of 800 msec.

Tracings B were recorded three weeks later. The atrial flutter still persists; a variable A-V ratio is present; thus the ventricular rate is faster than in the control tracing. The ventricular potentials of numerous spontaneous QRS's (those indicated by dark dots) are not sensed by the pacemaker. If the intervals between the few synchronized QRS's (clear circles) are measured, it is possible to rule out the presence of premature QRS's, which are not sensed by the pacemaker because they fall within its refractory period. In fact, a normal synchronization occurs during cardiac cycles of 440-480 msec. This indicates a pacemaker refractory period shorter than 440 msec. (see page 207). Therefore, the dark dots suggest an *abnormal sensing mechanism*. In this case, the abnormal mechanism is caused by a malfunction of the pacemaker electronic components, since all the non-sensed beats terminate cardiac cycles longer than 440 msec.

The non synchronized QRS's are always followed by automatic pacemaker impulses, some ineffective (arrows) and others with good ventricular capture (beats A). When the pacemaker does not sense spontaneous ventricular potentials, it behaves as during an asystolic pause, and, at the expiration of a stand-by interval of 800 msec., it delivers an automatic impulse. When it falls during a vulnerable period of ventricular excitability and far enough from the preceding non-synchronized QRS, the stimulus captures the ventricles (beats A). The ineffective spikes, however, always fall within the ventricular refractory period which follows the spontaneous QRS's. Thus, the tracings shown on the left page indicate a *malfunction of the sensing mechanism of a QRS-triggered pacemaker,* although they still suggest a *good automatic pacing capacity.*

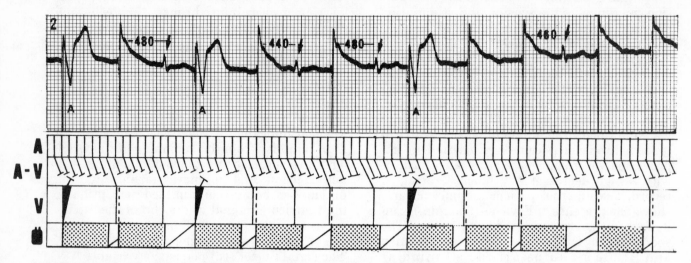

Fig. 44-A - Simulation of a QRS-synchronous pacemaker malfunction. The non sensed beats (arrows) fall within the pacemaker refractory period which, in this case, is 500 msec.

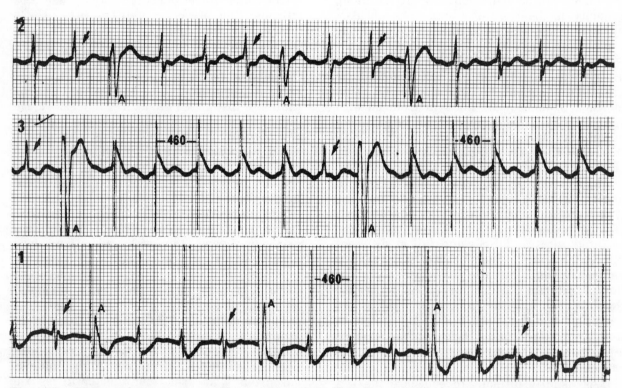

Fig. 44-B - QRS-synchronous pacemaker malfunction. The diagnosis is not certain because of the high ventricular rate and the presence of cardiac cycles very close to the maximal synchronizing limits of the pacemaker (400 msec.).

When a QRS-synchronous pacemaker does not sense spontaneous QRS's, the *pacemaker refractory period* must be measured before diagnosing a sensing mechanism malfunction. The pacemaker refractory period is that interval of time where the pacemaker is not able to sense spontaneous cardiac signals and, thus, is unable to synchronize.

As previously seen (see page 65), the refractory period of a QRS-synchronous "demand" pacemaker may vary according to different manufacturer, but it usually ranges between 350 and 500 msec. The refractory period is intentionally introduced, in this type of stimulators, to avoid the synchronization with early premature beats and to preset the length of the stand-by interval.

The tracing and diagram of fig. 44-A show a fine, undulated baseline and an irregular ventricular response, indicative of the presence of an atrial fibrillation. The spontaneous beats, synchronized with the QRS-triggered "demand" pacemaker, are occasionally followed by non-sensed QRS's (arrows). These, in turn, are followed in two occasions, by automatic beats with good ventricular capture (A).

A superficial examination of this tracing suggests a diagnosis of a sensing mechanism malfunction. Instead, this case illustrates a QRS-triggered pacemaker with a refractory period of 500 msec. Thus, each spontaneous QRS that falls within this time interval, from the delivery of the preceding artificial impulse, cannot be recorded by the pacemaker which is still refractory. In fact, all the QRS's indicated by the arrows fall within the pacemaker refractory period, while all the others are normally sensed and synchronized. The pacemaker function is, therefore, normal.

Occasionally, even the exact knowledge of the refractory period of a QRS-synchronous pacemaker may not be helpful in solving a doubious case of pacemaker malfunction. This is illustrated in fig. 44-B, where the rhythm is that of an atrial flutter with a fast ventricular rate (A-V ratio of 2:1). The great majority of spontaneous QRS's are normally synchronized by the ventricular-triggered "demand" pacemaker. Only occasionally spontaneous QRS's (arrows) are not sensed by the pacemaker (QRS's without spikes) and are followed by an automatic impulse with good ventricular capture (beats A). The shortest interval between two successive spikes synchronized with spontaneous QRS's is equal to 460 msec. Therefore, it may be safely assumed that the pacemaker refractory period must be below 460 msec. In this case it is equal to 400 msec.

All the non-sensed QRS's are very close to the critical limits of 400 msec., but are slightly more premature because of the small variations in the ventricular response often present during atrial flutter. Since these cardiac cycles are so short as to approach the critical limit of the pacemaker refractory period, it is not possible to diagnose the presence of a sensing mechanism malfunction. To solve the dilemma in such a case it would be advisable to slow the ventricular rate with drugs or carotid massage (see page 193), or to test the sensing mechanism with the chest wall stimulation technique (see page 183).

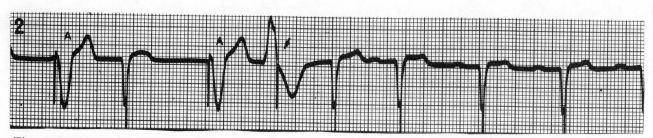

Fig. 45-A - QRS-synchronous pacemaker malfunction. All the pacemaker spikes are synchronized both with sinus and with extrasystolic QRS's but with some delay from the beginning of the ventricular repolarization.

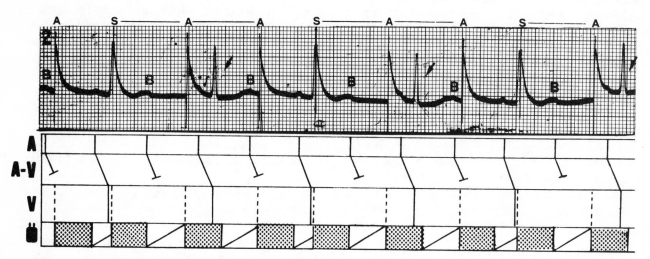

Fig. 45-B - QRS-synchronous pacemaker malfunction. A = pacemaker automatic impulses; S = spikes synchronized with sinus QRS's; B = P wave blocked within the A-V junction. The arrows indicate non sensed sinus QRS's which fall within the refractory period of the pacemaker.

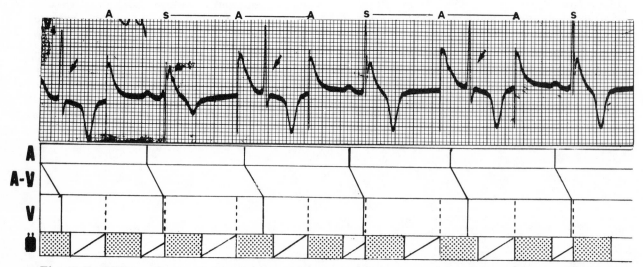

Fig. 45-C - QRS-synchronous pacemaker malfunction. Situation similar to the preceding figure. There is a loss of the stimulating function of the pacemaker with good residual sensing function.

The tracing of fig. 45-A is from a patient with a ventricular-triggered "demand" pacemaker. It shows sinus beats with prolonged A-V conduction (P-R = 0.26 sec.), pacemaker automatic beats (A) and a ventricular extrasystole (arrow). All the spontaneous QRS's clearly show synchronized spikes which indicate the type of pacing. However, it may be noted that the pacemaker spike is delivered with some delay from the beginning of spontaneous QRS's (the Q-spike interval is about 40 msec. in the sinus beats and 120 msec. in the ventricular extrasystole).

A delay in synchronization is considered an early sign of battery exhaustion. However, to have a diagnostic significance this delay must be present in all 12 electrocardiographic leads and it must have a value of at least twice the length of the normal synchronizing time of 20 msecs. It must be remembered, in fact, that the synchronized impulse is delivered only when the spontaneous ventricular potentials reach a voltage sufficient enough to be recorded by the pacemaker sensing mechanism.

Occasionally, the malfunction of a QRS-synchronous pacemaker may be manifested by a loss of stimulating capacity and lack of ventricular capture (pacing mechanism malfunction), while the unit may still be able to sense ventricular potentials and synchronize with them. This is what happens in fig. 45-B. A sinus rhythm is present with a second degree A-V block Mobitz type II (the blocked P waves are indicated with B). Some of the beats conducted to the ventricles are perfectly synchronized with the pacemaker (S). They are followed by a P wave blocked into the A-V junction and by a short asystolic pause. This is interrupted by a delivery of a pacemaker automatic impulse (S-A interval) which,

however, is not effective and does not capture the ventricles (notice the large deflection due to the voltage decay curve which simulates ventricular capture). At this point it is possible to diagnose a *pacing mechanism malfunction* because the impulses, falling in diastole, should depolarize the ventricles.

The following sinus beats are conducted to the ventricles (arrows) and are not sensed by the pacemaker. Attention must be paid not to diagnose a sensing mechanism malfunction. The non-sensed QRS falls 300 msec. from the delivery of the preceding artificial impulse, and, therefore, within the pacemaker refractory period. The unit behaves like it is facing an asystolic pause and, at the expiration of its own escape interval, it again delivers an automatic impulse (the A-A interval is equal to the SA interval). The next sinus beat conducted to the ventricles is sensed and synchronized in a normal fashion.

Fig. 45-C also shows pacemaker spikes which do not depolarize the ventricles even when falling in diastole and, therefore, during the normal excitability phase of the ventricles. The elevation of the isolectric line, which is induced by the voltage-decay curve of the ineffective unipolar impulse, simulates almost perfectly the morphology of automatic beats with ventricular capture. A bradycardic sinus rhythm is present with a good A-V conduction. Only every other sinus QRS is synchronized with the pacemaker (S). The QRS indicated by the arrow does not show a stimulus-artifact. Although the pacing mechanism is not functioning well, the pacemaker sensing function is still intact. The non-sensed QRS's, in fact, always fall within the pacemaker refractory period.

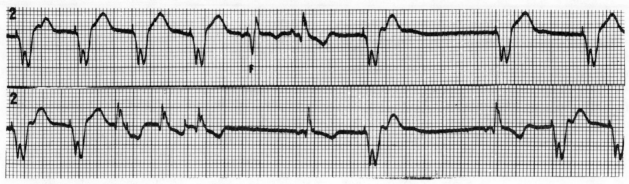

Fig. 46-A - QRS-inhibited pacemaker malfunction. Increased cardiac excitability threshold. The pacing is occasionally ineffective.

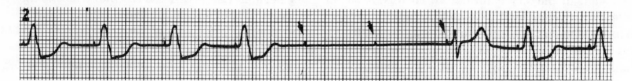

Fig. 46-B - QRS-inhibited pacemaker malfunction. Increased cardiac excitability threshold. Three impulses (bipolar stimulation) are not followed by ventricular capture.

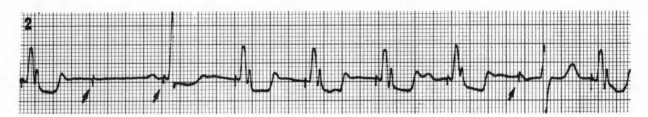

Fig. 46-C - QRS-inhibited pacemaker malfunction. Increased resistance secondary to cable fracture between the generator and the myocardium. The pacing is occasionally ineffective (arrow).

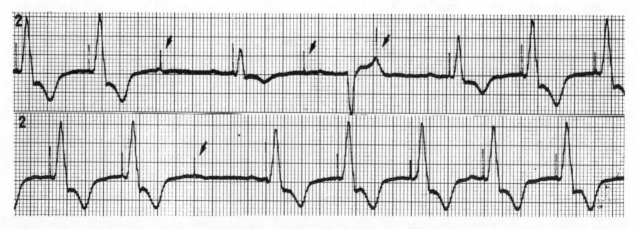

Fig. 46-D - QRS-inhibited pacemaker malfunction. Increased resistance in the electrode-myocardial junction. The arrows indicate ineffective stimuli.

QRS-INHIBITED PACEMAKER MALFUNCTION

As it is for the QRS-synchronous pacemaker, this type of unit has a more complex circuitry when compared to the more simple asynchronous pacemaker. Since the possibilities of malfunction are directly proportional to the number of electronic components of the pacemaker (with the exception of the simple battery exhaustion) it is not unusual to find situations like those presented in the following figures.

When using stimulators of the ventricular-inhibited type, the findings of pacemaker malfunctions may be similar to other types of pacemakers. For example, fig. 46-A and 46-B show a rather regular cardiac pacing accompanied by an occasionally absent ventricular capture. This may be caused by either an increased excitability threshold or by an increased myocardial resistance.

The *cardiac excitability threshold* is the minimal amount of current able to depolarize the ventricles. Regardless of the type or model of pacemaker used, each permanent unit will face a determined excitability threshold, below which the impulse will be too weak to depolarize the ventricles. When the excitability threshold is above the amount of current delivered by the stimulator, it determines the so-called "pacemaker exit block".

During an artificial pacing, the "excitability threshold" must not be confused with the "threshold potential", which is measured by the recording of the membrane potentials. The threshold potential is the membrane potential at which cardiac fibers are spontaneously depolarized. The myocardial fibers may be depolarized more easily (increased excitability) by either decreasing the excitability threshold or by increasing the threshold potential and by approaching the "resting potential".

The "excitability threshold" is usually expressed in terms of voltage or circuit intensity. Higher values are more easily obtained with an epicardial than with the endocardial stimulation, during a fasting or a sleeping state, with the use of 10% insulin and dextrose, KCL, NACL, and aldosterone. Lower values usually appear with exercise, KCL in a Ringer solution, adrenaline, ephedrine or methil-prednisone.

The higher the amount of current necessary to capture the heart, the higher its excitability threshold. "High threshold" means that a larger amount of current is necessary to capture the myocardium.

The threshold is influenced by a wide variety of factors. Among the most important are the type and location of the stimulating electrode, the impulse shape and the junction between the electrode and myocardium. Normally, the threshold increases rapidly in the first, second or third weeks following an artificial pacing, and it later levels on a plateau. Small variations may be present even months after the implantation and are induced either by pharmacologic or physiologic agents.

Unless a pacemaker has a high voltage output, exceeding twice the threshold values recorded at the moment of implantation, and is willing to pay a higher amount of energy, it is possible that it may encounter a high threshold and fail to capture the ventricles. Therefore, this may induce an "exit block" like the one presented in fig. 46-A and 46-B.

If the generator output is 5-6 times higher than the threshold, an eventual increase of threshold does not influence the stimulating capacity of the pacemaker. Units with values only 2-3 times higher than the threshold will usually require an increase in the output to overcome high excitability threshold.

An increase in the excitability threshold must not be confused with an increased *resistance* (normal value = about 500 ohms) of the *electrode-myocardial junction* (impedance). The resistance usually increases because of fibrous tissue surrounding the electrode tip, because of polarization and electrolysis of the positive pole of a bipolar catheter (or of a unipolar system stimulating with the positive pole), or in myocardial infarct involving tissue in the proximity of one or both electrodes (fig. 46-C and 46-D).

The excitability threshold may increase independently from the resistance. Usually, an increased resistance is thought of as increased threshold. While they are two well separated entities, *they present themselves electrocardiographically in the same way.* Both situations usually appear as an artificial stimulation with occasional loss of ventricular capture (rarely, the stimulation is totally ineffective), and both situations may be corrected by a simple increase of the generator voltage output. Thus, generators with variable output are preferred to those with fixed output.

Although it may be necessary to expose the catheter terminals and use sophisticated equipment, the diagnosis of an increased resistance is important because it may very often conceal a break in the cables connecting the generator to the myocardium. A large cable fracture may produce a very high or infinite resistance, and is usually recognized by obtaining a simple chest X-ray. On the other hand, in the presence of a small cable fracture, cable continuity is usually re-established by tissue fluids, which function as a bridge, and it may only be revealed by an unexplainable increase in the resistance.

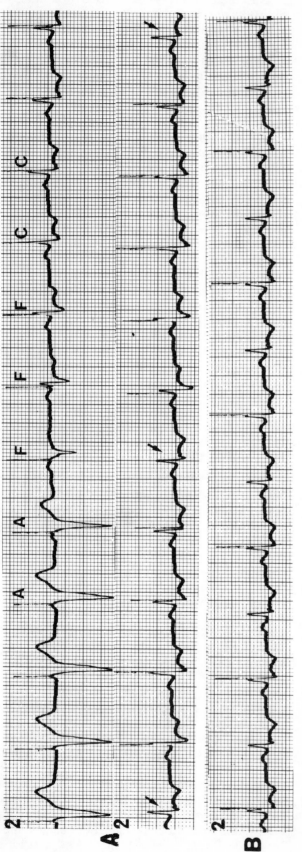

Fig. 47-A - **QRS-inhibited pacemaker malfunction.** The catheter tip has penetrated into the pericardial sac and the pacemaker senses the cardiac potential only late during ventricular depolarization (arrow). The pacing function is intact.

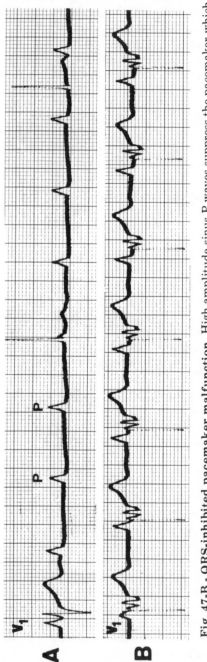

Fig. 47-B - **QRS-inhibited pacemaker malfunction.** High amplitude sinus P waves suppress the pacemaker which interprets the P waves as ventricular potentials.

The presence of a blocking circuit, which avoids the delivery of impulses during spontaneous ventricular activity, makes particularly hard the diagnosis of a *sensing mechanism malfunction* of a QRS-inhibited pacemaker. It is, therefore, useful to test the sensing function of this type of unit with the chest wall stimulation technique (see page 169).

Tracings of fig. 47-A illustrate a case of *abnormal sensing function* of a QRS-inhibited pacemaker, with an otherwise intact pacing capacity.

Tracing A shows a transition from a pacemaker automatic rhythm (A) into a sinus rhythm, with a normal A-V conduction (C), through several ventricular fusion beats (F). The morphology of fusion beats is progressively approaching that of sinus beats. It may be noticed that, when ventricular potentials of sinus origin are present, pacemaker spikes still fall within the QRS complexes. The pacemaker and the sinus rate are almost equal and this would suggest the presence of "pseudo-fusion beats" (see page 81).

With a careful examination of the sinus QRS complexes, it becomes clear that the pacemaker spikes show a progressive delay from the Q wave and "land" first within the ascending portion, then into the peak and within the descending branch of the R wave, until a QRS without spike (arrow in the second tracing) is reached. The pacemaker sensing mechanism is, therefore, malfunctioning and it is not triggered at the beginning, but at the end, of the spontaneous ventricular activation. In fact, only the QRS's indicated by the arrows inhibit the pacemaker, which otherwise delivers automatic impulses with a regular rate of 80/min.

The ineffective spikes first precede, are then simultaneous, and finally follow the sinus QRS's. This causes a sort of dissociation between the spontaneous and the artificial rhythm, and Wenckebach-type sequences between the R wave and the pacer spike. The R-stimulus intervals are progressively prolonged until the impulse delivery is completely blocked.

Tracing B, recorded a few days later, shows normal looking sinus QRS's alternating with complexes deformed by ineffective pacemaker spikes. Every other QRS inhibits the pacemaker, leading to a sort of a "2:1 pacemaker exit block". The malfunction was caused by the penetration of the catheter tip through the right ventricular wall and into the pericardial space. For this reason the pacemaker would only be suppressed by the ventricular signals of high voltage reached at the end of a spontaneous ventricular depolarization (abnormal sensing function), while the stimulating function remained unchanged.

Occasionally, high voltage P waves are interpreted, by a QRS-inhibited pacemaker, as ventricular potentials. Therefore, they may block the pacer impulse delivery. This is what happens in tracing A of fig. 47-B where, in spite of the presence of a QRS-inhibited pacemaker, a complete A-V block remains undisturbed and pacing is not performed. The sinus rhythm (rate = 80/min.), with P waves of high amplitude, continuously inhibits the pacemaker, which misinterprets the atrial signals as ventricular potentials. Tracing B shows the re-establishment of a normal ventricular pacing.

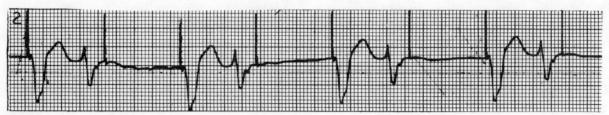

Fig. 48-A - Pacemaker arrhythmias. Ventricular bigeminy and asynchronous pacemaker.

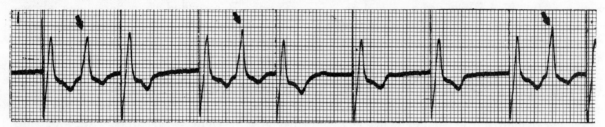

Fig. 48-B - Pacemaker arrhythmias. Interpolated ventricular bigeminy and asynchronous pacemaker.

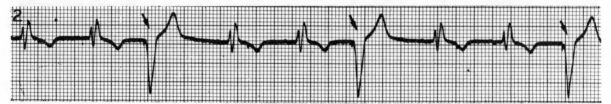

Fig. 48-C - Pacemaker arrhythmias. Ventricular trigeminy and asynchronous pacemaker.

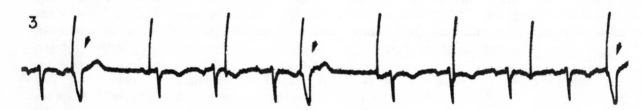

Fig. 48-D - Pacemaker arrhythmias. "Pacemaker on T phenomenon."

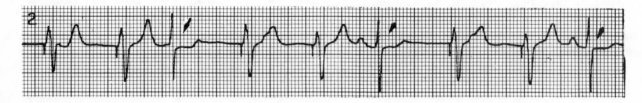

Fig. 48-E - Pacemaker arrhythmias. Ventricular trigeminy and QRS-inhibited pacemaker.

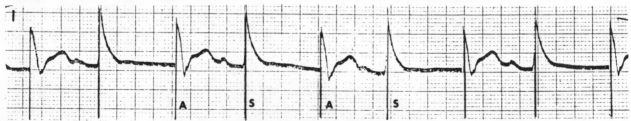

Fig. 48-F - Pacemaker arrhythmias. Ventricular bigeminy and QRS-synchronous pacemaker.

An irregular cardiac rhythm may be the consequence of an interaction between an artificial and a natural pacemaker. The most common situation is the "competition" between a pacemaker and a sinus rhythm. A "demand" pacemaker will maintain a regular cardiac rhythm only when it works in an automatic fashion and, therefore, when spontaneous cardiac activity is not present. In many of the tracings already examined, several bigeminal or trigeminal rhythms are maintained by the symbiosis of spontaneous and artificial impulses.

A short resume is presented on the left side page:

Fig. 48-A: "Ventricular bigeminy in the presence of an asynchronous pacemaker." The "couplets" are formed by a pacemaker beat and a ventricular extrasystole. The spike following the extrasystole is ineffective, because it lands into the ventricular refractory period.

Fig. 48-B: "Asynchronous pacemaker with interpolated ventricular extrasystoles." The pacemaker rhythm is regular and unaffected by the extrasystoles which are sandwiched between two pacemaker beats.

Fig. 48-C: "Ventricular trigeminy". The "triplets" are formed by two sinus beats and by a slightly premature pacemaker beat. The pacemaker is of the asynchronous type and shows competition with the sinus rhythm.

Fig. 48-D: "Pacemaker on T phenomenon". This is a malfunctioning asynchronous pacemaker in the presence of a sinus rhythm. The ventricular capture is only occasional, occurring when the impulses land into the descending branch of the T waves (see page 147).

Fig. 48-E: "Trigeminal rhythm in the presence of a QRS-inhibited pacemaker". The "premature beat" is of sinus origin and suppresses the pacemaker in a normal fashion.

Fig. 48-F: "Ventricular bigeminy and QRS-synchronous pacemaker". The "couplets" are formed by automatic pacemaker beats (A) alternating with synchronized sinus beats (S).

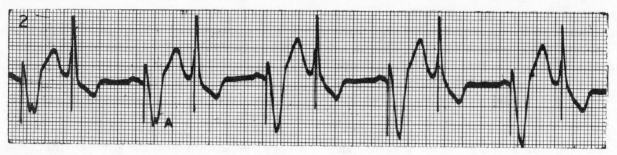

Fig. 49-A - Pacemaker arrhythmias. Ventricular bigeminy probably induced by "echo beats."

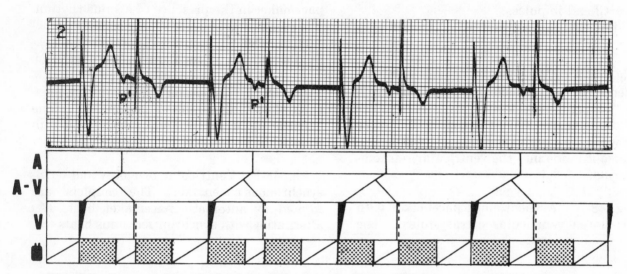

Fig. 49-B - Pacemaker arrhythmias. "Echo beats". The artificial impulse activates the atria in a retrograde fashion (P^1); it is "reflected" in the A-V junction and returns to the ventricles.

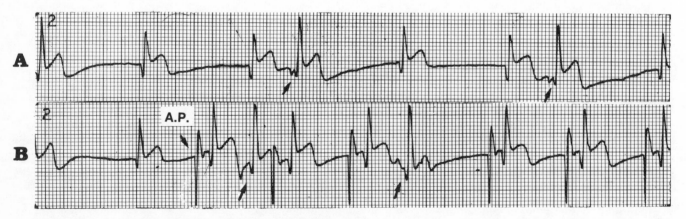

Fig. 49-C - Pacemaker arrhythmias. "Echo beats" during a junctional rhythm (A) and "inverse recipricol beats" during artificial pacing (AP) performed in tracing B.

PACEMAKERS AND ARRHYTHMIAS

"Echo beats"

The retrograde propagation of an artificial impulse through the A-V junction and into the atria is not rare in patients with artificial pacemakers. This is not only an electrocardiographic curiosity but it may occasionally cause the so-called *reciprocal rhythms* and *echo beats*. These may be present either with ventricular or atrial stimulators.

In fig. 49-A an automatic pacemaker beat alternates with a spontaneous QRS complex synchronized with a ventricular-triggered pacemaker. The synchronization is documented by the spikes within the spontaneous QRS's. The fixed coupling between the spontaneous and the artificial beat suggests a "re-entry" of the artificial impulse. While traveling in a retrograde fashion into the A-V junction, the impulse is "reflected" and it returns into the ventricles ("echo beats") and induces a bigeminal rhythm.

Another example of a pacemaker *reciprocal bigeminy* is presented in fig. 49-B. Each pacemaker automatic beat is followed by an obviously inverted P^1 wave (retrograde atrial activation) and by a spontaneous QRS, synchronized with a "demand" QRS-triggered pacemaker. The behavior of the artificial impulse is diagrammed below the figure. "Echo beats" appear when the retrograde V-A conduction is markedly delayed (in fig. 49-B the stimulus-P^1 interval is 0.44 - 0.48 sec.). In such a case, the pacemaker impulses, which are "reflected" into the A-V junction, find the ventricles excitable and produce a bigeminal rhythm.

Tracing A of fig. 49-C records a slow and regular junctional rhythm, controlling the ventricles probably because of a sinus arrest. The beats that are indicated by the arrows are spontaneous "echo beats" (reciprocal beats). Therefore, the junctional impulses are simultaneously directed to the ventricles and, more slowly, to the atria (P^1 waves with Q-P^1 intervals = 0.48 sec.); during the retrograde trip they are "reflected" and return to the ventricles which are again depolarized (QRS's indicated by the arrows).

This type of "junctional gymnastic" is still present during the atrial pacing performed in tracing B. Two P^1 waves are followed by "echo QRS's", indicated by the arrows. In this case, however, since the impulses reflected in the A-V junction originate from the atria (atrial pacing), the "echo beats" should be more accurately called "inverse reciprocal beats." (see "An Atlas of Cardiac Arrhythmias" by John A. Pupillo, M.D.)

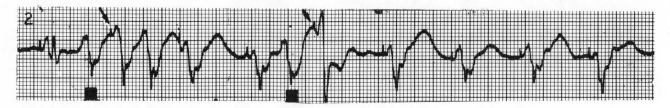

Fig. 50-A - Pacemaker arrhythmias. Repetitive phenomenon. The pacemaker spike induces repetitive ventricular contractions ("pacemaker on T phenomenon".)

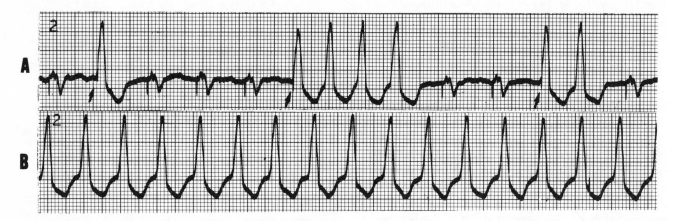

Fig. 50-B - Pacemaker arrhythmias. Repetitive phenomenon. The short bursts of repetitive ventricular extrasystoles are induced by the artificial impulse (A) and degenerate in a ventricular tachycardia (B).

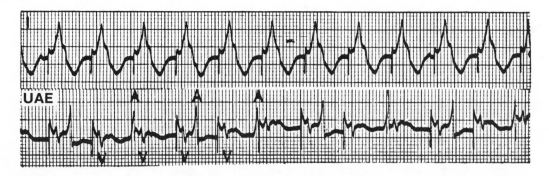

Fig. 50-C - Pacemaker arrhythmias. "Runaway pacemaker." L1 and the unipolar atrial electrogram (UAE) are not simultaneous; A = atrial waves; B = ventricular complexes.

Repetitive Phenomena

An artificial impulse falling within the relative refractory phase of the ventricle ("vulnerable period") may cause repetitive, and hemodynamically inadequate, ventricular contractions. This phenomenon is better known as *"pacemaker on T phenomenon"* and the artificial impulses may sometimes precipitate very dangerous arrhythmias (ventricular tachycardia and fibrillation), by "landing" on the peak of the T wave of a sinus beat or of an atrial or ventricular extrasystole. Repetitive phenomena seem to be favored by: a) myocardial hypoxia; b) abnormal electrolyte balance; c) myocardial damage secondary to coronary artery disease; d) acidosis and alkalosis; and, e) overdose of drugs which increase ventricular excitability.

The impulse indicated by the first arrow in fig. 50-A falls into a T wave of a ventricular extrasystole (dark squares), and produces a repetition of two ventricular extrasystoles, followed by automatic pacemaker beats. The next extrasystole is again followed by an artificial impulse with ventricular capture ("pacemaker on T phenomenon").

Repetitive phenomena, due to pacemaker impulses falling within the ventricular electrical diastole, may also be secondary to a mechanical stimulation of the ventricle. This usually happens when the intracavitary catheter is unstable and produces an endocardial irritation in excitable areas of the right ventricular chamber, such as the tricuspid valve and the postero-basal wall areas.

Tracing A of fig. 50-B exhibits ventricular extrasystoles, single, coupled, and repetitive which interrupt an otherwise regular pacemaker rhythm. The ectopic focus is always triggered by a pacemaker impulse falling far enough from the preceding QRS complex and, therefore, away from the ventricular vulnerable phase. Tracing B shows the rhythm degenerated into a ventricular tachycardia (150/min.). The arrhythmia was induced by a mechanical stimulation of the ventricle secondary to the catheter tip motion.

A rapid heart rate may follow an increased pacemaker delivery rate secondary to battery exhaustion. This phenomenon, which may also give rise to ventricular tachycardias and fibrillation, is not a repetitive depolarization due to a single pacemaker impulse, but is a consequence of a pacemaker malfunction. The pacer delivers high rate impulses with a reduced intensity, but which are still able to capture the ventricles. This phenomenon is known as a "runaway pacemaker."

A ventricular tachycardia due to a "runaway pacemaker" is presented in fig. 50-C and is documented with a separate recording of L1 and of the unipolar atrial electrogram (UAE). The unipolar atrial electrogram clearly shows the A-V dissociation between pacemaker QRS's (V waves with a rate of 125/min.), and the slower sinus P waves (A waves with a rate of 80/min.).

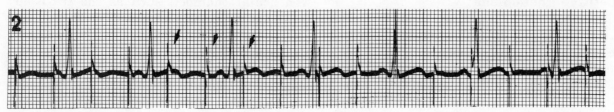

Fig. 51-A - Pacemaker arrhythmias. "Runaway pacemaker" and normal sinus rhythm. The pacemaker spikes are ineffective.

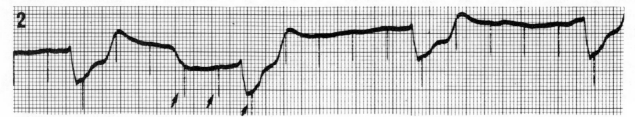

Fig. 51-B - Pacemaker arrhythmias. "Runaway pacemaker" and idio-ventricular rhythm.

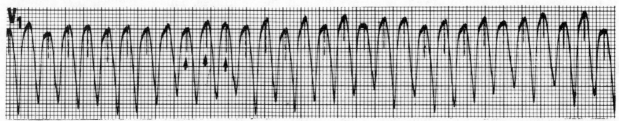

Fig. 51-C - Pacemaker arrhythmias. "Runaway pacemaker" and ventricular tachycardia. Each artificial impulse (rate = 300/min.) is followed by a QRS complex.

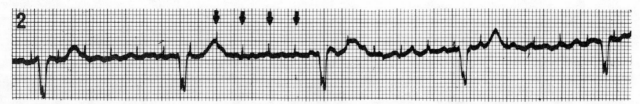

Fig. 51-D - Pacemaker arrhythmias. "Runaway pacemaker" and idio-ventricular rhythm. The arrows indicate ineffective spikes (210/min.) within a slow spontaneous ventricular rhythm.

PACEMAKER ARRHYTHMIAS

"Runaway Pacemaker"

This is a situation in which very high stimulation rates are reached with premature battery exhaustion. The improvement in the manufacturing of generators, the employment of high quality batteries, and a better isolation of the units from surrounding body fluids, have markedly reduced the number of cases of premature battery exhaustion, and therefore, of "runaway pacemakers." Furthermore, while a great majority of pacemakers signal the loss of battery power with an increase in the stimulation rate, in the newest type of pacemakers a decrease battery voltage is accompanied by a decrease in the stimulation rate.

During a routine control of a patient with an artificial pacemaker, the finding of an unstable pacing rate (faster or slower than those recorded in preceding tracings), is a good diagnostic criteria for electronic components malfunction and/or battery exhaustion. Once again, the importance of knowing all the details about the pacemaker being examined (usually specified in the manuals of different manufacturers) must be emphasized. It is also necessary to remember that the stimulation rate, measured by a simple ECG tracing, may not be accurate and comparable with preceding measurements. This is because of the variable frequency response and the paper speed of ECG machines. A change of 5 beats/min. in the pacing rate, with respect to the implantation rate, may call for the substitution of the generator pack. Therefore, it is advisable to measure the interval between two pacemaker impulses by using an electronic counter, which permits measurements of time intervals with an accuracy up to 0.1 msec.

The *runaway pacemaker* is usually a sudden event. The rate increase may be moderate (below 200/min.), or marked (rate 200-300/min. and above), and is accompanied by a reduced generator power. The impulse intensity is usually not high enough to capture the ventricles and this permits the reappearance of spontaneous rhythms. In some circumstances, however, the rapid impulses may stimulate the ventricles and produce lethal ventricular arrhythmias (ventricular tachycardia or fibrillation).

Fig. 51-A shows the spikes of a runaway pacemaker, with a rate of 150/min., and the reappearance of a sinus rhythm with a normal A-V conduction. None of the pacemaker impulses is followed by a ventricular response.

A similar situation is that of fig. 51-B, where a slow, agonal type ventricular rhythm, is dissociated from the fast stimulation rate (180/min.) of a runaway pacemaker.

Although a reduction of the spikes amplitude on the surface ECG may be associated with a decrease in voltage secondary to battery exhaustion, this is not a constant premonitory finding of a *runaway pacemaker*. It may be present in other situations such as respiratory motions, dipole magnitude, calibration of recording instruments, etc.

Fig. 51-C exhibits a ventricular tachycardia which is induced by a *runaway pacemaker*. The stimulation rate is 300/min., and is followed by a 1:1 ventricular response. Obviously, patients in such situations may show clear signs of reduced cardiac output.

The *runaway pacemaker* of fig. 51-D also fires at a very high rate (240/min.). The impulses, however, do not capture the ventricles and do not disturb the slow idioventricular rhythm.

REFERENCES

Dekker, E., Buller, J., Schuilenburg, R.M. (1965): *Aids to Electrical Diagnosis of Pacemaker Failure*, Amer. Heart J., 70:739.

Furman, S., Escher, D.J.W., Schwedel, J.B., Soloman, N., Rubinstein, B. (1964): *Motion Factors Producing Breaks in Implanted Cardiac Pacemaker Leads*, Surg. Forum, 15:248.

B.M. Beller, and G.A. Pupillo: *Potentially dangerous rate and amplitude control interaction in an externally battery powered demand pacemaker*, American Heart Journal, 81:717, 1971.

Hoffman, B.F., Cranfield, P.F. (1960): *The Electrophysiology of the Heart*, New York, McGraw.

Hoffman, B.F., Cranfield, P.F. (1964): *The Physiological Basis of Cardiac Arrhythmias*, Amer. J. Med., 37:670.

Judge, R.D., Preston, T.A., Luccesi, B.R., Bowers, D.L. (1966): *Myocardial Threshold in Patients with Artificial Pacemakers*, Amer. J. Cardiol., 18:83.

Kahn, D.R., Stern, A., Sigmann, J., Sloan, H. (1965): *An Emergency Method of Handling Broken Pacemaker Wires in Children*, Amer. J. Cardiol., 15:404.

Parsonnet, V., Gilbert, L., Zucker, R., Maxim, M. (1963): *Complications of the Implanted Pacemaker: A Scheme for Determing the Cause of the Defect and Methods for Correction*, J. Thorac. Cardiov. Surg., 45:801.

Sowton, E., Davies, J.G. (1964): *Investigations of Failure of Artificial Pacing*, Brit. Med. J., 1:1470.

Stein, E., Damato, A.N., Kosowsky, B.D., Lau, S.H., Lister, J.W. (1966): *Cardiovascular Response to Alterations in Heart Rate Above and Below the Sinus Rate*, Amer. J. Cardiol., 17:140.

Castellanos, Augustin, Jr., Lemberg, Louis, Rodriguez-Tocker, Lillia, and Berkovits, Barouh, V.: *Atrial Synchronized Pacemaker Arrhythmias: Revisited*, Amer. Heart J., 76:199, 1968.

McHenry, Malcolm, M., Nelson, Charles, G., Hopkins, Donald, M., and Smeloff, Edward, A.: *Permanently Implanted Transvenous Pacemakers*, Circulation, 38:324, 1968.

Sowton, E.: *Detection of Impending Pacemaker Failure*, Israel J. Med. Sci., 3:260, 1967.

Preston, T.A., Judge, R.D., Lucchesi, B.R., and Bowers, D.L.: *Myocardial Threshold in Patients with Artificial Pacemakers*, Amer. J. Cardiol., 18:83, 1966.

Preston, T.A., and Judge, R.D.: *High Myocardial Threshold to an Artificial Pacemaker: Report of a Fatal Case*, New Eng. J. Med., 276:297, 1967.

Parsonnet, V., Gilbert, L., Zucker, I.R., and Asa, M.M.: *Complications of the Implanted Pacemaker*, J. Thorac. Cardiov. Surg., 45:801, 1963.

Preston, T.A., Fletcher, R.D., Lucchesi, B.R., and Judge, R.D.: *Changes in Myocardial Threshold: Physiologic and Pharmacologic Factors in Patients with Implanted Pacemakers*, Amer. Heart J., 74:235, 1967.

Feldman, A.A.: *Excitability of the Human Heart on Endocardial Stimulation*, Clin. Res., 11:166, 1963.

Nash, D.T.: *Threshold of Cardiac Stimulation: Acute Studies*, Ann. N.Y. Acad. Sci., 111:877, 1964.

Sklar, H., Escher, D.J.W., Furman, S., and Schwedel, J.B.: *Energy Threshold for Right Ventricular Endocardial Stimulation as a Function of Pulse Duration*, Clin. Res., 13:220, 1965.

Furman, Seymour, Escher, Doris, J.W., Lister, John, and Schwedel, John, B.: *A Comprehensive Schema for Management of Pacemaker Malfunction*, Ann. of Surgery, 163:611, 1966.

Lister, J.W., Furman, S., Stein, E., Damato, A.N., Schwedel, J.B. and Escher, D.J.W.: *A Rapid Determination of Pacemaking Defects in Patients with Artificial Pacemakers*, Bull. N.Y. Acad. Med., 40: 982, 1964.

Parsonnet, V., Gilbert, L., Zucker, I.R., and Asa, M.M.: *Complications of the Implanted Pacemaker. A Schema for Determing the Cause of the Defect and Methods for Correction*, J. Thor. Cardiov. Surg., 45:801, 1963.

Pupillo, G.A.: « *Le Aritmie Cardiache* » *Testo-Atlante*, Vismar Edizioni Scientifiche, Roma, 1971.

Castellanos, A., Jr., and Lemberg, L.: *Arrhythmias Appearing After the Implantation of Synchronized Pacemakers*, Brit. Heart J., 21:747, 1964.

Katz, L.N., and Pick, A.: *Clinical Electrocardiography. Part I. The Arrhythmias*, Philadelphia, 1956, Lea & Febiger, Publishers.

Tavel, M.E., and Fisch, C.: *Repetive Ventricular Arrhythmia Resulting from Artificial Internal Pacemaker*, Circulation, 30:493, 1964.

Dressler, W., Jonas, S., and Rubin, R.: *Observations in Patients with Implanted Cardiac Pacemakers. IV. Repetitive Responses to Electrical Stimuli*, Am. J. Cardiol., 15:391, 1965.

Barold, S. Serge, Linhart, Joseph, W., and Samet, Philip: *Reciprocal Beating Induced by Ventricular Pacing*, Circulation, 38:339, 1968.

Rosenbleuth, A.: *Ventricular « echoes »*, Amer. J. Physiol., 195:53, 1958.

Moe, G.K., Preston, J.B., and Burlington, H.: *Physiologic Evidence for Dual A-V Transmission System*, Circulation Research, 4:357, 1956.

Kastor, J.A., and De Sanctis, R.W.: *Reciprocal Beating from Artificial Ventricular Pacemakers*, Circulation, 35:1170, 1967.

Bellet, S.: *Clinical Disorders of the Heart Beat, ed. 2.* Philadelphia, Lea & Febiger, 1963, p. 359.

Chapter VI

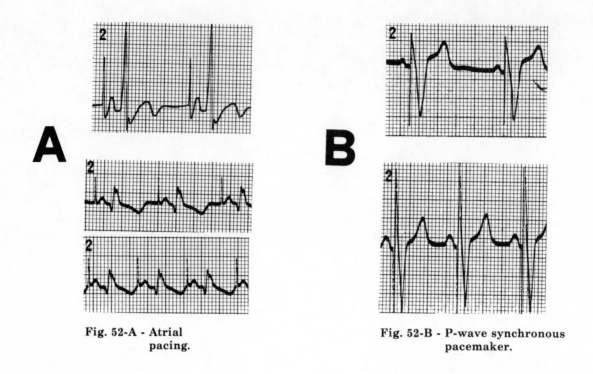

Fig. 52-A - Atrial pacing.

Fig. 52-B - P-wave synchronous pacemaker.

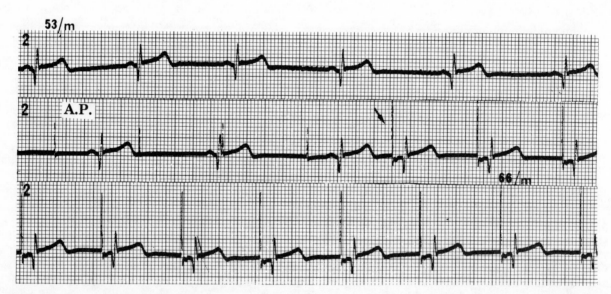

Fig. 52-C - Atrial pacing. Atrial pacing is started in the second tracing. The arrow indicates the moment in which the pacemaker impulses capture the atria.

PACEMAKERS IN SITUATIONS OTHER THAN A-V BLOCK

The electricial stimulation of the human ventricle represents the therapy of election of second and third degree A-V blocks, associated with bradycardic junctional or idio-ventricular rhythms. The main goals are: improved hemodynamic conditions, prevention of prolonged asystoles with Adams-Stokes syndrome, and the suppression of potential ectopic foci.

In recent years, the indications for the use of temporary or permanent artificial pacing have gradually spread to a larger number of clinical situations where dangerous arrhythmias are present in patients with otherwise intact A-V conduction systems. Obviously, the pharmacological armamentarium does not always offer a complete therapeutic solution. At the same time, more data have been accumulated on the combined efficacy of drugs and the electrical stimulation of the human atrium and ventricles.

ATRIAL PACING

The electrical stimulation of the atria is frequently used in the following situations: a) to improve the hemodynamic conditions of sinus bradycardias or S-A blocks, associated 1) with slow junctional or idio-ventricular rhythms, 2) with "sick S-A node syndromes", and 3) with the immediate post-operative period of cardiac surgery; b) to suppress atrial or ventricular extrasystolic foci; c) to control supraventricular tachyarrhythmias and, d) to evaluate the pre-operative and post-operative hemodynamic behavior and ventricular function of patients with valvular and/or coronary artery disease.

First of all, when examining an ECG of atrial pacing it is necessary not to confuse this type of stimulation with a ventricular pacing synchronous with the atria (P-wave syn-chronous pacemaker). *With atrial pacing, the spike always precedes the P wave* (the impulse depolarizes the atria) *and the QRS has a normal morphology* (fig. 52-A). In ventricular pacing synchronous with atrial potentials (P-wave synchronous pacemaker), the stimulus-artifact *follows the P-wave* and the QRS complex is aberrant for the anomalous ventricular depolarization caused by the artificial impulse (fig. 52-B).

In the majority of cases of atrial pacing, the atrial activation wave (P^1 wave) may be sharply different than that of sinus beats (P wave). The P^1 wave morphology depends on the position of the tip of the catheter, the stimulation site, and the propagation of the atrial activation wave. *P^1 waves follow immediately after the pacemaker spikes and precede the QRS complexes with an interval of time equal to a normal P-R interval.*

Since atrial pacing is almost exclusively performed as a temporary measure, the stimulation rate may be changed, within certain limits, in relation to the particular clinical situation being treated. The ventricular rate of the patient presented in fig. 52-C is artificially increased through atrial pacing. From the sinus bradycardia (53/min.) of the top tracing, the rhythm changes into a faster atrial rate which is under the control of artificial impulses (middle and bottom tracing). The first four spikes do not "capture" the atria, probably because of a non perfect electrode contact with the atrial wall. A slight increase of current intensity is enough to obtain a stable control of the atrial and ventricular rhythm. Note the greater amplitude of the spikes which are followed by P^1 waves (arrow) and the sudden increase of cardiac rate from 53/min. to 66/min. following atrial pacing.

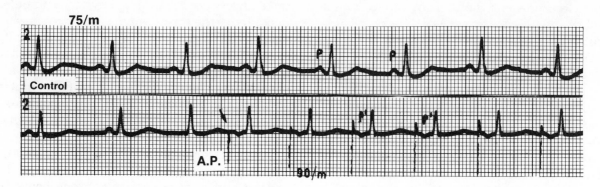

Fig. 53-A - Atrial pacing. The morphology of the pacemaker induced P[1] waves is sharply different from the P waves of sinus beats.

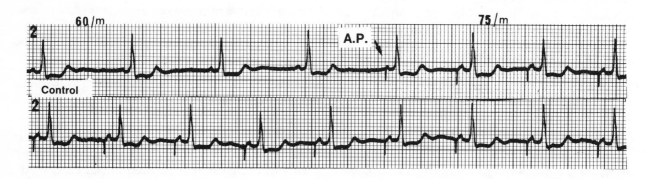

Fig. 53-B - Atrial pacing. The pacemaker induced P[1] waves and sinus P waves have similar configuration.

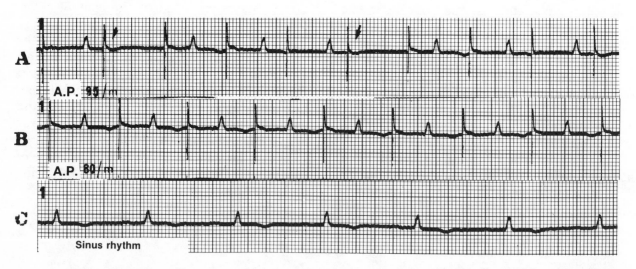

Fig. 53-C - Atrial pacing. C = sinus rhythm with P-R = 0.24 sec.; B = atrial pacing with a first-degree A-V block (P[1]-R = 0.32 secs.); A = atrial pacing with A-V Wenkebach (arrows indicate blocked P[1] waves).

A 1:1 change of both atrial and ventricular rate, following pacemaker impulses, and the appearance of P^1 waves are the cardinal criteria for a good "atrial capture". The morphology of P^1 waves is related to the position of the stimulating catheter and it may vary from one very similar to one entirely different than that of sinus beats. Usually, P^1 waves are easily recognized and may appear as negative, positive, or biphasic waves, and they all follow pacemaker spikes.

The preferred stimulating sites are usually the right atrium and the atrial wall close to the inferior vena cava. A stable pacing is also obtained by positioning the catheter into the coronary sinus. This, however, requires a certain operator ability. The right auricle is also a good pacing site but this requires a catheter manipulation, and usually the insertion of a metallic guide which must remain in place. Although it usually requires a greater current intensity and does not offer a great stability, the junctional area between the inferior vena cava and the right atrium is a satisfactory position for short time pacing, and therefore, is the most preferred pacing site.

The lower tracing of fig. 53-A shows the beginning of an atrial pacing (arrow). The spikes clearly precede the negative P^1 waves, which are markedly different from the sinus P waves of the control tracing, and are followed by a 1:1 ventricular response. The P^1-R interval is slightly longer than the P-R interval of sinus beats.

The atrial pacing performed in fig. 53-B is indicated by the sudden increase of cardiac rate; in this case, the artificially induced P^1 waves are very similar to the sinus P wave of the control tracing. This indicates a normal atrial activation front, which occurs when the tip of the catheter is situated next to the superior vena cava and, therefore, to the S-A node.

Tracing A of fig. 53-C shows a regular artificial stimulation (95/min.) which, on a superficial examination, seems totally ineffective and independent from a somewhat irregular spontaneous rhythm. P or P^1 waves are not clearly recognized and the R-R intervals are irregular.

A closer examination of tracing B shows a synchronization between pacemaker spikes and QRS complexes (each spike precedes a QRS complex of 360 msec.). This is indicated by a slight elevation of the baseline, immediately following each pacemaker impulse (P^1 wave). The tracing, therefore, shows an atrial pacing with a first degree A-V block. It is now easy to understand the situation of tracing A, which also shows an atrial pacing, with a good atrial capture and a second degree A-V block with Wenckebach periods. The P^1-R interval becomes progressively longer until an impulse is blocked in the A-V junction. Therefore, the spike is followed by a P^1 wave but not by a QRS (arrows). The pause is terminated by an artificial impulse with the shortest P^1-R interval (see page 118). Tracing C records the patient in a sinus rhythm. The QRS's are regular (60/min.) and preceded by sinus P waves and prolonged P-R intervals.

The atrial pacing in this patient reveals a progressive fatigue of the A-V conduction tissue when facing increased atrial rates. Only a slight increase of the atrial rate (from 75-95/min.), induces a second degree A-V block. Atrial pacing, therefore, appears to be a useful diagnostic tool in testing the functional capacity of the A-V junction.

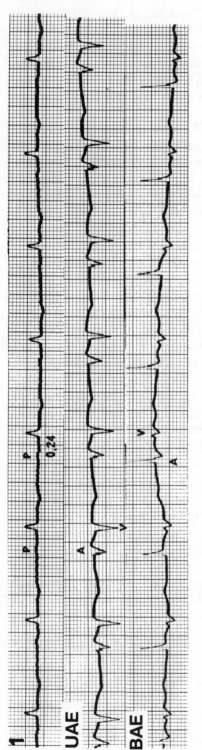

Fig. 54-A - Sinus bradycardia with prolonged P-R interval. Control tracing, surface ECG (lead L1), unipolar atrial electrogram (UAE) and bipolar atrial electrogram (BAE).

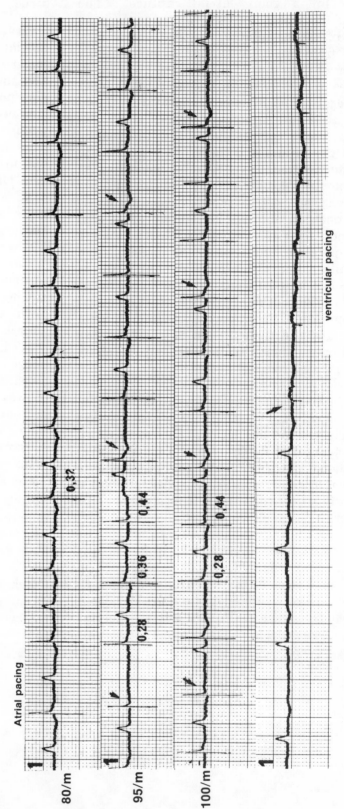

Fig. 54-B - Atrial pacing. 80/min. = first degree A-V block; 95/min. = second degree A-V block with 4:3 Wenkebach periods; 100/min. = 3:2 A-V Wenkebach. The bottom tracings show a ventricular pacing.

Before deciding for an atrial pacing it is useful to test the conduction capacity of the A-V junction. The conduction velocity through the A-V junction may be markedly reduced, and this may induce the operator to prefer a different stimulation site (for example ventricular pacing) to maintain the desired cardiac rate.

Tracings of fig. 54-A are obtained from the same patient of fig. 53-C. They show a sinus bradycardia with a prolongation of the P-R interval (0.24 sec.). Although P waves are not easily recognized on the surface ECG, the rhythm is of sinus origin, as it is documented by the unipolar (UAE) and bipolar atrial electrograms (BAE).

When atrial pacing is started with a low rate (80/min.), a marked prolongation of the P^1-R interval (0.32 sec.) can be noticed. This is secondary to an already fatigued A-V conduction (see the prolonged P-R of the upper tracing of fig. 54-B). At faster pacing rates (95/min. and 100/min.), the A-V conduction further deteriorates and a second degree A-V block, with Mobitz type II sequences, appear (second and third tracings). The presence of Wenckebach periods of 4:3 and 3:2, therefore, indicates the upper limits of conduction capacity of the A-V junction (the arrows indicate blocked P^1 waves). In this case, an effective atrial pacing cannot be performed with rates faster then 80/min. without compromising the regularity of the ventricular rate. Therefore, a ventricular pacing is performed (bottom tracing of fig. 54-B).

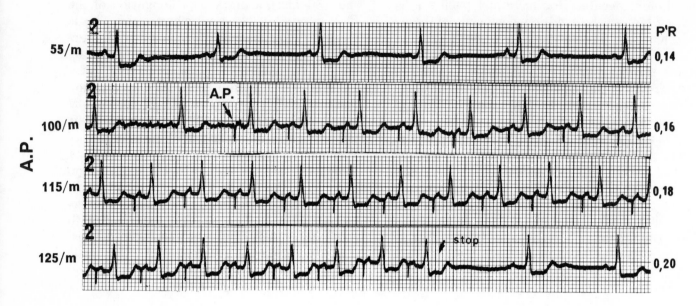

Fig. 55-A - Atrial pacing. Notice the increment of the P^1-R interval with increasing atrial pacing rates.

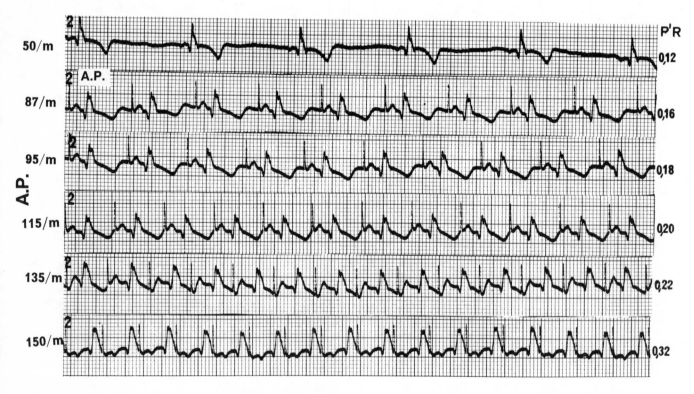

Fig. 55-B - Atrial pacing. The P^1-R interval goes from 0.12 sec. (control tracing) to 0.32 sec. at an atrial pacing rate of 150/min. The ventricular response is of 1:1.

An increased sinus rate induced by exercise, pharmacological agents, or neurohumoral stimuli, is always associated with a slight shortening of the P-R interval. This is in sharp contrast with what happens during atrial pacing. *An increased atrial rate secondary to atrial pacing is constantly accompanied by a prolongation of the P^1-R interval.* It is a common opinion that the behavior of the A-V junction, during atrial pacing of a supine, resting patient, is due to a lack of intervention of sympathetic amines; they, instead, increase the A-V conduction velocity during sinus and supraventricular tachycardias (spontaneous or induced by physical exercise). Furthermore, the recordings of intracavitary electrograms and of His bundle potentials have clearly shown that the delay is not within the myocardium-atrial electrode junction, but is located in different areas of the A-V conduction tissue.

Atrial pacing, therefore, offers a simple and practical way to evaluate the functional capacity of the A-V junction in basal conditions. The possibility of establishing "normal A-V conduction values at different atrial pacing levels", the reproducibility of the findings at distance of time, the early demonstration of latent A-V conduction disturbances, and the study of the efficacy of drugs on the A-V junction, have made atrial pacing a routine technique in the evaluation of cardiac patients with conduction abnormalities and arrhythmias.

The control tracings of fig. 55-A show a bradycardia (57/min). The P-R interval (0.14 sec.) and the QRS duration are within normal limits. Atrial pacing at different levels (100/min. . . . . 125/min.) is performed in the second, third, and last tracing. During the entire stimulation a prompt atrial capture is obtained with a 1:1 ventricular response. The P^1-R interval is slightly prolonged with increasing pacing rates. It goes from a value of 0.14 sec., in the control tracing, to 0.16 - 0.20 sec. with faster atrial rates. With cessation of atrial pacing, a sinus control is promptly re-established (bottom tracing).

A progressive increase of the P^1-R intervals is obtained during the atrial pacing of fig. 55-B. In spite of the prolonged P^1-R intervals, the 1:1 ventricular response, during the faster atrial rates (150/min.), indicates a good conduction capacity of the A-V junction.

A prolongation of the P^1-R interval is considered normal for atrial pacing rates above 100/min. The appearance of Wenkebach type A-V conduction at atrial pacing rates of 100/min. or less, is considered a definite abnormal response (see page 155).

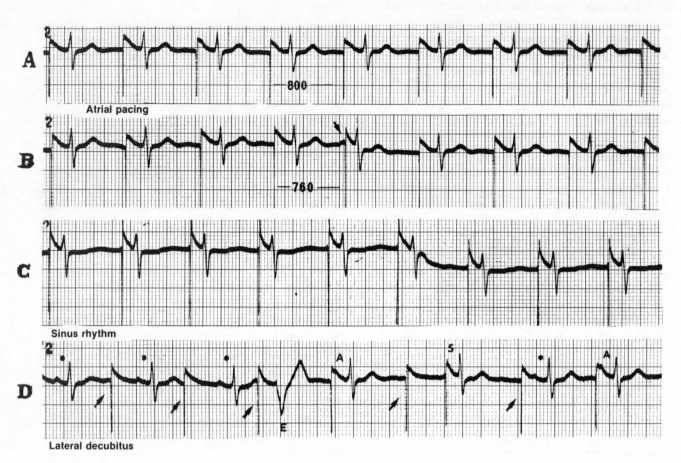

Fig. 56-A - Permanent atrial pacing. See text.

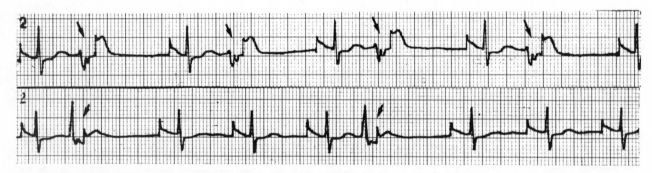

Fig. 56-B - Permanent atrial pacing. The retrograde atrial conduction of the ventricular extrasystoles is demonstrated by the pacemaker synchronization with premature P¹ waves (arrows).

ATRIAL PACING

One of the greatest ambitions of pacemaker manufacturers is the realization of a permanent, "demand type", atrial pacing system which would use only an intracavitary atrial catheter. So far, the efforts in maintaining a stable permanent catheter within the right atrial cavity have not been successful.

The opposite page shows two cases of permanent atrial pacing, through a venous catheter connected to a QRS-synchronous type pacemaker (see page 53). Instead of sensing ventricular potentials and delivering the impulse within the ventricular refractory period, the pacemaker senses P wave potentials and delivers the synchronized impulse within the atrial refractory period. In the absence of atrial activity, or in the presence of an asystolic pause which is longer than the *pacemaker escape interval*, the unit starts a fixed rate atrial pacing.

Tracing A of fig. 56-A shows a regular atrial pacing with a rate of 75/min. (the interval between two stimuli is equal to 800 msec.). Each spike is followed by a P[1] wave with a P[1]-R interval of 0.20 sec. and a normal QRS complex. The pacemaker spike is sharply delineated on the isolectric line and "captures" the atria with a fixed, automatic pacing rate.

Tracing B shows an almost identical situation except for a slightly premature impulse (760 msec. from the preceding spike). The spike is not followed by a P[1] wave, but *falls within* a spontaneous P wave. The pacemaker, therefore, "senses" sinus P wave potentials, and delivers an impulse 20 msec. after the beginning of the spontaneous atrial activation.

Tracing C shows the same patient with a normal sinus rhythm (80/min.), that is slightly faster than the automatic pacemaker rhythm (75/min.). All the spikes are ineffective because they fall 20 msec. after the beginning of the P wave. Notice the difference of the P wave-spike relation and of the length of the P-R intervals (tracing A and C).

After the implantation of the permanent pacemaker, the control tracing (D), which is recorded in a left lateral decubitus, shows evident signs of pacemaker malfunction, secondary to instability of the catheter within the atrial chamber. The impulses indicated by the arrows are ineffective, not synchronized with the atrial signals, and are unable to capture the atria. Notice the "simulation of of a P[1] wave" by the voltage-decay curve. The dots indicate sinus beats, while "A" are automatic impulses with atrial capture. "S" indicates the only sinus beat synchronized with the pacemaker, as suggested by the prematurity of the spike within the otherwise regular delivery of impulses and by the spike falling within the initial portion of the sinus P wave. "E" indicates a single extrasystole.

Tracings of fig. 56-B present an atrial rhythm induced by an artificial stimulator. Each spike is followed by a P[1] wave and by a ventricular complex. Sinus beats are not present; the "demand" mechanism of the permanent atrial pacemaker is revealed by the numerous multifocal ventricular extrasystoles indicated by the arrows. Although the retrograde P waves of the ventricular extrasystoles are not clearly visible, their presence is revealed by the pacemaker spikes following each extrasystole. Being synchronized with atrial potentials, the unit senses the atrial waves and discharges the impulse within the atrial refractory period. This is proved also by the slight prematurity of the synchronized impulses within the extrasystolic P[1] waves.

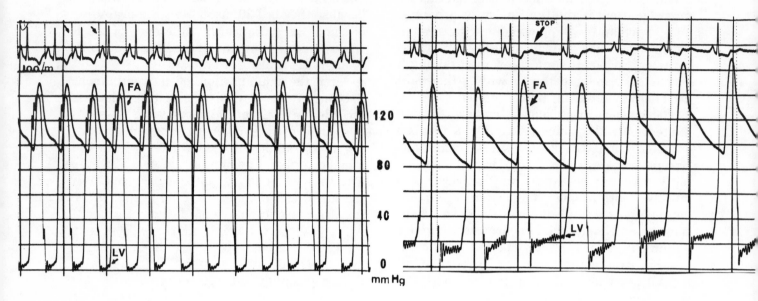

Fig. 57-A - Atrial pacing. Atrial pacing is employed in the evaluation of left ventricular function. LV = left ventricle; FA = femoral artery.

Fig. 57-B - Atrial pacing. Notice the increase in left ventricular endiastolic (LV) and femoral artery pressures (FA) with the cessation of atrial pacing.

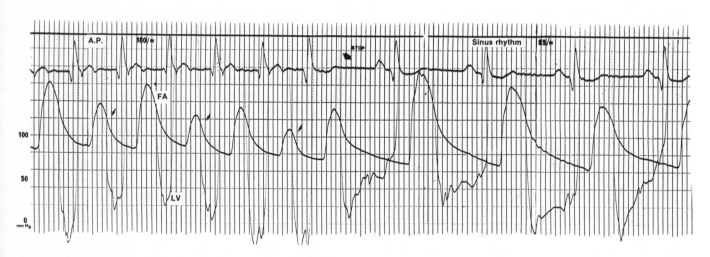

Fig. 57-C - Atrial pacing. A "pulsus alternans" is present during a rapid atrial pacing (FA = femoral artery; LV = left ventricle).

Atrial pacing is commonly used in the hemodynamic evaluation of cardiac function of patients with valvular and coronary artery disease. The technique allows one to evaluate: a) the conduction capacity of the A-V junction; b) the behavior of left ventricular and peripheral pressures under increased cardiac rates; c) the cardiac output before, during, and after atrial pacing; d) the ventricular function curves at rest, and with changes of endiastolic pressure induced by atrial pacing; e) the behavior of the ventricular contractility during angina pectoris induced by atrial pacing, and, f) the pre and post-operative pressure gradients and ventricular function curves in patients with valvular lesions.

Tracings of fig. 57-A and 57-B illustrate how some of this information is obtained during the hemodynamic study of a patient with coronary artery disease. Three cardiac parameters are recorded simultaneously during atrial pacing: a) surface ECG; b) left ventricular pressure (LV) and, c) femoral artery pressure (FA).

In fig. 57-A the cardiac rate (100/min.) is under the control of an artificial pacemaker, and a spike (arrows) precedes each P^1 wave. The values of left ventricular and femoral pressure curves can be derived from the pressure scale (0.200 mm Hg).

When atrial pacing is stopped (fig. 57-B) a sinus rhythm, previously suppressed by the faster artificial rate, reappears promptly. The asystolic pause between the last atrial paced beat and the first spontaneous beat determines a long diastolic ventricular filling time, and a sudden volume overload on the left ventricular chamber. The myocardium behaves according to its own state of compliance and contractility. In this case the cessation of atrial pacing induces a sudden increase of both the left ventricular endiastolic and peripheral artery pressures.

Since atrial pacing induces volume and pressure changes, it allows the construction of left ventricular function curves. This is done by utilizing the pressure values, like those presented in fig. 57-A and 57-B, and cardiac outputs obtained before, during, and after atrial pacing. The function curves are then compared to control curves of normal patients, and used to diagnose abnormalities of myocardial contractility.

Sometimes, during an atrial pacing, abnormal left ventricular hemodynamic behaviors are suggested by the appearance of a "pulsus alternans" at a faster cardiac rate. The first part of fig. 57-C records a femoral artery "pulsus alternans", during fast (180/min.) atrial pacing rates (note the spike preceding the P^1 wave and the prolongation of the P^1-R interval during pacing). With the cessation of atrial pacing (arrow) and the reappearance of a sinus rhythm with a normal P-R interval (85/min.), the peripheral and the left ventricular diastolic pressures appear sharply increased. This is caused by a better ventricular diastolic filling and by an improved left ventricular systolic pressure and left ventricular work.

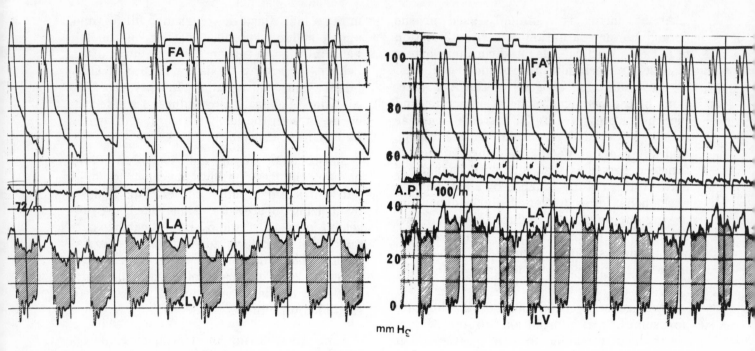

Fig. 58-A - Control tracing of a patient with a pure mitral stenosis. LV = left ventricle; LA = left atrium; FA = femoral artery.

Fig. 58-B - Atrial pacing. Same patient of fig. 58-A during atrial pacing. Notice the increased pressure gradient across the stenotic mitral valve.

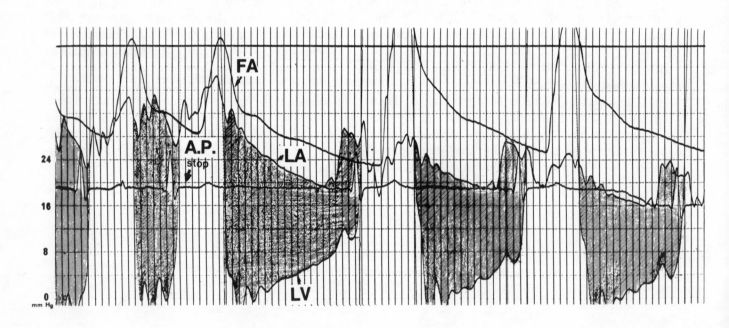

Fig. 58-C - Atrial pacing. The sudden cessation of atrial pacing is followed by a longer ventricular diastolic filling period and by a sudden fall of the pressure gradient (same patient of fig. 58-A and 58-B).

Atrial pacing is easily performed and it is reproducible. Since its introduction, an increasing amount of experience and control values have been accumulated. Thus, it is today preferred to physical exercise in the hemodynamic evaluation of patients with coronary or valvular diseases. The increased cardiac rates obtained through atrial pacing may also be utilized in the hemodynamic evaluation of patients with valvular diseases. In addition to giving data about the conditions of the myocardium, atrial pacing allows one to evaluate the rate related changes of pressure gradients across the diseased valves.

Fig. 58-A and 58-B show a simultaneous recording of left ventricular (LV), femoral artery (FA), and left atrial (LA) pressures in a patient with mitral stenosis. The surface ECG is recorded at the center of the tracing and the pressure values are read from the mm. of Hg. scale. The pressure gradients between the left atrium and ventricles (shaded area) are first measured with a control sinus rate of 72/min. (fig. 58-A), and then during atrial pacing with a rate of 100/min. (fig. 58-B). The increase in the valvular gradient (10 mm. of Hg.), during atrial pacing, is associated with a drop in left ventricular and femoral artery pressures. This is secondary to a sudden pressure rise in the left atrium, an incomplete left ventricular diastolic filling, and, therefore, a reduced ventricular systolic volume.

The pressure tracings of fig. 58-C belong to the same patient, and are recorded during atrial pacing. The pressure scale is now 0-40 mm. of Hg. Notice the prolonged left ventricular diastolic filling phase which appears immediately after the cessation of atrial pacing, and before the first sinus beat. Furthermore, sudden fall of left atrial and peripheral pressures can be observed. This is caused by an improved left atrial emptying, during the diastolic pause, and by a ventricle which responds to the Frank-Starling law.

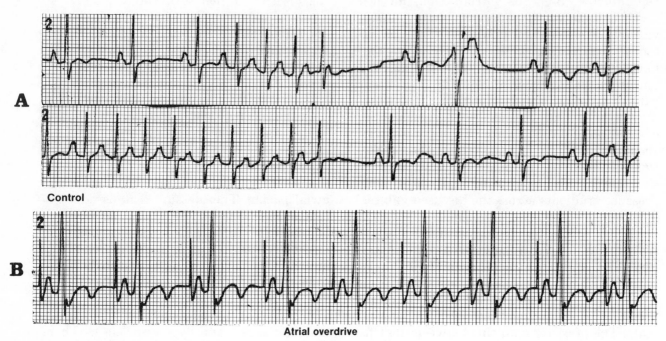

Fig. 59-A - Overdrive atrial pacing. Episodes of paroxysmal atrial tachycardia (A) are controlled with atrial pacing (B).

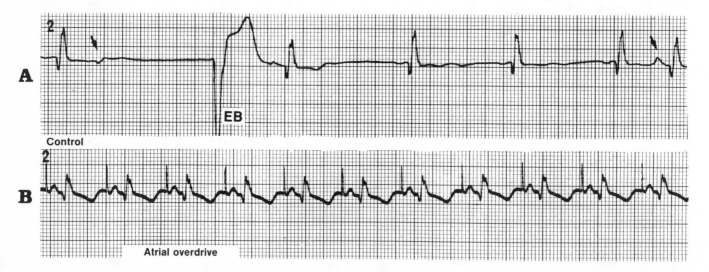

Fig. 59-B - Overdrive atrial pacing. Tracing A shows a bradycardic rhythm, atrial extrasystoles (arrows) and an asystolic pause with an escape ventricular beat (EB). The rhythm is controlled by an overdrive atrial pacing of 95/min. (B).

Sometimes a ventricular or a supraventricular cardiac arrhythmia may be accompanied by inadequate hemodynamic conditions and the arrhythmia may not be easily controlled with drugs. Temporary or permanent electrical pacing of the heart, alone or associated with drugs, is today a well established mode of therapy. It is usually called "overdrive pacing" of the heart.

Overdrive pacing means electrical capture of the human atrium or ventricle, performed with the intention to stabilize an irregular, ectopic cardiac rhythm which may easily degenerate into a more dangerous arrhythmia or which induces inadequate hemodynamic conditions. If the conduction through the A-V node is still good and unimpaired by drugs, the *overdrive pacing* is performed in the atrium; if the A-V conduction is compromised, the stimulating electrode is then placed into the ventricle.

To be able to suppress the ectopic focus, the rate selected for overdrive must be at least 15-20 beats/min. faster than the rate of the spontaneous rhythm. Occasionally, when in presence of ectopic rhythms which may easily degenerate into ventricular tachycardia and/or fibrillation, it is necessary to use overdrive pacing rates of 100 or more beats/min. to suppress the ectopic focus. *Overdrive* is usually a temporary pacing modality and is used in conjunction with drugs. When the rhythm is controlled, the stimulation rate is slowly reduced until it is discontinued. Occasionally, with recurrent arrhythmias, it may be necessary to implant a permanent pacemaker.

Tracing A of fig. 59-A shows a supraventricular tachycardia which repetitively overcomes an unstable sinus rhythm. Several bouts of paroxysmal atrial tachycardias, with a ventricular response of 1:1 (rate = 180/min.), begin and end abruptly and alternate with a sinus rhythm (the arrow indicates a ventricular extrasystole). Since the A-V conduction is still good, an *overdrive atrial pacing*, with a rate of 90/min, is performed. This successfully suppresses the atrial ectopic focus and, therefore, leads to improved and more stable hemodynamic conditions (B).

Tracing A of fig. 59-B illustrates a bradycardic atrial rhythm, interrupted by atrial extrasystoles (arrows). One of the extrasystoles (first arrow) is blocked within the A-V junction and causes a long asystolic pause ending in a ventricular escape beat (Ve). *The atrial overdirve pacing*, with a rate of 95/min., suppresses the extrasystolic focus and maintains a faster and regular cardiac rate (tracing B).

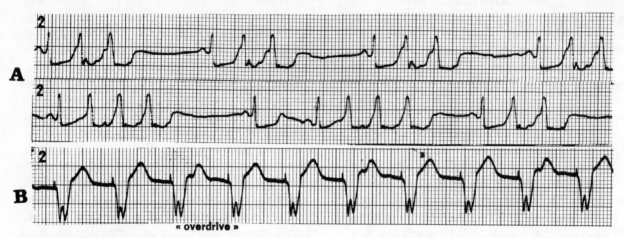

Fig. 60-A - Overdrive ventricular pacing. A regular ventricular pacing, with a rate of 85/min. (B), controls the unstable cardiac rhythm secondary to a ventricular trigeminy and quadrigeminy (A).

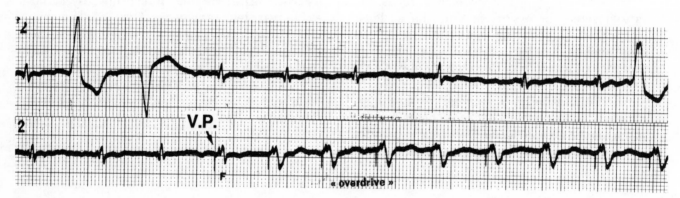

Fig. 60-B - Overdrive ventricular pacing. The fast ventricular pacing (100/min.) of the bottom tracing suppresses the multifocal ventricular extrasystoles present during atrial fibrillation (upper tracing).

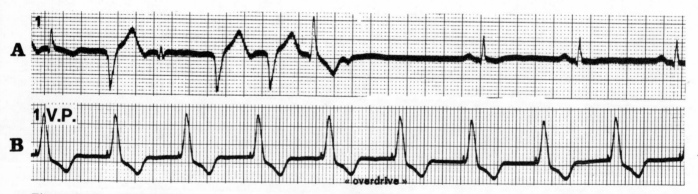

Fig. 60-C - Overdrive ventricular pacing. Tracing A shows a bradycardic sinus rhythm with frequent multifocal ventricular extrasystoles. The ventricular rhythm is stabilized with an overdrive ventricular pacing (B).

When the basic rhythm is of sinus origin and the A-V conduction is still intact, the preferred site for "overdrive pacing", and suppression of an ectopic focus, is naturally the atrium. However, overdrive pacing is performed in the ventricles, when it is necessary to improve the myocardial contractility with drugs which may decrease the A-V conduction (for ex. digitalis), or when the atria cannot be captured because of the presence of a flutter or fibrillation, or when the two conditions are associated.

To be effective, the overdrive of an ectopic focus must be performed at a "critical rate". This means a pacing rate which suppresses the arrhythmia but which, at the same time, maintains an adequate hemodynamic status.

Several ventricular extrasystoles are present in tracing A of fig. 60-A; the coupling of the extrasystoles with sinus beats determines trigeminal and quadrigeminal sequences, separated by prolonged asystolic intervals. In this patient, a *ventricular overdrive* (B) in association with digitalis therapy was preferred to an atrial overdrive pacing in maintaining a stable cardiac rate.

Fig. 60-B shows a rapid *overdrive ventricular pacing* (100/min.), to maintain a regular ventricular rate in a patient with atrial fibrillation and multifocal ventricular extrasystoles. The beat indicating the beginning of overdrive pacing is a fusion beat (F). Later, the ventricles are constantly controlled by the pacemaker.

Tracing A of fig. 60-C shows bursts of multifocal ventricular extrasystoles interrupting a slow sinus rhythm. Bradycardic rhythms of any origin are a good setting for the appearance and degeneration of ectopic foci, particularly in patients with digitalis therapy (as in the case in question).

Tracing B shows a regular rhythm maintained by an *overdrive ventricular pacing*. The stimulation rate is 75/min. and the extrasystolic foci are completely suppressed. The faster and more stable ventricular pacing rate shortens the interval of time in which the heart is vulnerable to ectopic impulses (and suppresses the extrasystoles).

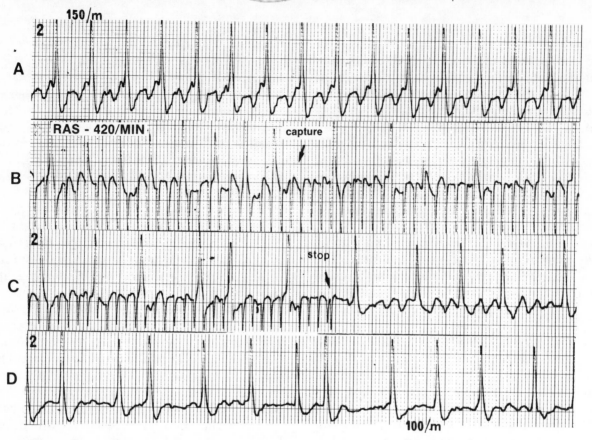

Fig. 61-A - Rapid atrial stimulation. See text.

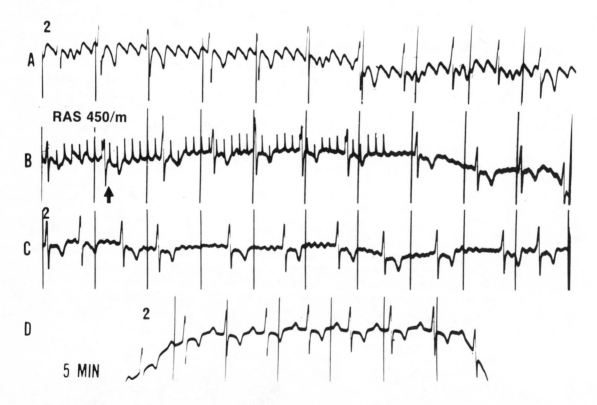

Fig. 61-B - Rapid atrial stimulation. See text.

RAPID ATRIAL STIMULATION

Rapid atrial stimulation (RAS) is a new technique which permits one to suppress supraventricular tachyarrhythmias by rapid artificial pacing of the atria. Artificial impulses are delivered from an external generator at rates usually faster than those of the tachyarrhythmic focus. The artificial impulses may interrupt a circular movement within the atria, or a "re-entry" mechanism between the atria, A-V junction, and the ventricles, or they may suppress a single ectopic focus. Because of their fast rate, they will induce an atrial fibrillation, thereby reducing the ventricular response. In an elevated percentage of cases, after the cessation of a RAS, a sinus rhythm reappears, usually after short periods of atrial fibrillation.

Therefore, the main goal of this technique is to *reduce the fast ventricular rates*, which are usually associated with atrial tachyarrhythmias, *within acceptable hemodynamic ranges*. This is obtained either by taking advantage of the spontaneous A-V block induced by the increased atrial rates (from atrial flutter to atrial fibrillation), or with the conversion of the arrhythmia into a normal sinus rhythm.

The RAS is performed by inserting a catheter into the right atrium (to avoid the accidental stimulation of the ventricles, (the catheter position must be documented either with an intracardiac electrogram or with fluoroscopy) and by connecting it to an external generator capable of high pacing rates (up to 1000 impulses/min.). The RAS is started with a pacing rate slightly faster than the spontaneous atrial rate, and usually in short bursts. The "atrial capture" by the artificial impulses is manifested by a decreased amplitude of the atrial waves and by an irregular ventricular response.

Fig. 61-A shows a RAS performed on a patient with an atrial flutter (atrial rate = 300/min.) and a fast and regular ventricular rate of 150/min. (A-V ratio of 2:1). Tracing B shows the artificial impulses of RAS, with a rate of about 450/min., which determine a slight alteration of the F waves morphology. The ventricular rate in the first portion of the tracing (R-R intervals) is equal to that of the control tracing (A). This means that the artificial impulses have not yet captured the atria. Suddenly (arrow), the R-R intervals become irregular and this is associated with a finer undulation of the baseline. This indicates that the RAS has taken command over the atrial flutter and, therefore, controls both the atrial and ventricular rhythms (the atrial F waves = 300/min. change into f waves = 450/min.). At this point the operator maintains the RAS for a period of time which may go from a few seconds to a few minutes and then abruptly terminates the stimulation. In the case presented, when the RAS is suddenly stopped (tracing C), the atrial rhythm continues to be a stable atrial fibrillation with a ventricular response of 100/min. (tracing D). Fig. 61-A does not show a conversion of the atrial tachyarrhythmia into a sinus rhythm; however, a reduction of the fast ventricular rate into an acceptable slower rate, is obtained. The atrial flutter is changed into a more stable atrial fibrillation and the ventricular rate is reduced from 150/min. to 100/min.; furthermore, the atrial fibrillation permits a better control of the ventricular rate with digitalis therapy.

Figure 61-B presents another case of atrial flutter. This time a high degree of A-V block is present and therefore the ventricular rate is not too fast (A). The RAS is performed with the purpose of converting the arrhythmia into a normal sinus rhythm. The stimulation rate at which atrial capture is obtained (arrow) is equal to 420 impulses/min. (B). After stopping the RAS, a short period of atrial fibrillation takes place (C) and is followed, after a few minutes, by the reappearance of a normal sinus rhythm (D). The maintainance of a normal sinus rhythm, obtained with RAS, depends on numerous factors; the use of antiarrhythmic drugs, the state of myocradial oxygenation, the atrial pressure and dimensions, and the presence of systemic diseases. However, with unstable atrial rhythms, RAS may be used repetitively for days or weeks, without discomfort for the patient (by leaving the catheter in the atrium), until the optimal pharmacologic control is finally achieved.

Except for atrial fibrillation, where the elevated atrial rate does not allow for atrial capture, rapid atrial stimulation usually controls many supraventricular tachyarrhythmias and obtains the same results of external electric cardioversion. CWS has the following advantages: a) general anesthesia is not necessary; b) there is an absence of pain for the patient; c) there is an absence of post conversion arrhythmias; d) digitalis may be maintained before the stimulation; and, e) RAS or atrial pacing may be performed several times simply by leaving the catheter in the atrium.

This last possibility is particularly important because it avoids the need for repetitive external electrical shocks (external cardioversion) in particularly ill patients, and offers an alternative to those patients who do not tolerate drugs well. Furthermore, the stimulating catheter may also be used for recording intracavitary electrograms, thereby increasing the diagnostic ability of the physician in the presence of complicated arrhythmias.

Among the most important disadvantages: the necessity of fluoroscopic control and the possibility of rapid stimulation of the ventricles, if the catheter tip suddenly crosses the tricuspid valve during RAS.

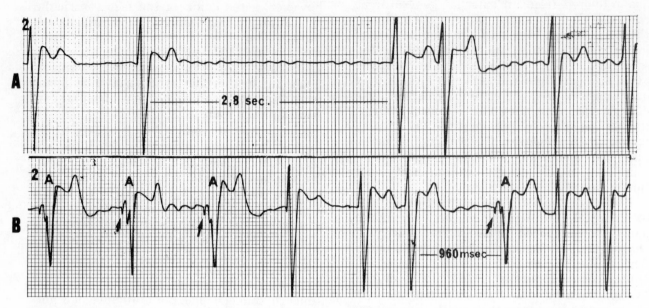

Fig. 62-A - Ventricular pacing. Prolonged asystolic pauses (2.8 sec.) during an atrial fibrillation (tracing A) are controlled with the use of a ventricular-inhibited pacemaker.

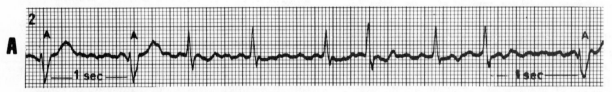

Fig. 62-B - Ventricular pacing. A QRS-inhibited "demand" pacemaker occasionally emerges (beats A) during an atrial fibrillation.

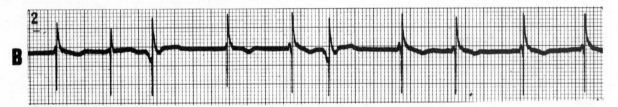

Fig. 62-C - Ventricular pacing. A QRS-synchronous "demand" pacemaker is present during an atrial fibrillation.

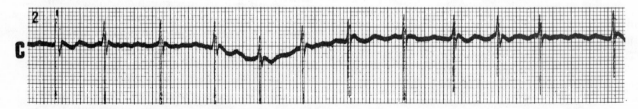

Fig. 62-D - Ventricular pacing. Each ventricular complex of the atrial fibrillation is synchronized with a QRS-synchronous pacemaker.

QRS-triggered and QRS-inhibited "demand" pacemakers are often used in patients with persistent atrial tachyarrhythmias. This is particularly true when using drugs like digitalis which, while improving myocardial contractility, decrease the conduction velocity through the A-V junction.

Persistent atrial flutter and fibrillation are typical examples of the indication for ventricular pacing. High amounts of digitalis are necessary in some patients to control the ventricular rate of atrial flutter and fibrillation and, at the same time, to treat the underlying heart disease of which the arrhythmia is one of the manifestations. Therefore, the therapeutic dilemma between improved hemodynamic conditions on one side (positive inotropic effect) and the presence of drug related asystolic pauses on the other side (negative dromotropic effect), may be solved with the use of a "demand" ventricular pacemaker.

Tracing A of fig. 62-A illustrates an atrial fibrillation with a ventricular response characterized by prolonged asystolic pauses (note the 2.8 sec. interval without ventricular contractions) and the presence of a high degree of A-V block in a patient with heart failure and chronic digitalis therapy. The temporary suspension of digitalis while improving the A-V conduction, it would cause a deterioration of the heart failure. The delicate therapeutic balance of the patient was maintained with the use of a *QRS-inhibited "demand" pacemaker* (tracing B) which would stimulate the ventricles only after long asystolic pauses. The escape interval is set at 960 msec. and, after its expiration, the pacemaker delivers automatic impulses (beats A) with good ventricular capture (the spikes are almost invisible and are indicated by the arrows).

A similar situation is presented in fig. 62-B. During the atrial fibrillation the automatic beats of a *QRS-blocking "demand" pacemaker* appear at the end of 1 second intervals without ventricular activity.

At the operator's request, a *QRS-synchronous pacemaker* may also be used in situations similar to those already presented. In fig. 62-C and 62-D the QRS-synchronous pacemaker spikes are buried within the spontaneous QRS's of an atrial fibrillation (ventricular refractory phase). Automatic beats are not present since the stand-by pacemaker function is never requested.

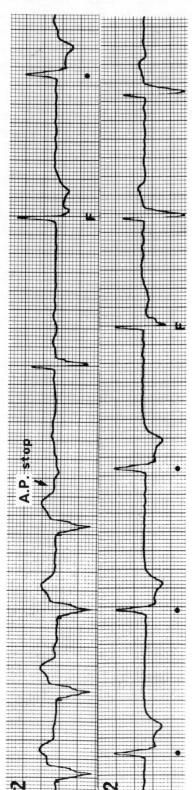

Fig. 63-A - Ventricular pacing. The stimulation is intentionally discontinued (arrow) and this reveals an atrial fibrillation with a high degree of A-V block and ventricular escape beats (dots). F = ventricular fusion beat.

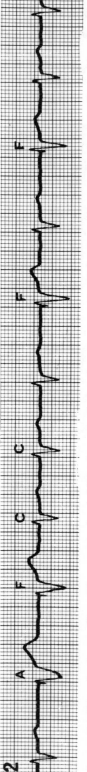

Fig. 63-B - Ventricular pacing. The ventricular-inhibited pacemaker maintains a cardiac rhythm in symbiosis with impulses coming from an atrial fibrillation; F = ventricular fusion beat.

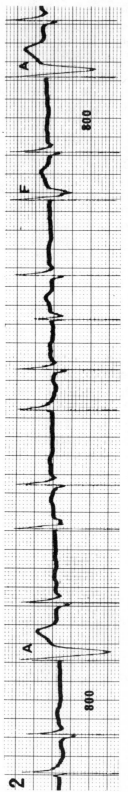

Fig. 63-C - Ventricular pacing. The ventricular-triggered pacemaker captures the ventricles only at the end of asystolic pauses of 800 msec.

The intentional interruption of the temporary pacing, in the upper tracing of fig. 63-A, causes the reappearance of a spontaneous rhythm which clearly indicates the A-V conduction pathology. The baseline is finely undulated because of atrial fibrillation and the spontaneous QRS's have different morphologies. The regular beats, indicated by the dots, are idio-ventricular escape beats induced by the presence of a high degree of A-V block; all others are due to impulses from the fibrillating atria which are capable of crossing the A-V junction, except for the two fusion beats indicated by the letter "F". The slow ventricular rate, the presence of prolonged pauses between two consecutive QRS complexes, the presence of ventricular escape beats, and the need for digitalis therapy are some indications for ventricular pacing in the presence of atrial fibrillation.

Atrial fibrillation is again treated with a combination of electric and digitalis therapy in fig. 63-B. Beats "F" are ventricular fusion beats; their morphology is in between that of the spontaneous QRS's indicated with "C" (impulses conducted to the ventricles) and that of automatic pacemaker beats. Note the morphology of beat "A" which is the only pacemaker automatic beat with complete ventricular capture.

In fig. 63-C a "demand" QRS-synchronous pacemaker controls and maintains a good ventricular rhythm in the presence of an atrial fibrillation. The great majority of spikes are synchronized with spontaneous QRS's and fall into the ventricular refractory period. Only when the atrial impulses do not cross the A-V junction for a time interval of 800 msec. or longer, does the pacemaker deliver an automatic impulse (A) which captures the ventricles (F = ventricular fusion beat).

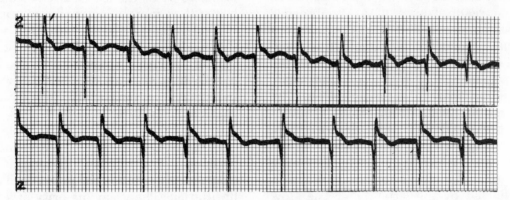

Fig. 64-A - Ventricular pacing. A QRS-synchronous pacemaker is present during an atrial flutter with a rapid ventricular response.

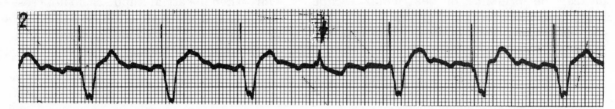

Fig. 64-B - Ventricular pacing. An atrial flutter is present and the ventricles are controlled by a QRS-inhibited pacemaker. Only one of the atrial impulses reaches the ventricles (arrow).

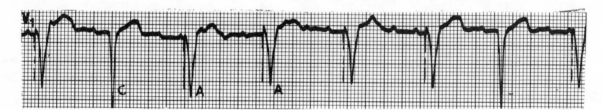

Fig. 64-C - Ventricular pacing. Beats C are due to atrial impulses conducted to the ventricles. All the others are pacemaker automatic beats within the atrial flutter.

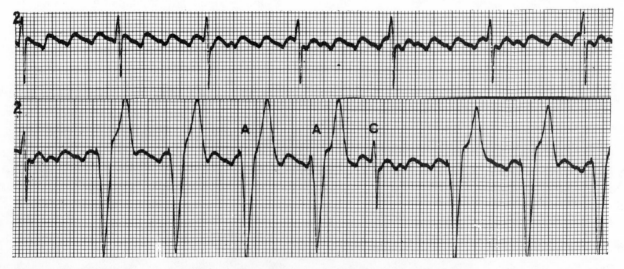

Fig. 64-D - Ventricular pacing. C = conducted beats; A = pacemaker automatic beats.

Four cases of persistent atrial flutter are presented in the figures on the opposite page. These cases were unresponsive to the usual therapeutic measures of drugs and electric cardioversion and were thus treated with a permanent demand pacemaker.

Fig. 64-A shows an atrial flutter with an elevated ventricular response. Pacemaker automatic beats are not present because of the adequate ventricular rate; all the spikes are synchronized with spontaneous QRS's. The stimulator is of the *QRS-synchronous type*.

In the presence of an atrial flutter, the ventricular rhythm of fig. 64-B is under control of pacemaker automatic beats (A). Only one of the F waves filters through the A-V junction and depolarizes the ventricles (arrow). By inhibiting the pacemaker and blocking the delivery of the impulse, the spontaneous QRS reveals the "demand" nature of the *QRS-inhibited pacemaker*.

Letters "C" of fig. 64-C and 64-D indicate beats that are conducted to the ventricles in the presence of an atrial flutter. Both patients have stand-by pacemakers of the *QRS-inhibited type*. In fig. 64-D, spontaneous QRS's are easily recognized (beats C), whereas in fig. 64-C, their configuration is very similar to pacemaker automatic beats (A). The conducted beats do not have a stimulus-artifact before the QRS.

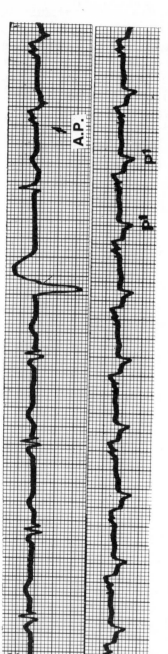

Fig. 65-A - Ventricular pacing and A-V dissociation. Notice the retrograde conduction to the atria of the artificial impulses (P¹).

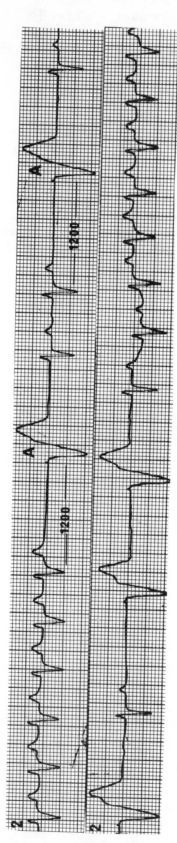

Fig. 65-B - Ventricular pacing and "sick S-A node syndrome". See text.

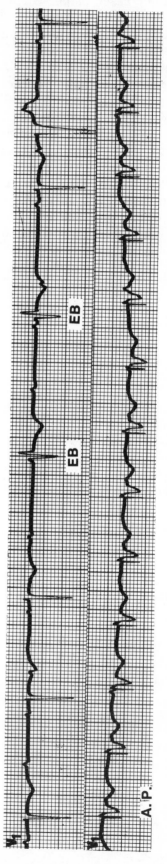

Fig. 65-C - Ventricular pacing and "chaotic atrial tachycardia". EB = ventricular escape beats.

Tracings of fig. 65-A present an A-V dissociation between a sinus and a junctional rhythm, in a patient who was on digitalis and diuretic therapy and was ultimately treated with temporary ventricular pacing. Notice the P waves partially obscured by QRS complexes in the upper tracing ("pseudo-fusion"), the prompt ventricular response to artificial impulses (arrow), and the presence of P^1 waves indicating retrograde atrial activation (lower tracing).

Paroxymal supraventricular tachyarrhythmias are occasionally sustained by a decreased efficiency of the sino-atrial node. The irregular delivery of impulses from the S-A node and the presence of atrial and junctional ectopic foci may lead to a syndrome characterized by paroxymal episodes of supraventricular tachycardia, followed by asystolic pauses long enough to be usually symptomatic *("sick S-A node syndrome")*. The presence of a stand-by ventricular pacemaker is very useful in such circumstances. The pacer is triggered when a post-tachycardic asystolic pause is not spontaneously terminated by a junctional escape beat.

In fig. 65-B several sequences of a fast and unstable atrial rhythm are counterpointed by automatic beats of a *QRS-inhibited "demand" pacemaker*. It is clearly shown that the automatic beats (A) always close long asystolic pauses (1200 msec.) without spontaneous cardiac activity; during the bouts of supraventricular tachycardia the pacemaker is, instead, continuously suppressed (sick S-A node syndrome).

The upper tracing of fig. 65-C shows a chaotic atrial rhythm characterized by numerous and rapid atrial activation waves, coming from different ectopic foci and associated with an occasional second degree A-V block and ventricular escape beats (EB). The irregular ventricular rate is corrected by ventricular pacing (90/min.). The lower tracing shows a stable control of the ventricular rate by artificial impulses while the atrial ectopic foci are still firing rapidly.

REFERENCES

Haft, Jacob, I., Kosowsky, Bernard, D., Lau, Sun, H., Stein, Emanuel, Damato, Anthony, N.: *Termination of Atrial Flutter by Rapid Electrical Pacing of the Atrium*, Amer. J. Cardiol., 20:239, 1967.

Zeft, Howard, J., Cobb, Fred, R., Waxman, Menashe, B., Hunt, Noel, C., Morris, James, J.: *Right Atrial Stimulation in the Treatment of Atrial Flutter*, Annals of Intern. Med., 70:447, 1969.

Lister, John, W., Cohen, Lawrence, S., Bernstein, William, H., and Samet, Philip: *Treatment of Supraventricular Tachcardias by Rapid Atrial Stimulation*, Circulation, 38:1044, 1968.

Massumi, R.A., Kistin, A.D., and Tawakkol, A.A.: *Termination of Reciprocating Tachycardia by Atrial Stimulation*, Circulation, 36:637, 1967.

Zipes, Douglas, P., Wallace, Andrew, G., Sealy, Will, C., and Floyd, Walter, L.: *Artificial Atrial and Ventricular Pacing in the Treatment of Arrhythmias*, Ann. Intern. Med., 70:885, 1969.

Bruce, R.A., Blackmon, J.R., Cobb, L.A., and Dodge, H.T.: *Treatment of Asystole or Heart Block During Acute Myocardial Infraction with Electrode Catheter Pacing*, Amer. Heart J., 69:460, 1965.

Benchimol, A., and McNally, E.M.: *Atrial Pacing During Selective Coronary Angiography*, Brit. Heart J., 29:264, 1968.

Silverman, L.F., Mankin, H.T., and McGoon, D.C.: *Surgical Treatment of an Inadequate Sinus Mechanism by Implantation of a Right Atrial Pacemaker Electrode*, J. Thorac, Cardiov. Surg., 55:264, 1968.

Cohen, L.S., Buccino, R.A., Morrow, A.G., and Braunwald, E.: *Recurrent Ventricular Tachycardia and Fibrillation Treated with a Combination of Beta-adrenergic Blockade and Electrical Pacing*, Ann. Intern. Med., 66:945, 1967.

Furman, S., Escher, D.J.W., and Solomon, N.: *Stand-by Pacing for Multiple Cardiac Arrhythmias*, Ann. Thorac. Surg., 3:327, 1967.

Kastor, J.A., De Sanctis, R.W., Harthorne, J.W., and Schwartz, G.H.: *Transvenous Atrial Pacing in the Treatment of Refractory Ventricular Irritability*, Ann. Intern. Med., 66:939, 1967.

Sowton, E., Leatham, A., and Carson, P.: *The Suppression of Arrhythmias by Artificial Pacemaking*, Lancet, 2:1098, 1964.

Heiman, D.F., and Helwig, J.: *Suppression of Ventricular Arrhythmias by Transvenous Intracardiac Pacing*, J.A.M.A., 195:1150, 1966.

Lew, H.T., and March, H.W.: *Control of Recurrent Ventricular Fibrillation by Transvenous Pacing in the Absence of Heart Block*, Amer. Heart J., 73:794, 1967.

McCallister, B.D., McGoon, D.C., and Connolly, D.C.: *Paroxysmal Ventricular Tachycardia and Fibrillation without Complete Heart Block: Report of Case Treated with a Permanent Internal Cardiac Pacemaker*, Amer. J. Cardiol., 18:898, 1966.

Moss, A.J., Rivers, R.J., Griffith, L.S.C., Carmel, J.A., and Millard, E.B.: *Transvenous Left Atrial Pacing for the Control of Recurrent Ventricular Fibrillation*, New Eng. J. Med., 278:928, 1968.

O'Brien, K.P., Higgs, L.M., Glancy, D.L., Epstein, S.E.: *Hemodynamic Accompaniments of Angina. A Comparsion During Angina Induced by Exercise and by Atrial Pacing*, Circulation, 39:735, 1969.

Khaja, F., Parker, J.O., Ledwich, R.J., West, R.O., Armstrong, P.W.: *Assessment of Ventricular Function in Coronary Artery Disease by Means of Atrial Pacing and Exercise*, Amer. J. Cardiol., 26:107, 1970.

Linhart, J.W., Hildner, F.J., Barold, S.S., Lister, J.W., Samet, P.: *Left Heart Hemodynamics During Angina Pectoris Induced by Atrial Pacing*, Circulation, 40:483, 1969.

Balcon, R., Hoy, J., Malloy, W., Sowton, E.: *Hemodynamic Comparison of Atrial Pacing and Exercise in Patients with Angina Pectoris*, Brit. Heart J., 31:168, 1969.

Linhart, Joseph, W.: *Myocardial Function in Coronary Artery DiDsease Determined by Atrial Pacing*, Circulation, 44:204, 1971.

Linhart, J.W.: *Pacing Induced Changes in Stroke Volume in the Evaluation of Myocardial Function*, Circulation, 43:253, 1971.

Lister, J.W., Stein, E., Kosowsky, B.D., Lau, S.H., Domato, A.N.: *Atrioventricular Conduction in Man. Effect of Rate. Exercise. Isoproterenol and atropine on the PR Interval*, Amer. J. Cardiol., 16:516, 1965.

Sonnenblick, E.H., Morrow, A.G., Williams, J.F., Jr.: *Effects of Heart Rate on the Dynamics of Force Development in the Intact Human Ventricle*, Circulation, 33:945, 1966.

Ross, J.J., Linhart, J.W., Braunwald, E.: *Effect of Changing Heart Rate in Man by Electrical Stimulation of the Right Atrium: Studies at Rest, During Exercise, and with Isoproterenol*, Circulation, 32:549, 1965.

Dimond, E.G., Dunn, M., Brosius, F. (1960): *Management of Arrhythmias in Acute Myocardial Infarction*, Progr. Cardiov. Dis., 3:1.

Glass, H., Shaw, G., Smith, G. (1963): *An Implantable Cardiac Pacemaker Allowing Rate Control*, Lancet, 1:684.

Harris, A., Bluestone, R. (1966): *Artificial Pacing for Slow Heart Rates Following Acute Myocardial Infarction*, Brit. Heart J., 28:631.

Judge, R.D., Wilson, W.S., Siegel, J.H. (1964): *Hemodynamic Studies in Patients with Implanted Cardiac Pacemakers*, New Eng. J. Med., 270:1391.

Julian, D.G., Valentine, P.A., Miller, G.G. (1964): *Disturbances of Rate, Rhythm and Conduction in Acute Myocardial Infarction*, Amer. J. Med., 37:915.

Kaujser, L., Sowton, G.E. (1966): *The Influence of Heart Rate on Maximum Working Capacity in Patients with Artificial Pacemakers*. In Press.

Pupillo, G.A.: « *Le Aritmie Cardiache* » *Testo-Atlante*, Vismar Edizioni Scientifiche, Roma, 1971.

J.W. Linhart, and G.A. Pupillo: *Left ventricular end-diastolic pressure elevation in angina pectoris with normal left ventricular function* (presentato per pubblicazione).

Chapter VII

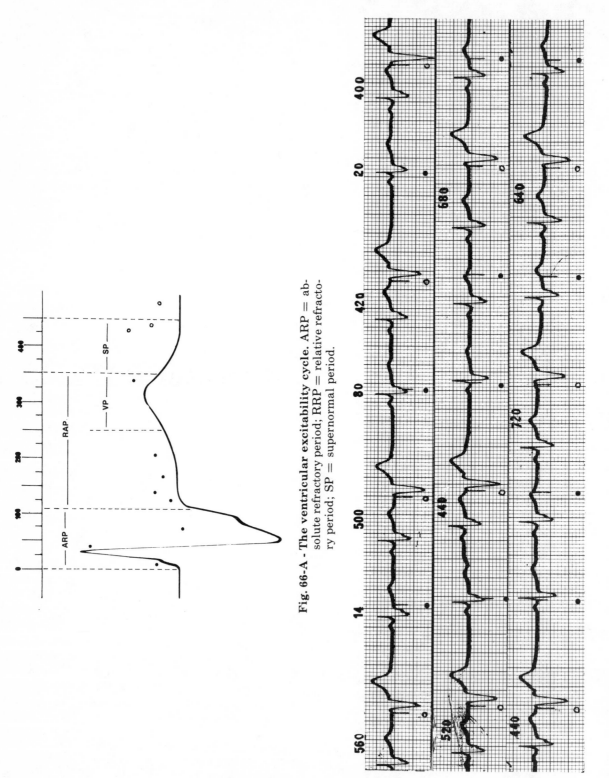

Fig. 66-A - The ventricular excitability cycle. ARP = absolute refractory period; RRP = relative refractory period; SP = supernormal period.

Fig. 66-B - Pacemakers and ventricular excitability. The numbers indicate the Q-spike intervals. Dark circles indicate ineffective pacemaker impulses; clear circles indicate impulses with ventricular capture.

With the widespread use of artificial pacemakers there has been a rapidly increasing knowledge about the natural electrophysiological events of the human heart. At the same time, through the simple analysis of ECG tracings it has become quite easy to measure several specific cardiac parameters such as *conduction, excitability,* and *automaticity.* ECG tracings showing competition between spontaneous and artificial pacemaker rhythms, the evidence of signs of battery exhaustion, the possibility of titrating the intensity and stimulation rate (with temporary pacemakers), offer a gratuitous possibility to analyze the different phases of ventricular and atrial excitability, and to study some of the new and interesting aspects of automaticity and conduction in the human heart.

PACEMAKERS AND VENTRICULAR EXCITABILITY

Before the advent of artificial stimulators, the different phases of the excitability cycle of the human atrium and ventricle were studied by merely relying upon spontaneous events, such as the presence of extrasystoles with variable coupling intervals, or the interaction between a sinus and a parasystolic rhythm. The tracings presented in the next few pages clearly show how easy and useful it is to obtain a great deal of information about the atrial and ventricular excitability phases, by the simple and careful examination of an ECG tracing where artificial pacing is associated with spontaneous cardiac activity.

The QRS complex, the ST segment, and the T wave of spontaneous beats, recorded on the surface ECG, represent the biolectric expansion of a complete cycle of the ventricular excitability. Therefore, it is possible to correlate the different phases of ventricular excitability with the electrocardiographic curves recorded. The diagram in fig. 66-A shows:

a) the isolectric period preceding the QRS which represents the resting phase of myocardial excitability (also called *diastolic phase)*;

b) immediately after depolarization, the ventricular myocardium is totally unexcitable. This phase, which lasts almost 0.10 sec., corresponds to the *absolute ventricular refractory period* (ARP) where a stimulus, no matter how intense, does not produce a propagated response. The QRS complex recorded during this phase is the result of ventricular activation forces; it translates the biolectric process of ventricular contraction with a slight anticipation on the mechanical event;

c) the absolute refractory period is followed by the relative refractory period (RRP). This is the phase where the myocardial excitability gradually recovers and where a stimulus may, in particular circumstances, again activate the ventricles. During this phase an area called *vulnerable period* (VP) can be recognized, where a single stimulus may produce more than one propagated response (salvos of extrasystoles, ventricular tachycardia, and fibrillation). The relative refractory period is represented on the surface ECG by the ST segment, the ascending branch, the peak, and a small portion of the descending branch of the T wave;

d) the recovery of ventricular excitability is therefore followed by a short phase in which the myocardium is hyperexcitable and during which even a subliminal stimulus may produce a propagated response. This particular phase, which involves part of the descending branch of the T wave, the isolectric line and part of the U wave, usually lasts 90-180 msec., and is called *supernormal excitability period* (SP);

e) the supernormality phase is finally followed by a complete myocardial resting state, (represented by the isolectric line of the surface ECG) during which the ventricles wait for an impulse to initiate a new cycle.

Tracings of fig. 66-B show a sinus rhythm, conducted to the ventricles with a right bundle branch block, in competition with a slow rhythm (53/min.) of an asynchronous pacemaker. The great majority of artificial impulses are not effective and ventricular capture is only occasional.

By measuring the Q-stimulus intervals, which goes from the beginning of the QRS to the artificial impulse, it may be observed that only the impulses falling 400 msec. or farther from the spontaneous ventricular depolarization are capable of capturing the ventricles (either during the supernormal excitability phase or during the diastolic phase). Premature impulses (between 0-400 msec.), however, are not effective because they fall into the absolute ventricular refractory phase. The effective stimuli are indicated with a clear circle, while those which are unable to activate the ventricles are indicated by a dot (they are also diagrammed in fig. 66-A). It is impossible to identify the stimuli which capture the ventricles during the supernormal excitability phase, because the pacing intensity is above the diastolic excitability threshold (see page 149). This tracing demonstrates how a common iatrogenic parasystole of an asynchronous pacemaker offers the possibility of studying the excitability phases of the human ventricle.

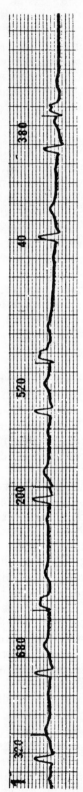

Fig. 67-A - Pacemakers and ventricular excitability. Every other impulse captures the ventricles because it falls within the period of normal excitability.

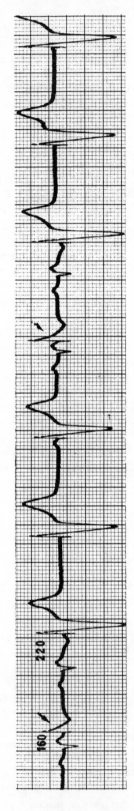

Fig. 67-B - Pacemakers and ventricular excitability. The arrows indicate ineffective impulses falling within the ventricular absolute refractory period.

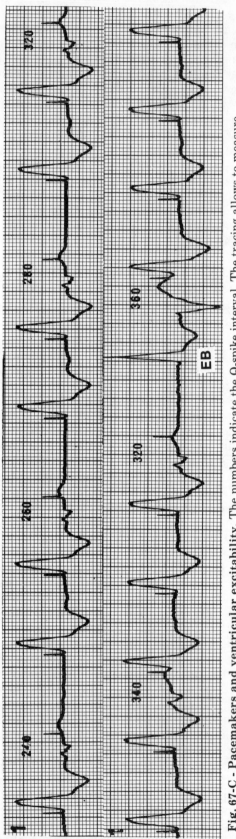

Fig. 67-C - Pacemakers and ventricular excitability. The numbers indicate the Q-spike interval. The tracing allows to measure the ventricular excitability phases.

Fig. 67-A shows a ventricular trigeminy. The two regular beats of the "triplets" are of sinus origin (60/min.), while the premature beats are induced by artificial impulses of an asynchronous pacemaker with a slow pacing rate (46/min.). Because of their time-table, the pacemaker spikes fall in different areas of the sinus cycle. When they land within the ascending branch or close to the peak of the T waves (Q-stimulus interval 380 msec.), they are not effective because they find the ventricles in the *absolute refractory phase*. When the Q-stimulus interval is 380 msec., or longer, it induces a propagated response. Note the complete compensatory pause after the artificial premature beat, due to a sinus P wave blocked within the A-V junction.

Three artificial impulses with good ventricular capture alternate with two sinus beats with normal A-V conduction in fig. 67-B. In both cases, the first of the two sinus beats is followed by an ineffective spike 160 and 220 msec. after the beginning of the spontaneous ventricular depolarization and, therefore, during the *absolute refractory phase*. The spike following the second sinus beat falls far enough from the QRS and captures the ventricles during a normal excitability phase.

In fig. 67-C several ventricular extrasystoles interrupt an asynchronous pacemaker rhythm. The pacemaker obviously does not sense the potentials of sinus beats and, therefore, delivers an impulse immediately after each premature beat. Since the extrasystoles have variable coupling intervals with the pacemaker beats, the spikes happen to fall progressively farther from the beginning of the extrasystolic QRS's (note the Q-stimulus intervals in the upper tracing). When the Q-stimulus interval reaches 340 msec. (lower tracing) the impulse depolarizes the ventricles and the extrasystole is sandwiched between two automatic pacemaker beats. When the Q-stimulus intervals are below 340 msec. the impulses are not effective, because the ventricles are in the *absolute refractory phase*. The second ventricular extrasystole of the lower tracing is followed by a ventricular escape beat (EB) (note the pacemaker spike over the peak of the R wave), by a ventricular extrasystole from a different ectopic focus, and finally by a ventricular capture beat caused by the pacemaker impulse falling into the phase of *ventricular excitability* (Q-stimulus interval equals 360 msec.).

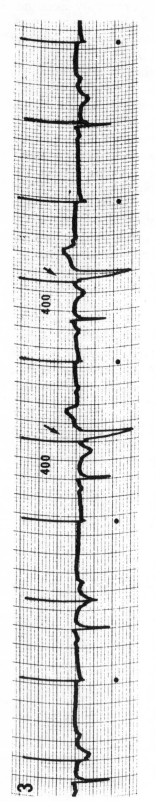

Fig. 68-A - Pacemakers and ventricular excitability. The supernormal phase. Only the impulses indicated by the arrows capture the ventricles since they fall in the supernormal excitability phase. Although they fall in electrical diastole, all the other impulses are not effective.

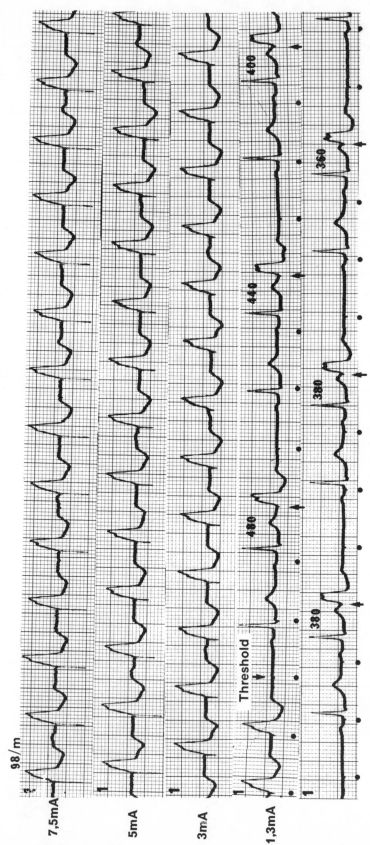

Fig. 68-B - Pacemakers and ventricular excitability. The supernormal phase. Ventricular capture ceases to be constant at stimulation intensity of 1.3 mA. Only impulses falling within the supernormal phase depolarize the ventricles (arrows).

PACEMAKERS AND THE SUPERNORMAL EXCITABILITY PHASE OF THE HUMAN VENTRICLE

Artificial cardiac pacing has helped in identifying that *supernormal excitability phase* of the human ventricle which had been previously denied by several authors. The fundamental criteria in the identification of a supernormality phase is that the *current intensity* applied to the myocardium must be *below the excitability threshold* for that particular ventricle. The supernormal phase cannot be separated from a normal excitability period if the impulse intensity is higher than the excitability threshold.

As explained before (see page 166) the phase of supernormality follows that of relative refractoriness and, during this period of hyperexcitability, even subliminal impulses are capable of provoking a propagated response. This phase is usually found when measuring the cardiac excitability threshold at the moment of implantation of a permanent pacemaker (when the stimulus intensity is very low). It has often been observed in tracings showing pacemaker malfunctions.

Fig. 68-A shows an obvious pacemaker malfunction. None of the impulses of the asynchronous pacemaker are capable of capturing the ventricles, except for those indicated by the arrows. The spikes indicated by the dots do not depolarize the ventricles, although they all fall in diastole, far from the preceding QRS and, therefore, within the resting phase of the myocardium (when it is normally excitable). Therefore, all the impulses, regardless of their amplitude on the surface ECG (unipolar pacing), are below the excitability threshold of that ventricle. Note that the two impulses which capture the ventricles (arrows) "land" just at the end of the T-wave, about 400 msec. from the preceding sinus QRS. Therefore, they are effective only because they fall in that area of the cardiac cycle where the *ventricular supernormality phase* is located. During this phase of the cardiac cycle even subliminal stimuli (below the diastolic excitability threshold) are capable of producing a propagated response.

In the human ventricle, the supernormality phase seems to coincide not with the U wave, as it has been sustained by some authors, but with an area which expands in diastole up to 200 msec. from the end of the T wave. Supernormal excitability is seen only with an anodic stimulation and it is not demonstrable with a catodic stimulation. It is also found with a bipolar pacing but it is due only to the anode-electrode, as it has been demonstrated by the separate use of both electrodes. The measurements obtained indicate that during the supernormality phase the excitability threshold is almost 15% lower than during the diastolic period.

Tracings of fig. 68-B demonstrate how the *supernormality phase* can be localized during the excitability threshold measurements routinely performed at the moment of implantation of a permanent pacemaker. The stimulation rate (98/min.) is the same during all recordings; the impulse intensity, instead, is gradually decreased.

From 7.5 mA to 3mA each artificial impulse is followed by a normal ventricular response; 1.3 mA intensity is followed by a sudden loss of ventricular capture. Here the stimulation is bipolar and the impulse amplitude is, at this point, so small that the identification of the spikes is not easy; the impulses are indicated by dots (ineffective) and by arrows (effective).

At this point, it is possible to know the excitability threshold for that particular ventricle and for the area of myocardium in contact with the electrode (threshold = 1.3 mA). In fact, the majority of spikes, although they fall within areas of normal cardiac excitability, do not cause a ventricular response (because they are below threshold). Only those falling 360 to 480 msec. from the preceding sinus QRS (arrows) capture the ventricles. The effective spikes land at the end of the ventricular repolarization, in that area where the ventricular *supernormal excitability phase* is located.

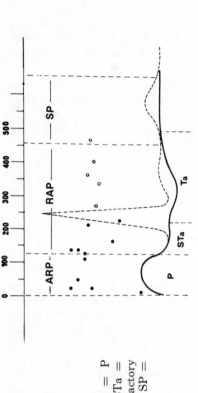

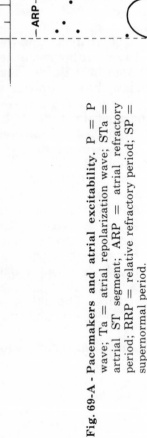

Fig. 69-A - Pacemakers and atrial excitability. P = P wave; Ta = atrial repolarization wave; STa = atrial ST segment; ARP = atrial refractory period; RRP = relative refractory period; SP = supernormal period.

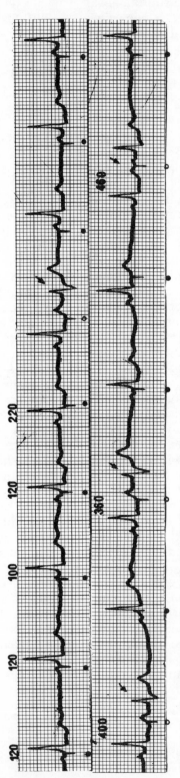

Fig. 69-B - Pacemakers and atrial excitability. Only the impulses indicated by clear circles capture the atria. All others are ineffective because they fall within the absolute refractory phase. The numbers represent the intervals of time between the beginning of the P wave and the spike.

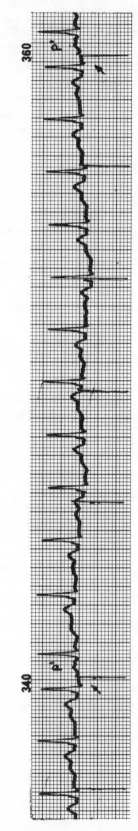

Fig. 69-C - Pacemakers and atrial excitability. Arrows indicate the impulses which polarize the atria (P¹).

The increasing use of atrial pacing has made possible a precise identification and measurement of the excitability phases of the human atrium. Atrial depolarization and repolarization include the following (fig. 69-A):

a) *an absolute refractory period (ARP)*, which corresponds to the P wave of the surface ECG, and during which an impulse does not produce a propagated response;

b) *a relative refractory period* (RRP), during which a slight deflection of the isolectric line appears on the surface ECG, and may be particularly evident in a complete A-V block. The deflection follows the P wave and is conventionally called Ta wave, (which means atrial T wave). It is preceded by the STa segment, so called in analogy to the ventricular ST segment. The STa segment is recorded during the P-R interval and the first part of the QRS complex, while the Ta wave is overimposed on the final portion of the QRS complex and the beginning of the ventricular T wave. The Ta wave appears like a deflection of opposite direction, but enclosing an area similar to that of the P wave, (the atrial gradient is equal to zero);

c) *a period of supernormal excitability (SP)*, which starts within the ascending branch of the Ta wave and extends somewhat into the isolectric line. During this period, even an impulse with an intensity lower than the excitability threshold is capable of activating the atria. Therefore, the entire atrial excitability cycle involves and surpasses the QRS complex and a good part of the ST segment of the ventriculogram. The electrical atrial systole, also called PTa, corresponds to the QT interval of the ventriculogram and its duration fluctuates generally between 200 and 400 msec. The atrial activity is usually overimposed of about 200 msec. to the ventricular one.

The interaction between a normal sinus rhythm and an atrial pacing, presented in fig. 69-B, enables one to study the excitability and refractory phases of the atria. The sinus rhythm (60/min.) is slightly faster than the artificial pacing (53/min.). The pacemaker spikes, therefore, march through the entire cardiac cycle of sinus origin. The great majority of artificial impulses are not effective (the spikes which do not capture the atria are indicated by dots). Only when they land far enough from the beginning of P waves, and the P-stimulus intervals are longer than 340 msec., do they depolarize the atria. Note that the impulses indicated by a clear circle are followed by a P^1 wave, with a prolonged P^1-R interval, and by a premature QRS within the regular sinus cycles. The effective impulses fall within the normal excitability phase of the atria *(atrial diastolic resting phase)*, while the others fall within the *absolute refractory period* and do not produce a propagated response.

Therefore, by measuring the different P-spike intervals on the tracing, it may be stated that the atrium is refractory up to a maximal limit of 340 msec. (which on the surface ECG, includes the P waves, the P-R interval, the entire QRS complex and a good portion of the ST segment). Furthermore, it may be noted that three of the four "premature beats" (arrows) show prolonged P^1-R intervals and QRS's with a right bundle branch block configuration. The intraventricular conduction defect is in relation to the prematurity of the atrial waves, which finds the His-Purkinje system still partially refractory. The last of the effective impulses (P-S interval equals 460 msec.) has a normal P^1-R interval and a QRS similar to a sinus one; this impulse falls far enough from the preceding sinus beats and finds the atrium, the A-V junction, and ventricles in a state of normal conduction and excitability.

Fig. 69-C presents again a slow atrial pacing associated with a somewhat rapid sinus rhythm. Only the impulses which are indicated by the arrows, and with P-S intervals (P-stimulus) of 340-360 msec., are capable of capturing the atria. Note the different morphology of the premature P^1 waves which indicate an ectopic origin of the atrial waves. All other impulses are not effective because they fall into the absolute atrial refractory period.

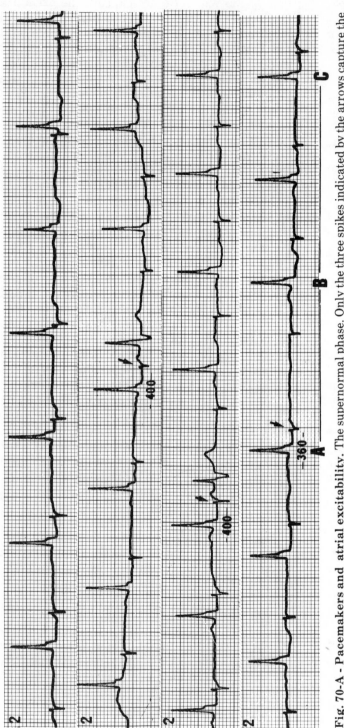

Fig. 70-A - Pacemakers and atrial excitability. The supernormal phase. Only the three spikes indicated by the arrows capture the atria during the supernormal excitability phase. Two of them are also followed by a slightly aberrant QRS complex. Although falling in diastole, the remaining spikes are not effective.

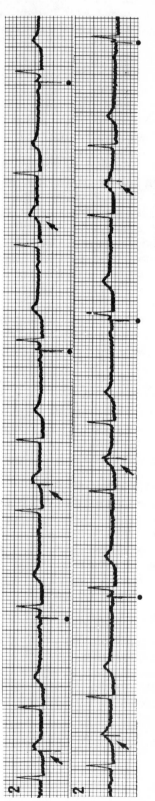

Fig. 70-B - Pacemakers and atrial excitability. The arrows indicate the impulses which capture the atria. Notice the prolonged P'-R intervals.

Again, it must be emphasized that to be able to localize a supernormality phase, either atrial or ventricular, and to separate it from a normal excitability phase, it is necessary that the artificial stimulation has an intensity below the excitability threshold of the atrium and/or ventricle being examined. In the cases shown on the preceding page, while it has been possible to separate the atrial excitability from the refractory phase, a supernormal excitability phase could not be localized because of the presence of impulses with an intensity higher than the excitability threshold.

Tracings of fig. 70-A show a short but indicative sequence, taken from a 10 hour recording, in a patient with a temporary atrial pacemaker. Even with a superficial examination of the tracing, it is immediately evident that the pacemaker impulses (small spikes with a rate of 60/min.) are delivered within a bradycardic sinus rhythm and, in the majority of cases, are not effective. It may be observed that such impulses "scan" all the areas of atrial excitability. Since the sinus rate is slightly slower than the pacemaker rate, the impulses scan the entire isoelectric line moving through QRS's, P waves, etc. The impulses do not capture the atria when a normal response to atrial pacing would be expected (during the atrial diastolic resting phase). The intensity of the stimuli is not high and it is below the atrial excitability threshold. This is because of a floating catheter tip into the atrial chamber and lack of a good contact with the atrial wall.

Three artificial impulses (arrows), however, land 360-400 msec. from the preceding P wave. Only these three impulses depolarize the atria. Two of the (arrows) are followed by a premature P^1 wave, by a slightly prolonged P^1-R interval, and by QRS complexes with right bundle branch block configuration (since the premature impulses find the right bundle not completely repolarized). The incomplete compensatory pause suggests a premature depolarization also of the S-A node.

The impulse indicated in the last tracing captures the atria. However, it is not followed by a ventricular depolarization because it is more premature than the other two conducted impulses (P-stimulus interval = 360 msec.) and it is blocked within the A-V junction. Note that this impulse also causes an in-

complete compensatory pause (AB< BC) which indicates that the P^I wave has prematurely depolarized the sinus node.

Therefore, in this tracing, the indispensable prerequisite for the identification of a hyperexcitability phase is satisfied by the presence of *subliminal impulses*. Consequently, it may be stated that the impulses which activate the atria must necessarily fall within a *phase of supernormality of the atrial excitability*. In the case presented, the supernormal phase is situated between 350-400 msec. from the beginning of the P-wave. Because of the better visibility of the QRS complexes, the measurements can also be made from the beginning of the Q wave (instead of the P wave) to the stimulus, and the supernormal atrial phase will be then situated 230-280 msec. from the beginning of the ventricular depolarization.

An alternative interesting explanation of this tracing (although slightly more sophisticated) involves the so called *Wedesky facilitation*. According to this theory, the *"electrotonic propagation"* to the atria of ventricular potentials of the sinus QRS, which precede the effective impulse, will decrease the atrial excitability threshold and will enable the capture by the subliminal pacemaker impulse. The Wedesky facilitation has been extensively studied in the human ventricles and the A-V junction, but very little is known about its presence into the atria (see page 165).

The atrial trigeminy of fig. 70-B is formed by two sinus beats and by a premature beat caused by artificial impulses which capture the atria (arrows). The stimulation rate is very slow and the effective impulses fall almost invariably close to the peak of the T-wave. Furthermore, the impulse is followed by a marked prolongation of the P^1-R interval and by a normal appearing QRS; note that the P-R of sinus beats is also slightly prolonged. The ineffective impulses are indicated by the dots. They almost always fall within the P-R interval of the sinus beat and therefore, into that phase of atrial repolarization which is electrically silent. However, in this case it cannot be stated that the effective stimuli fall into the atrial supernormality phase because of unavailability of impulses which, although falling in diastole, do not depolarize the atria, and thereby indicate a subliminal intensity.

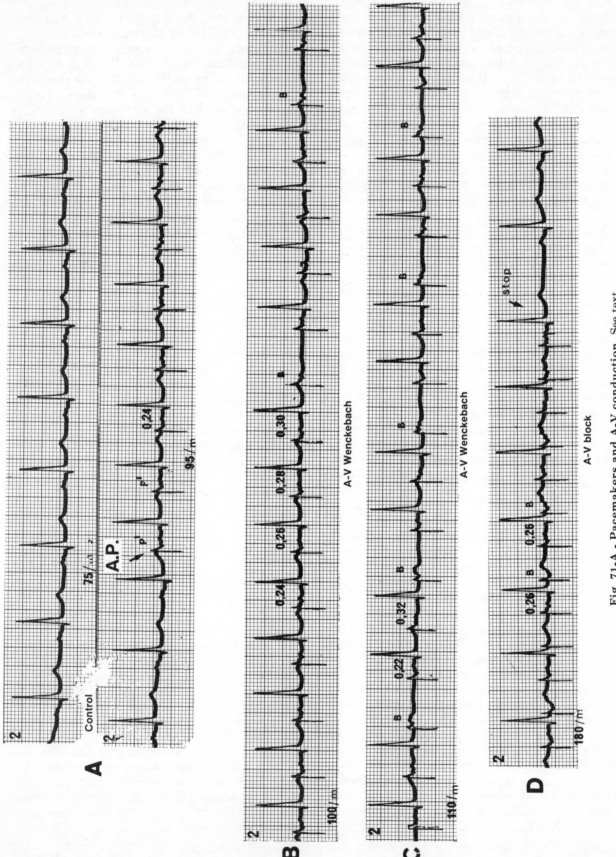

A-V Wenckebach

A-V Wenckebach

A-V block

Fig. 71-A - Pacemakers and A-V conduction. See text.

Anterograde A-V conduction

With the electrical stimulation of the atria, it is also possible to evaluate the behavior of the A-V junction when facing artificially induced rapid atrial rates. It is well known that *atrial pacing usually induces a gradual and progressive prolongation of the P^1-R interval with increasing atrial rates* (see page 118). This is exactly the opposite of what happens with increased atrial rates following physical exercise or neuro-humoral stresses. Increased P-R intervals during atrial pacing is considered normal when it happens with elevated atrial rates (usually above 120/min.); otherwise, it may suggest a latent, abnormal function of the A-V junction, which may later become evident with the appearance of A-V blocks.

Tracings of fig. 71-A offer a beautiful synthesis of the behavior of the A-V junction toward rapid atrial rates obtained through artificial pacing. In "A" a control sinus rhythm is present, with a rate of 75/min. and a P-R interval of 0.16 sec. In the second tracing, the atrial pacing (AP), with a rate of 95/min., is followed by a prompt atrial capture. Note the different morphology of the P^1 waves, the ventricular response of 1:1 and the prolongation of the P^1-R interval (0.24 sec.) over the control (0.16 sec.), indicating a first degree A-V block.

In "B" the stimulation rate is increased to 100/min. A progressive prolongation of the P^1-R interval (0.24. . .0.30 sec.) is present until a P^1 wave is blocked within the A-V junction. The sequence starts again with a beat which is conducted to the ventricles with the shortest P^1-R interval (0.20 sec.) and which again becomes prolonged in the following beats until it reaches another blocked P^1 wave (the blocked P^1 waves are indicated with B). Therefore, atrial pacing produces Wenkebach sequences for the presence of a second degree A-V block Mobitz Type II. It may also be observed that only a further, slight increase in the atrial pacing rate (110/min.), induces ventricular bigeminy caused by a 3:2 Wenkebach. Every third P^1 wave is blocked within the A-V junction while the other two show a P^1-R interval respectively of 0.24 and 0.32 sec. (tracing C).

A further increase in the atrial rate (tracing D) and the progressive A-V block is transformed into a stable 2:1 A-V block (Mobitz type II). When atrial pacing is discontinued (arrow), a prompt sinus rhythm reappears, with a rate and a P-R interval similar to the control tracing.

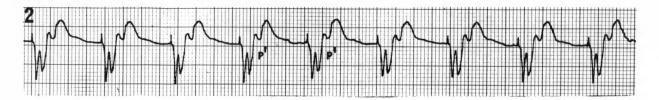

Fig. 72-A - Pacemakers and retrograde V-A conduction. The artificial impulses capture both ventricles and the atria (P^1). They travel in a retrograde fashion through the A-V junction.

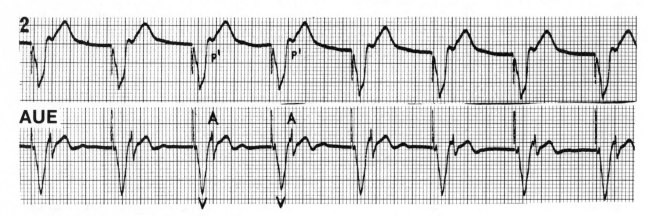

Fig. 72-B - Pacemakers and retrograde V-A conduction. The retrograde ventriculo-atrial conduction and the atrial capture are documented by the P^1 waves of the surface ECG and by the A waves of the unipolar atrial electrogram (UAE).

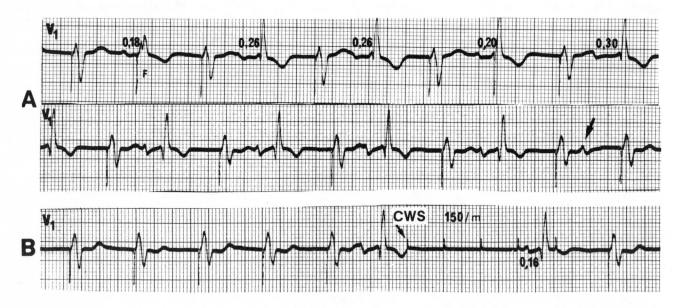

Fig. 72-C - Pacemakers and "concealed" retrograde V-A conduction. The P-R intervals of sinus beats alternating with pacemaker beats (tracing A), are longer than the P-R intervals (0.16 sec.) of chest wall stimulation (CWS). The delayed anterograde A-V conduction is due to the "concealed" retrograde penetration of the pacemakers impulses through the A-V junction.

Retrograde V-A conduction

Occasionally, a pacemaker impulse which depolarizes the ventricles may penetrate the A-V junction in a retrograde fashion and activate the atria. The retrograde atrial activation wave is recognizable on the surface ECG as a small, negative P^1 wave immediately following the pacemaker QRS (fig. 72-A).

Retrograde V-A penetration may also be present when the A-V junction is not capable of a good anterograde conduction (page 22). For this to happen it is necessary that a "unidirectional A-V block" is present and that the artificial impulse travels through a differential retrograde V-A conduction pathway.

When P^1 waves are not clearly evident on the surface ECG, their presence may be documented by simultaneous or sequential recording of intracavitary electrograms. The two tracings of fig. 72-B show the sequential recording of a surface lead (lead 2) and of an atrial unipolar electrogram (AUE). Each pacemaker QRS complex (indicated by V in the AUE), is followed by an atrial activation wave (indicated with A in the AUE and with P^1 in lead 2). The Q-P interval, which indicates the ventriculo-atrial conduction time, is equal to 0.20 sec. and it is within normal limits. Notice that this patient was treated for the presence of a high degeee of A-V block in the anterograde conduction of the sinus impulse.

In the majority of cases, however, the artificial impulse will die within the A-V junction. The interruption of its retrograde journey will be indicated by the behavior of the immediately following sinus impulse. The sinus impulse which follows the pacemaker beat may find the A-V junction totally or partially refractory and, thus, may be either blocked or conducted to the ventricles with a marked delay, This indirectly proves a *concealed retrograde V-A conduction* of the artificial impulse.

Tracing A of fig. 72-C shows a bigeminal rhythm caused by alternating pacemaker capture beats and sinus beats that are conducted to the ventricles. The P-R intervals of the sinus beats vary in length from 0.18 sec. in the fusion beat (F), to a maximum of 0.30 sec. (the last P-R of the first tracing). The second tracing records a P wave blocked within the A-V junction. Here, the P wave is indicated by the arrow and is not followed by a QRS.

Tracing B illustrates the technique of chest wall stimulation (see page 169), which was performed with the intention of suppressing the ventricular-inhibited pacemaker and to measure the length of the P-R intervals of sinus beats, undisturbed by pacemaker impulses. CWS (arrow), performed with a rate of 150/min., promptly suppresses the pacemaker. the external impulses, interpreted as intracavitary potentials, are indicated by small positive artifacts. The sinus beat appearing during CWS shows a P-R interval of 0.16 sec., which indicates the normal A-V conduction time of sinus impulses.

The longer duration of the P-R intervals of the sinus rhythm, symbiotic with that of the artificial pacemaker, is due to the *retrograde concealed V-A penetration* of artificial impulses into the A-V junction and a consequent A-V delay of the anterograde sinus impulses. When the pacemaker is suppressed, the CWS unveils the true P-R interval of the sinus beats (0.16 sec.).

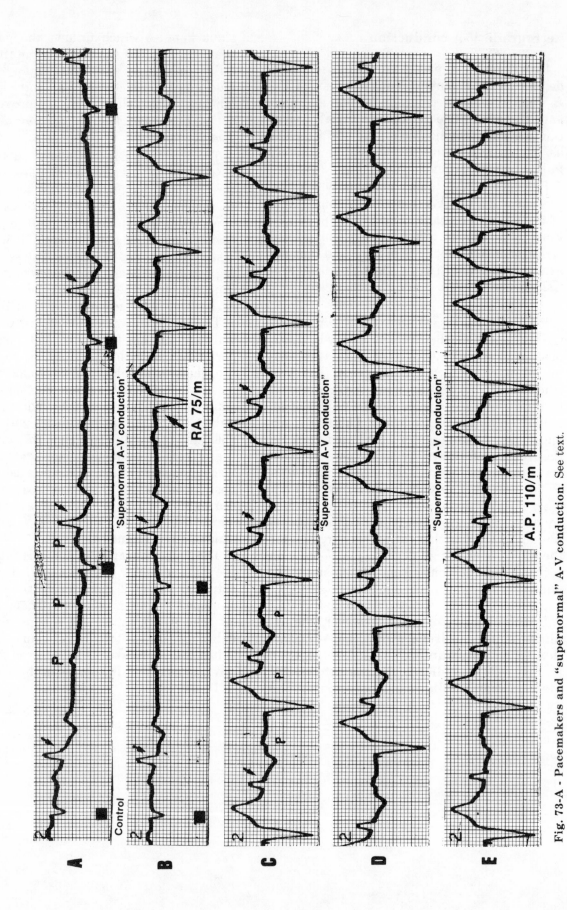

Fig. 73-A - Pacemakers and "supernormal" A-V conduction. See text.

PACEMAKERS AND THE ATRIO-VENTRICULAR CONDUCTION

Supernormal A-V conduction

The presence of a supernormal A-V conduction explains an occasional unusual behavior of the A-V junction, when atrial impulses are able to reach the ventricles also in the presence of a complete A-V block. Since the A-V conduction is depressed or suppressed in the presence of an A-V block, the term "supernormal" does not indicate an A-V conduction faster than normal, but an A-V conduction "better" than that expected in that particular situation.

In tracing A of fig. 73-A a sinus rhythm is present with a rate of 100/min., and P waves are blocked within the A-V junction. The ventricular rhythm, slow and independent from the sinus rhythm, is maintained by an idioventricular spontaneous pacemaker (QRS indicated by dark squares). It is clearly visible that, in spite of the presence of the A-V block, only the P waves immediately following the idioventricular QRS's are able to cross the A-V junction and activate the ventricles (QRS indicated by the arrows). These findings indicate the existence of a supernormality phase in the A-V conduction, which becomes manifest through the intervention of either the ventricular potentials or the mechanical effect of the immediately preceding ventricular contraction.

In tracing B a "demand" ventricular pacing is initiated (QRS-inhibited pacemaker) with a rate of 75/min. (arrow). After four regular pacemaker beats, QRS complexes of sinus origin reappear and, in tracing C and D, determine a ventricular bigeminy. The pacing rate is halved by the spontaneous QRS's which suppress the pacemaker (arrows). Again, the sinus P wave which activates the ventricles is always the one immediately following the pacemaker automatic QRS's, while the next P wave is blocked within the A-V junction.

Therefore, the ventricular potentials, or the mechanical effect of the ventricular contraction induced by the pacemaker, seem to "lubricate" the A-V conduction and "facilitate" the conduction of the next sinus impulse. Only a considerable increase of the stimulation rate (tracing E) seems to eliminate this unusual phenomenon.

A true supernormal phase has not been clearly demonstrated for the A-V junctional tissues, while other facts have been considered, one of these being the intervention of phasic neuro-humoral factors, especially in the presence of particularly slow ventricular rates, dissociated from a faster sinus rhythm. During a slow idio-ventricular rhythm, the ventricular systolic volume may be increased and may induce an increased vagal activity from the arterial baro-receptors, during each ventricular systolic wave.

It has been suggested that a vagal reflex may explain the well known phenomenon of "ventriculo-phasic sinus arrhythmia", which is often present during complete A-V block. It consists in a slight premature delivery of a sinus impulse immediately after a ventricular contraction. The same concept may be applied to the A-V conduction in explaining the presence of a supernormal phase. Furthermore, this would explain why, in a certain number of cases, after the insertion of an artificial pacemaker for advanced A-V blocks, a normal or intermittent A-V conduction may reappear. The differences of opinion have been conciliated by indicating the phenomenon as *"ventriculo-phasic A-V supernormality"*.

The time necessary for the vagal reflex to influence the A-V junction, and decrease the conduction velocity of the next impulses, seems to be longer than 600 msec. (R-P interval longer than 600 msec.). Any sinus or atrial impulse with a R-P interval shorter than 600 msec. will propagate better than one with a longer R-P interval. The cholinergic activity in the S-A node and in the A-V junction is at a minimum just before each vagal stimulation. It is at this point that a penetration of the A-V conduction system seems more probable than in any other area of the cardiac cycle.

This period of "increased" or "less depressed" conduction capacity is considered an evidence of a *"supernormal phase of the A-V conduction."*

The interval of 600 msec. from the idio-ventricular QRS, which precedes the vagal influence on the A-V junction, would include: a) the time between the QRS and the systolic wave reaching the arterial baroceptors; b) the conduction time in the baroceptors nerves, CNS delay and afferent vagal conduction time and, c) the time between the vagal stimulus and its physiologic effect on the A-V junction. In the case presented, all the atrial impulses, conducted to the ventricles during the supernormal phase, always fall after R-P intervals shorter than 600 msec. from the preceding idio-ventricular or artificial beat.

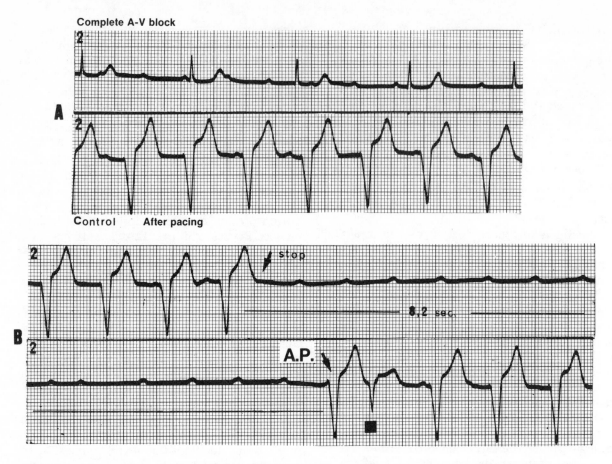

Fig. 74-A - Pacemakers and cardiac automaticity. The sudden cessation of artificial pacing (B) is followed by a prolonged asystolic pause (8.2 sec.) secondary to "overdrive suppression."

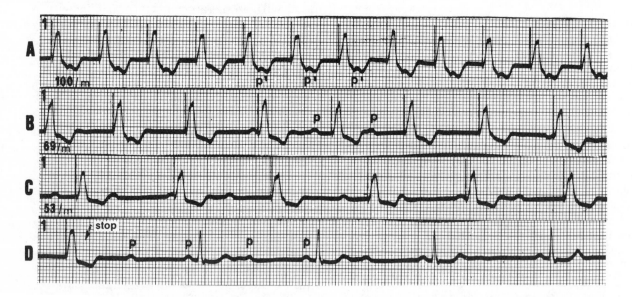

Fig. 74-B - Pacemakers and cardiac automaticity. The tracings show the correct way to interrupt an artificial pacing and, thus, avoiding the "overdrive suppression"; notice the prompt reappearance of a sinus rhythm with a second degree A-V block.

PACEMAKERS AND THE CARDIAC AUTOMATICITY

Overdrive Supression

Artificial cardiac stimulation is also of great help in understanding the *automatic function* of natural pacemakers. A well known electrophysiological phenomenon is that of a faster spontaneous cardiac pacemaker, delivering a great number of impulses per minute, which suppresses a slower and subsidiary cardiac pacemaker. Pharmacologic agents such as Atropine and Isoproterenol utilize this capacity to suppress, for example, a bradycardic ventricular parasystolic focus, often present during an acute myocardial infarct.

Artificial pacing, also, can suppress spontaneous cardiac automaticity. For example, a fast ventricular pacing suppresses a slow idioventricular rhythm associated with a complete A-V block. After pacing, a spontaneous rhythm may reappear only after a more or less prolonged asystolic interval. This phenomenon is called *overdrive suppression* and is sometimes used, as a therapy, to intentionally suppress ectopic foci which may conceal and/or degenerate in more dangerous arrhythmias. Not unusually, patients with bradycardic rhythms (with or without a complete A-V block) also have ventricular unifocal or multifocal extrasystoles which can easily degenerate into ventricular tachycardia or fibrillation. The ectopic foci may be suppressed by the high ventricular rates obtained through atrial or ventricular pacing ("overdrive pacing"; see page 129).

Overdrive suppression, therefore, must be kept in mind when a cardiac rhythm is entirely controlled either by a temporary or a permanent artificial pacemaker. This is also true when it may be necessary to interrupt an artificial pacing (for example, to substitute a malfunctioning generator, to diagnose the presence of spontaneous cardiac activity, to relocate a stimulating electrode, etc.). It must also be remembered that, because of the "overdrive suppression", a prolonged ventricular asystole may also be induced by a sudden dislocation of a stimulating catheter.

Tracing A of fig. 74-A is of a patient artifically paced because of a complete A-V block and a junctional bradycardic rhythm (ventricular rate = 42/min.). The sudden cessation of the temporary ventricular pacing (tracing B), during the implantation of the permanent pacemaker, induces a dramatic episode of prolonged ventricular asystole. Note that sinus P waves (100/min.) are present while ventricular spontaneous activity is totally absent; the overdrive suppression was also associated with episodes of Adams-Stokes syndrome. When artificial pacing is restarted (last tracing), a ventricular extrasystole is present (dark square) after the first pacemaker automatic beat; most likely, this is mechanically induced by the tip of the catheter after the first ventricular contraction. Pacing is bipolar (the spikes are almost invisible) and the pacemaker is a QRS-inhibited type (the extrasystole, in fact, suppresses the temporary pacemaker).

Independently from its duration, a *temporary cardiac pacing must not be interrupted abruptly.* As shown in fig. 74-B, pacing must be gradually slowed down till complete cessation. Note that a stimulation rate of 100/min. (A), with complete ventriculr capture and retrograde atrial depolarization (P^1), is gradually lowered to a rate of 69/min. (B). Sinus P waves reappear before a pacing rate of 53/min. (C). When the artificial stimulation is interrupted, a sinus rhythm with a second degree A-V block promptly reappears without prolonged asystolic pauses (D).

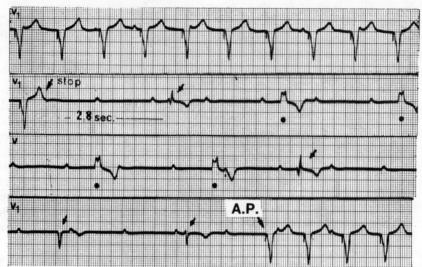

Fig. 75-A - Pacemakers and cardiac automaticity. "Overdrive suppression."

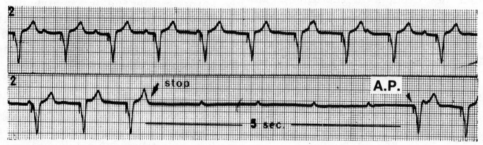

Fig. 75-B - Pacemakers and cardiac automaticity. "Overdrive suppression."

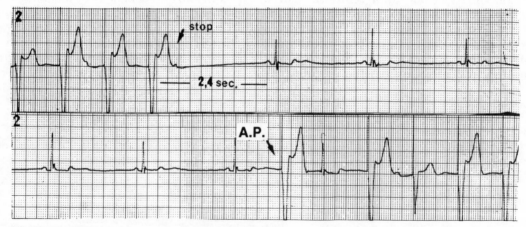

Fig. 75-C - Pacemakers and cardiac automaticity. "Overdrive suppression."

PACEMAKERS AND THE CARDIAC AUTOMATICITY

Overdrive Suppression

The reason why the automaticity of natural cardiac pacemakers, either primary or secondary, is suppressed by rapid impulses (natural or artificial) is still *intensively* investigated and is still a matter of speculation. With the production of experimental ventricular asystoles, it has been observed that the length of the *asystolic interval,* which is the interval between the last artificial impulse and first spontaneous beat, is related to the stimulation rate; it will be longer, the higher the stimulation rate is before its interruption. The length of the asystolic interval may be shortened by Digitalis and by Isoproterenol, and may be lengthened by Pronestyl.

It has also been observed that a good myocardium has a very important role in the immediate restoration of a spontaneous activity, and that the degree of inhibition of a spontaneous pacemaker automaticity does not involve only the first beat, but also the restoration of a spontaneous rhythm with a rate closer to the pre-stimulation rate. Usually, the pre-stimulation rate will be reached after numerous cardiac cycles ("warming up effect"), probably as a result of a gradual loss of inhibition of the spontaneous pacemaker.

The tracings on the opposite page again show three cases of *overdrive suppression,* determined by the sudden interruption of artificial pacing. In fig. 75-A, the interruption of a temporary pacing is followed, after an asystolic pause of about 3 secs., by a double idio-ventricular bradycardic rhythm, independent from a sinus rhythm for the presence of a complete A-V block. Note the two different morphologies of spontaneous QRS's, one of ventricular (dots) and one of low junctional origin (arrows).

In fig. 75-B the interruption of artificial pacing is not followed by a spontaneous ventricular activity (only sinus P waves are present) and pacing is restored after an aystolic interval of 5 sec. Some surgeons take advantage of prolonged asystolic pauses, intentionally obtained by interrupting a temporary pacing, during implantation of permanent pacemakers. The asystolic ventricles facilitate the suturing of the epicardiac electrodes.

Fig. 75-C illustrates the reappearance of a bradycardic sinus rhythm after the interruption of an artificial pacing. The asystolic interval is 2.4 sec. Sometimes, in the same patient, the asystolic interval may change from moment to moment and, occasionally, a malfunctioning pacemaker may induce a sudden emergence of idio-ventricular contractions or precipitate a lethal asystolic pause.

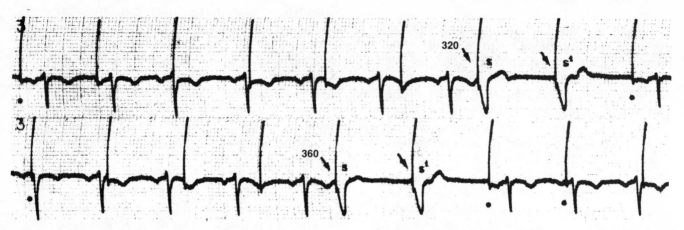

Fig. 76-A - Pacemakers and cardiac automaticity. "The Wedensky effect" facilitates ventricular capture by the subliminal impulses (S^1) which follow the capture during the supernormal excitability phase (S).

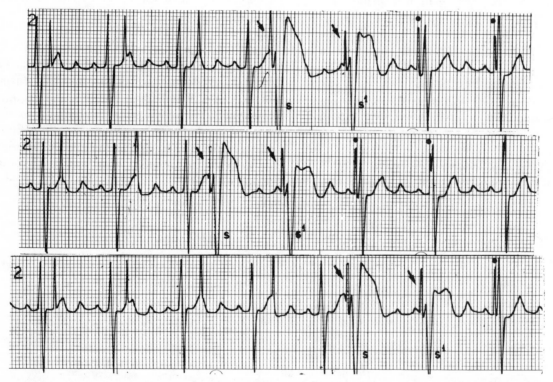

Fig. 76-B - Pacemakers and cardiac automaticity. The repetitive ventricular capture by otherwise ineffective artificial impulses (S^1) is due to a lowered excitability threshold ("Wedensky effect").

"The Wedenski effect"

The sinus rhythm of fig. 76-A is disturbed by the presence of asynchronous pacemaker spikes. The competition with the sinus rhythm is only occasional (arrows) and the presence of undoubtly ineffective impulses (dots) clearly indicates a pacemaker malfunction. The spikes pointed by dots, through falling in full diastole, do not capture the ventricles and are pathognomonic of pacemaker malfunction. The other stimuli land too close to the preceding QRS, and one cannot be sure whether their ineffectiveness is due to the normal ventricular refractory phase or to a pacemaker malfunction.

The first of the two impulses capturing the ventricles (indicated with "S" in both tracings) lands 320-360 msec. from the preceding QRS, over the terminal portion of the T wave and, therefore, in that area where the supernormal excitability phase is located. The subliminality of the impulses (demonstrated by the presence of ineffective spikes in full diastole) is the conclusive element in demonstrating the supernormality phase. The true meaning of this tracing is in the ventricular capture beat following the "supernormal" beat (indicated with "S^1"). As illustrated, an "S^1" beat is regularly present in both tracings following the "S" beat. The subliminal impulse, therefore, captures the ventricles, not only during the supernormality phase (S), but also immediately after it. (S^1).

Something very similar is shown in fig. 76-B where a pacemaker malfunction is present during an atrial flutter with a 4:1 A-V block. The pacemaker impulses are not effective, except for the spikes indicated by the arrows. The impulses indicated by the dots document an intensity below the excitability threshold, because they fall in diastole and should capture the ventricles. The first of the two effective spikes (S) must, therefore, fall during the ventricular supernormal phase. The following pacemaker impulse (S^1), although below threshold is also able to capture the ventricles. Therefore, it can be safely assumed that in both circumstances, the *ventricular potentials of the subliminal impulse which falls into the supernormality phase (S), "facilitate" the ventricular capture by the following artificial stimulus (S^1) which, since it falls in diastole and it is below the threshold, should not be effective.* Furthermore, this phenomenon occurs after periods of relatively prolonged ineffective pacing.

The electrophysiology behind the "repetitive ventricular capture of subliminal impulses" delivered by a malfunctioning pacemaker is the following: "each *effective impulse* (in this case, the effective impulse is the one which falls in the supernormal phase) *decreases the cardiac excitability threshold to a level, and for a length of time, such as to enable the next subliminal impulse* (artificial or spontaneous) *to capture the ventricles.*"

This electrophysiologic mechanism is also known as the *Wedenski effect* and is a clinical variant of what has been elegantly demonstrated in vitro. The *Wedenski effect* is the demonstration of a prolonged stimulating effect of electrical current. It consists of a decreased excitability threshold (first demonstrated in the isolated nerve and later in the Purkinje fibers) which follows a "strong" electrical stimulus (higher than threshold). With the advent of artificial pacemakers, the Wedenski effect has been also observed in the human heart. It has been documented that a subliminal impulse can produce a propagated response if it is preceded by a high intensity stimulus. In the cases presented in fig. 76-A and 76-B, the "strong" stimulus is the effective spike falling into the supernormal phase.

The Wedenski effect helps in understanding the mechanism of some of the complex cardiac arrhythmias, and may be at base of some of the ventricular arrhythmias appearing in patients with artificial pacemakers. It must not be confused with the "Wedenski facilitation" and with the "Wedenski inhibition," also named by the Author who first described them.

The *"Wedenski facilitation"* involves the impulse conduction. It has been shown that when the impulse transmission through an isolated nerve is blocked, with the use of cold or compression, the afferent impulses cannot go through the area of blockage but they decrease the electrical threshold beyond the block. It was thought that this phenomenon was caused by a propagation of "electrotonic potentials" beyond the area of blockage. If the impulse is transmitted in a normal fashion, however, there is not enough time for electrotonic propagation; if the impulse is blocked, the electrotonic effect may appear for some distance beyond the blocked area.

It has been suggested that the "Wedenski facilitation" explains the ventricular pre-excitation in the Wolff-Parkinson-White syndrome and the ventricular capture of ineffective pacemaker spikes (below excitability threshold), which fall immediately after a blocked P wave. This would be due to electrotonic propagation of current from the atria by the blocked P wave.

The *"Wedenski inhibition"* also involves the A-V junction and may be, in someway, compared to the "concealed A-V conduction" of supraventricular impulses. However, the clinical extrapolation of all these three phenomenons still need further documentation.

REFERENCES

Albert, H.M., Pittman, B., and Robichaux, P.: *Cardiac Stimulation Threshold*, Ann. N. Y. Acad. Sci., 111:889, 1964.

Burchell, H.B.: *Analogy of Electronic Pacemaker and Ventricular Parasystole, with Observations of Refractory Period, Supernormal Phase and Synchronization*, Circulation, 27:878, 1963.

Burchell, H.B., Connolly, D.C., and Ellis, F.H.: *Indications and Results of Implanting Cardiac Pacemakers*, Amer. J. Med., 37:764, 1964.

Castellanos, A., Jr., Lemberg, L., Jude, J.R., and Berkovits, B.V.: *Repetitive Firing occurring During Synchronized Electrical Stimulation of the Heart*, J. Thorac. Cardiovasc. Surg., 51:334, 1966.

Chardack, W.M.: *Heart Block Treated with an Implanted Pacemaker*, Progr. Cardiovasc. Dis., 6:507, 1964.

Davies, J.G., and Sowton, E.: *Electrical Threshold of the Human Heart*, Brit. Heart J., 28:231, 1966.

Dressler, W., and Jonas, S.: *Observations in Patients with Implanted Pacemakers. II Effective Refractory Period and Full Recovery Time of the Ventricular Myocardium Calculated from Clinical Tracings*, Amer. Heart J., 67:724, 1964.

Dressler, W., Jonas, S., and Kantrowitz, A.: *Observations in Patients with Implanted Pacemakers. I Clinical Experience*, Amer. Heart J., 66:325, 1965.

Dressler, W., Jonas, S., and Rubin, R.: *Observations in Patients with Implanted Cardiac Pacemaker. Repetitive Responses to Electrical Stimuli*, Amer. J. Cardiol., 15:391, 1964.

Dressler, W., Jonas, S., and Schwartz, E.: *Supernormal Phase of Myocardial Excitability in Man*, Circulation, 32 (Suppl. 2): 79, 1965.

Drury, A.N.: *The Ellective Refractory Period, Full Recovery Time, and Premature Response Interval Depression of Artificial Pacemakers by Extraneous Impulses*, Amer. Heart J., 73:24, 1967.

De Saint Pierre, G., Cammilli, L., and Pozzi, R.: *Studio sulle modalità di risveglio dei segnapassi ventricolari in letargo*, Folia Cardiol., 22:393, 1963.

Edelist, A., Langendorf, R., Pick, A., and Katz, L.N.: *Physiologic and Pharmacological Studies in Stokes-Adams Disease Patients During the Use of an Artificial Cardiac Pacemaker. Effect of Rapid Stimulation on Inherent Rate of Spontaneous Cardiac Pacemakers*, Circulation, 28:710, 1963.

Gaskell, W.L.: *On the Innervation of the Heart, with Special Reference to the Heart of the Tortoise*, J. Physiol., 4:43, 1883.

Langendorf, R., and Pick, A.: *Concealed Conduction. Further Evaluation of a Fundamental Aspect of Propagation of Cardiac Impulse*, Circulation, 13:381, 1956.

Lemberg, L., Castellanos, A., Jr., and Berkovits, B.V.: *Pacemaking on Demand in A-V Block*, J.A.M.A., 191:12, 1965.

Linenthal, A.M., and Zoll, P.M.: *Quantitative Studies of Ventricular Refractory and Supernormal Periods in Man*, Trans. Ass. Amer. Phys., 75:258, 1962.

Pick, A., Langerdorf, R., and Katz, L.N.: *Depression of Cardiac Pacemakers by Premature Impulses*, Amer. Heart J., 41:49, 1951.

Soloff, L.: *Iatrogenic Parasystole and Interpolated Premature Ventricular Beats*, Amer. Heart J., 63:563, 1962.

Zimmerman, H.A., Bersano, E., and Dicosky, C.: *The Auricular Electrocardiogram*, Illinois, Charles C. Thomas, 1968.

Moe, G.K., Preston, J.B., and Burlington, H.: *Physiologic Evidence for dual A-V Transmission System*, Circulation Research, 4:357, 1956.

Lister, J.W., Delman, A.D., Stein, E., Grunwald, R., and Robinson, G.: *Dominant Pacemaker of the Human Heart: Antegrade and Retrograde Activation of the Heart*, Circulation, 35:22, 1967.

Castillo, C., and Samet, P.: *Retrograde Conduction in Complete Heart Block*, Brit. Heart J., 29:553, 1967.

Scherf, D.: *Retrograde Conduction in Complete Heart Block*, Dis. Chest, 35:320, 1959.
of Ventricular Muscle in the Intact Unanaesthesised Cat and Rabbit, Quart. J. Exper. Physiol., 26:181, 1936-37.

Feldman, D.S., and Kantrowitz, A.: *Electrical Characteristics of Human Ventricular Myocardium Stimulated in Vivo*, Clin. Res., 11:22, 1963.

Hoffman, B.F., and Cranefield, P.F.: *The Physiologic Basis of Cardiac Arrhythmias*, Amer. J. Med., 37:670, 1964.

Hoffman, B.F., Kao, C.Y., Suckling, S.E.: *Refractoriness in Cardiac Muscle*, Amer. J. Physiol., 190:473, 1957.

Lemberg, L., Castellanos, A., Jr., and Berkovits, B.V.: *Pacemaking on Demand on A-V Block*, J.A.M.A., 191:12, 1965.

Linenthal, A.J. and Zoll, P.M.: *Quantitative Studies of Ventricular Refractory and Supernormal Periods*, Trans. Ass. Amer. Physicians, 75:285, 1962.

Linenthal, A.J., and Zoll, P.M.: *Ventricular Fusion Beats and Myocardial Conduction Time in Man; Their Significance for Anomalous Atrioventricular Excitation*, Circulation, 28:758, 1963.

McHenry, P.I., and Knoebel, S.B.: *Supernormal Excitation of the Human Heart*, J. Indiana State Med. Ass., 58:125, 1965.

Preston, T.A., Judge, R.D., Bowers, D.L., and Morris, J.D.: *Measurement of Pacemaker Performance*, Amer. Heart J., 71:92, 1966.

Soloff, L.A.: *Iatrogenic Parasystole and Interpolated Premature Ventricular Beats*, Amer. Heart J., 63:563, 1962.

Soloff, L.A., and Fewell, J.W.: *The Supernormal Phase of Ventricular Excitation in Man: Its Bearing on the Genesis of Ventricular Premature Beats and a Note on Atrioventricular Conduction*, Amer. Heart J., 59:869, 1960.

Walker, W.J., Elkins, J.T., and Wood, L.W.: *Effects of Potassium in Restoring Myocardial Response to Subthreshold Cardiac Pacemakers*, New Eng. J. Med., 271:597, 1964.

Arbell, E.R., Langerdorf, R., Pick, A., and Katz, L.N.: *The Effect of Atrial Depolarization on the Response to subthreshold Ventricular Stimulation. Presented at the Second Conference on Paired Stimulation and Post-extrasystolic Potentiation in the Heart*, The Rockefeller University, May 12, 1967.

Castellanos, A., Jr., Lembergm, L., Gomez, A., and Berkovits, B.V.: *Effects of Acitylstrophanthidin on Post Coronary Ligation Diastolic Stimulation*, Clin. Res., 16:26, 1968.

Castellanos, A., J., Lemberg, L., Johnson, D., and Berkovits, B.V.: *Repetitive Firing Occurring During Synchronized Electrical Stimulation*, J. Thorac. Cardiovasc. Surg., 51:334, 1966.

Castellanos, A., Jr., Lemberg, L., Johnson, D., and Berkovits, B.V.: *The Wedensky Effect in the Human Heart*, Brit. Heart J., 28:276, 1966.

De Saint Pierre, G., Toscani, A., Pozzi, R., and Cammilli, L.: *L'azione di un nuovo derivato adrenalinico (Alupent) nei confronti del risveglio dei segnapassi idioventricolari in letargo, studiata mediante una nuova tecnica*, Settim. Med., 51:1189, 1963.

Hoffman, B.F., and Singer, D.: *Effects of Digitalis on Electrical Activity of Cardiac Fibers*, Prog. Cardiovasc. Dis., 7:226, 1964.

Linenthal, A.J., and Zoll, P.M.: *Quantitative Studies of Ventricular Refractory and Supernormal Periods in Man*, Trans. Ass. Amer. Phys., 75:285, 1962.

Castellanos, A., Jr., Lemberg, L., and Gosselin, A.: *Double Artificial Ventricular Parasystole. Iatrogenic Arrhythmia for the Study of Excitability and Conductivity in the Human Heart*, Cardiologia, 47:273, 1965.

Castellanos, A., Jr., Lemberg, L., and Jude, J.R.:

Chapter VIII

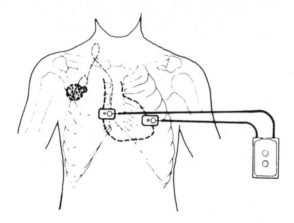

Fig. 77-A - Chest wall stimulation. The position of the stimulating electrodes on the thoracic wall.

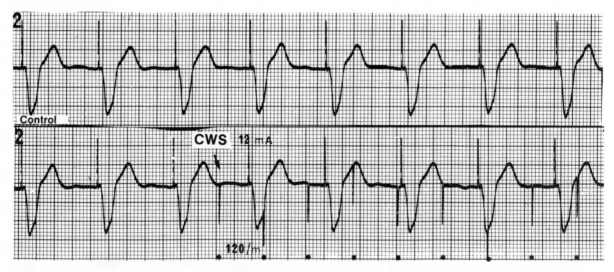

Fig. 77-B - Chest wall stimulation and asynchronous pacemaker. The external impulses (dots) do not influence the activity of the permanent pacemaker.

PROVOCATIVE TESTS IN THE EVALUATION PACEMAKERS FUNCTION

A. Chest wall stimulation (CWS)

The *chest wall stimulation* technique (CWS) is a provocative test, which has been introduced in the functional evaluation of artificial pacemakers. The test is easy to perform and is of remarkable usefulness. It consists essentially in the delivery of electrical impulses over the external thoracic wall of a patient with an implanted artificial pacemaker. The external impulses do not influence the cardiac activity and do not disturb the patient. They are sensed by the pacemaker which interprets them as cardiac potentials and, therefore, responds according to its own characteristics.

Technique

A control ECG tracing, usually L2 and V1, must always be recorded before the application of CWS. Two small electrodes (precordial suction cups serve the purpose) are applied on the anterior thoracic wall in the areas where usually V1, V4, V5 are recorded. One must establish good electrode contact with the thoracic wall and avoid cutaneous resistance by using a conductive paste and by inducing a small erythema with a gentle rub of the area. The thoracic electrodes are, then, connnected to an external asynchronous generator which can deliver impulses of variable intensity and rate and controlled by an external switch.

After measuring the heart rate in the control tracing, CWS is initiated with a rate 10-20 beats/min. above the control rate. The response to chest wall stimulation is recorded, if possible, in the lead where the direction of the external impulses is opposite to that of the implanted pacemaker impulses. In this way the activity of both stimulators is easily recognized. The direction of the external stimuli may be modified either by reversing the connection of the negative and positive poles of the external pacemaker or by selecting a different ECG lead or a different stimulation site on the thoracic wall. The external stimulation intensity is gradually increased until a response is obtained from the internal pacemaker or up to a maximum of 25 mA. Occasionally, it may be necessary to test different areas of the parasternal and precordial wall before locating the optimal stimulation site and obtain a response. This is done in order to avoid faulty execution of CWS technique and misdiagnose an internal pacemaker malfunction.

When the patient has a permanent pacemaker with a bipolar intracavitary catheter it may be necessary to deliver chest wall potentials strong enough to be sensed and able to trigger the demand mechanism. In particularly difficult cases, it may be useful to position the external electrodes along the main frontal plane of the impulse vector, which may be easily calculated from the surface ECG.

The majority of patients do not notice the stimuli on the chest wall up to current intensity of 12 mA. In those rare cases when it is necessary to use high intensity, the impulses may be noticed by the patient, but they are usually well tolerated.

It must be clearly stated that the technique of chest wall stimulation (CWS) does not give any information when studying an asynchronous type of pacemaker. This type of pacemaker does not have a sensing mechanism of spontaneous cardiac potentials and therefore, its firing time-table will remain undisturbed by the external impulses.

The bottom tracing of fig. 77-B shows a CWS performed in a patient with an asynchronous type of pacemaker. The external chest wall stimuli can be recognized on the surface ECG because of their different rate and polarity (they are indicated by the dots) and by comparing them to permanent pacemaker impulses. Of course, the CWS is ineffective and does not alter the behavior of the implanted pacemaker.

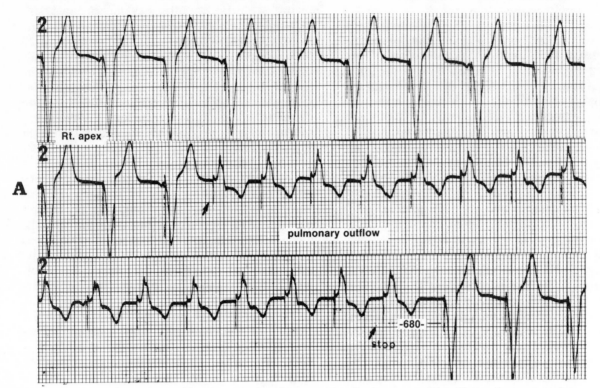

Fig. 78-A - Right ventricular apical and pulmonary outflow tract pacing. Notice the suppression of the QRS-inhibited right apical pacemaker by the faster impulses of a second catheter located in the pulmonary outflow tract.

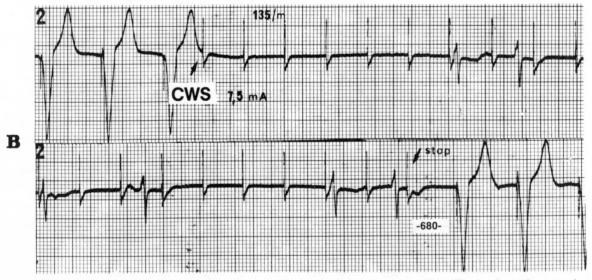

Fig. 78-B - Chest wall stimulation (CWS) and QRS-inhibited pacemaker. The implanted pacemaker is suppressed by the faster external impulses which are interpreted as ventricular potentials. This allows for the reappearance of a slow spontaneous rhythm.

CWS AND THE QRS-INHIBITED PACEMAKER

The technique of chest wall stimulation (CWS) can be usefully applied in the study of "demand" ventricular-inhibited pacemakers. This type of pacemaker is "suppressed" by spontaneous cardiac potentials, and, since the impulse delivery is blocked, the pacemaker does not interfere with the recording of the spontaneous ECG. The stimuli applied on the thoracic wall are interpreted by the QRS- inhibited pacemaker as cardiac potentials and, as such, they inhibit the delivery of pacemaker impulses.

CWS performed in patients with ventricular-inhibited pacemakers permits the analysis of the following parameters: *a)* evaluation of the "sensing function" and of the "stand-by interval"; *b)* evaluation of residual cardiac activity; *c)* morphologic examination of the spontaneous ECG; *d)* study of cardiac arrhythmias; *e)* measurement of pacemaker refractory period; *f)* identification of the "pacemaker click";

The following tracings will illustrate how the CWS technique can be usefully employed in the study of the parameters listed above. The measurement of the pacemaker refractory period and the identification of pacemaker clicks will be discussed in separate chapters (see page 203).

A. *Evaluation of the sensing function and of the stand-by interval.*

Tracings of fig. 78-A and 78-B clearly show the identical behavior of a QRS-inhibited pacemaker toward intracardiac external chest wall potentials. The tracings are recorded from a patient with a QRS-inhibited permanent pacemaker who is first stimulated with an intracavitary catheter, located in the pulmonary outflow tract (A), and then through chest wall stimuli (B). They permit the evaluation of the pacemaker sensing mechanism.

The upper tracing of fig. 78-A shows a regular artificial pacing (90/min.) with no evidence of spontaneous cardiac activity. The QRS complexes show a good ventricular capture and indicate a right ventricular apical pacing (see page 5). The artificial stimulation is performed with a permanent pacemaker of the ventricular-inhibited type.

The arrow in the second tracing indicates the beginning of cardiac pacing through a sec-ond catheter located in the pulmonary outflow tract. Note that the sudden change of cardiac rate (110/min.) is accompanied by QRS's of different morphology, caused by the different intracavitary stimulation site.

The impulses of the second pacemaker (asynchronous) are sensed by the permanent pacemaker (QRS-inhibited) which behaves as if in the presence of a spontaneous ventricular tachycardia, and it remains suppressed during the entire period of the faster pacing (lower tracing). The 680 msec. interval between the end of rapid pacing and the reappearance of the automatic rhythm is the *escape interval* of the permanent pacemaker. This tracing, therefore, shows how it is possible: a) to test the permanent pacemaker *sensing mechanism;* b) to evaluate the *stand-by function* and c) to measure the *escape or stand-by interval* of the pacemaker, even in the absence of spontaneous cardiac potentials.

The same data can be obtained through the technique of *chest wall stimulation* (CWS). This is illustrated in fig. 78-B where CWS offers the possibility of *recording the presence of residual cardiac activity.*

The arrow of the upper tracings indicates the beginning of CWS; the faster external stimuli can easily be recognized and show a polarity opposite to that of the permanent pacemaker spikes. Notice how the permanent pacing is promptly interrupted by CWS (indicating a good pacemaker sensing mechanism) and is promptly restored at the end of external stimulation. The recording of several spontaneous QRS's of the patient indicate the presence of an atrial fibrillation, with a slow ventricular response for the presence of a high degree of A-V block.

An acute observer may notice that the duration of the stand-by interval, measured by the last external impulse to the first permanent pacemaker impulse in fig. 78-B, is shorter than that of fig. 78-A. However, it must not be forgotten that, during CWS the QRS-inhibited pacemaker may sense either the external or the spontaneous QRS potentials. In fact, the interval between the last spontaneous QRS and the first permanent pacemaker impulse is equal to that of fig. 78-A (680 msec.). Thus, the last chest wall impulse is not effective because it falls within the pacemaker refractory period (see page 203).

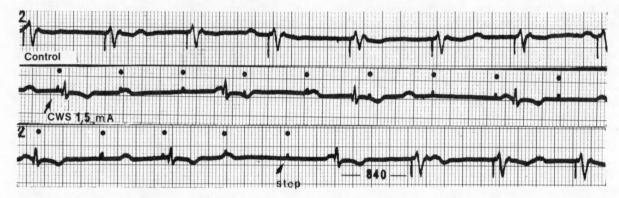

Fig. 79-A - CWS and QRS-inhibited pacemaker. The external impulses (dots) suppress the pacemaker and allow for the reappearance of a sinus rhythm with a complete A-V block.

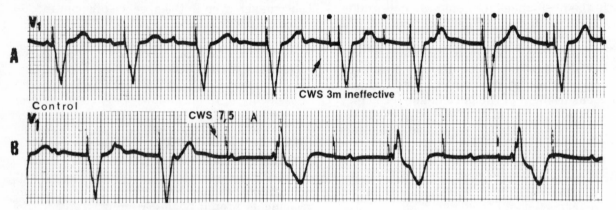

Fig. 79-B - CWS and QRS-inhibited pacemaker. Tracing A shows ineffective impulses with a 3 mA intensity. The pacemaker inhibition is obtained promptly with impulses of 7.5 mA and delivered in a different area of the thoracic wall (B).

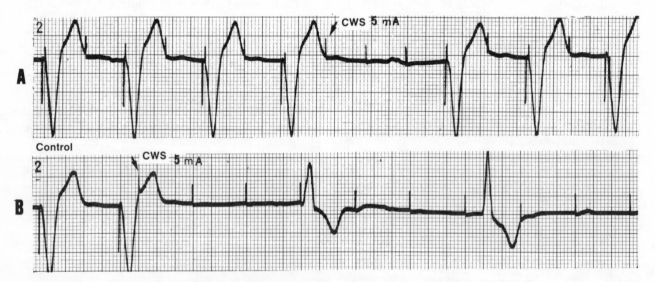

Fig. 79-C - CWS and QRS-inhibited pacemaker. The suppression of the permanent pacemaker is first intermittent (A) and then continuous when the CWS is performed in the optimal chest wall location (B).

CWS AND THE QRS-INHIBITED PACEMAKER

A. *Evaluation of the sensing function and of the stand-by interval*

Occasionally, when only a very small amount of current is employed to deactivate an implanted QRS-inhibited pacemaker, the chest wall impulses may not be clearly visible on the surface ECG in that particular lead being recorded. In the middle tracing of fig. 79-A, the external impulses are indicated by dots; although a minimal amount of current intensity is being used (1.5 mA), chest wall stimulation completely suppresses the pacemaker activity (compare with the control tracing) and shows an underlying sinus rhythm with a third degree A-V block. The underlying spontaneous pacemaker shows QRS complexes with a normal morphology and must, therefore, be localized in the A-V junction. The bottom tracing shows how the permanent pacemaker automatic stimulation is promptly restored when CWS is discontinued. Also, in this tracing, the pacemaker stand-by interval can be measured by the last spontaneous QRS complex to the first automatic impulse (840 msec.).

When a cardiac rhythm is totally controlled by a QRS-inhibited pacemaker and no spontaneous cardiac activity is present, the pacemaker works constantly in an automatic fashion, and therefore, with a fixed rate pacing. Since this situation is very common there is no way of knowing that: a) in case of reappearance of spontaneous QRS's the pacemaker will sense the ventricular potentials and will inhibit the impulses delivery (presence of a good sensing function), and b) in the presence of a pacemaker malfunction, the cardiac rhythm will be maintained by an adequate residual cardiac activity.

Before the advent of CWS in the examination of patients with permanent pacemakers, information was obtained with drugs which increase cardiac automaticity (isoproterenol, noradrenalin, metaraminol, etc). Because of the safety and simplicity of execution and because it is easily reproducible at distance of time, the chest wall stimulation technique has now totally replaced the use of drugs in the evaluation of ventricular-inhibited pacemaker function.

Tracing A of fig. 79-B shows the beginning of a chest wall stimulation (the external stimuli have the same direction of the internal pacemaker spikes and they are indicated by dots) which does not, as it would be expected, suppress the QRS-inhibited pacemaker. Before diagnosing a sensing mechanism malfunction it is better to test other areas of the thoracic surface, using impulses of greater intensity. The CWS of tracing B is, in fact, performed in a different area of the thoracic wall and with slightly stronger stimuli (7.5 mA). This time the expected result is obtained and a sinus rhythm with a high degree of A-V block emerges with the suppression of the permanent pacemaker.

Occasionally a CWS will inactivate a permanent pacemaker in an intermittent fashion, this will happen when one of the chest wall electrodes lies very close to the optimal site of stimulation (fig. 79-C tracing A). In such a case only a slight change of the stimulating site will allow for a complete inactivation of the implanted pacemaker (fig. 79-C tracing B).

173

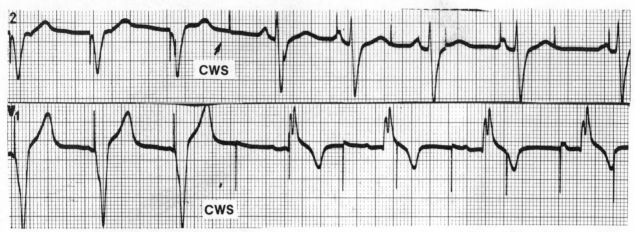

Fig. 80-A - CWS and QRS-inhibited pacemaker. During CWS the QRS morphology of spontaneous beats may be examined in more than one lead.

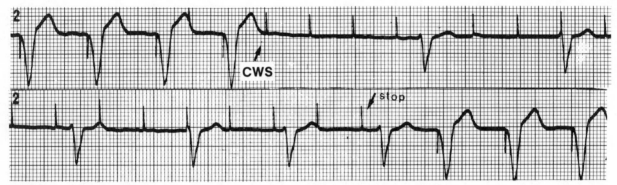

Fig. 80-B - CWS and QRS-inhibited pacemaker. An atrial fibrillation is revealed by the suppression of the permanent pacemaker through CWS.

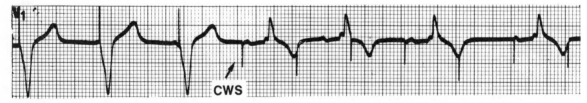

Fig. 80-C - CWS and QRS-inhibited pacemakers. A sinus rhythm with a complete R.B.B.B. reappears with the suppression of the internal pacemaker through CWS.

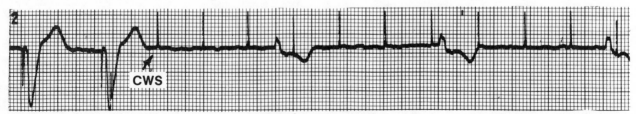

Fig. 80-D - CWS and QRS-inhibited pacemaker. An atrial fibrillation with a complete A-V block and a slow idioventricular rhythm are revealed by CWS.

B. *Evaluation of residual cardiac activity.*

To maintain a permanent pacemaker continuously suppressed, it is necessary that the external stimulation rate of a CWS be faster than that of the implanted pacemaker. This eventually will enable the reappearance of a spontaneous rhythm, which had been suppressed by the automatic permanent pacing. Therefore, if a spontaneous rhythm reappears promptly, a CWS can be employed for the morphologic examination of spontaneous QRS's, by obtaining a 12 leads electrocardiogram.

Tracings of fig. 80-A are not simultaneous and are recorded in lead 2 and V1. They clearly show the reappearance of a sinus rhythm during CWS, in a patient with a QRS-blocking permanent pacemaker (first three beats in both tracings) the morphologic examination of sinus beats shows a normal P-R interval and a complete R.B.B.B., associated with a left axis deviation (left anterior hemiblock).

An atrial fibrillation (finely undulated isolectric line and irregular ventricular response) appears with the suppression of a ventricular-inhibited pacemaker during chest wall stimulation (fig. 80-B). Furthermore, it is possible to observe that, while the first spontaneous QRS appears after a long asystolic pause, the conduction through the A-V node of atrial impulses improves in the following beats.

The knowledge of the presence of spontaneous cardiac activity, revealed by CWS in patients with QRS-inhibited pacemakers, is of extreme importance to avoid fatal asystolic pauses in case of pacemaker malfunction. When it is demonstrated, with CWS, that spontaneous cardiac activity is either not present or it is markedly bradycardic, it may be wise to change the generator before a complete battery failure for that type of unit. The half life of most ventricular-inhibited demand pacemakers varies between 18 months and 4 years. The newly developed lithium-powered generators may last up to 12 years.

In fig. 80-C, the sinus rhythm with R.B.B.B., which appears with the suppression of a demand QRS-inhibited pacemaker by CWS, has an adequate rate for good cardiac hemodynamics.

In figure 80-D, however, an atrial fibrillation (notice the finely undulated isolectric line), with a complete A-V block and a slow idio-ventricular rhythm, appears after the suppression of a QRS-inhibited pacemaker with chest wall stimulation.

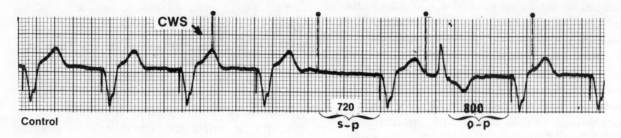

Fig. 81-A - CWS and QRS-inhibited pacemaker. The S-P interval is slightly shorter than the Q-P interval. Dots indicate the chest wall stimuli.

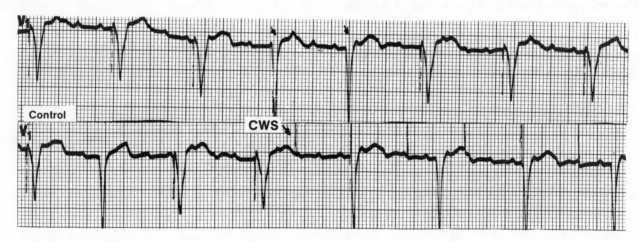

Fig. 81-B - CWS and QRS-inhibited pacemaker. An atrial flutter with a stable 4:1 A-V block is revealed by a CWS.

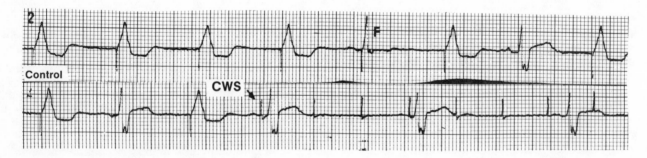

Fig. 81-C - CWS and QRS-inhibited pacemaker. The patient's spontaneous activity is a bradycardic sinus rhythm. F = fusion beat.

B. *Presence of residual cardiac activity.*

In the presence of spontaneous QRS's, a calibrated chest wall stimulation enables one to analyze the behavior of a QRS-inhibited pacemaker both with external and intracavitary potentials. This permits testing the sensing capacity of the pacer to chest wall and spontaneous cardiac voltages. Occasionally it is possible to find a difference between the length of the automatic "stand-by" interval, which follows the suppression of the pacemaker by an external impulse, and the interval following the pacemaker inhibition by a spontaneous QRS (fig. 81-A). This difference does not indicate a pacemaker malfunction and it is called "histeresis". From the surface ECG it is difficult to know exactly at what point, from the beginning of the spontaneous QRS, the ventricular potentials trigger the blocking circuit of the pacemaker. It is quite common to find differences up to 100 msec. between the "external stimulus-pacemaker spike interval" (S-P interval) and the "spontaneous QRS-pacemaker interval" (Q-P interval), even in the presence of a perfectly functioning pacemaker.

In fig. 81-A for example, the CWS is intentionally performed with a rate lower than that of the permanent pacemaker. The first impulse is not effective because it falls within the pacemaker refractory period (see page 203);

the second impulse, instead, inhibits the pacemaker and is followed by an escape interval of 720 msec. (S-P interval); the third impulse is again early and is not sensed by the permanent pacemaker. At this point, a spontaneous QRS is sensed by the demand pacemaker and is followed by a stand-by interval (Q-P interval) of 800 msec. The interval is conventionally measured from the beginning of the QRS to the pacemaker spike. The fourth external impulse is again ineffective because of its prematurity and because it falls within the pacemaker refractory period.

An atrial flutter, with QRS complexes very similar to QRS-inhibited pacemaker beats, is present in the top tracing of fig. 81-B. The CWS, performed in the bottom tracing, eliminates all the pacemaker beats and indicates the presence of a stable 4:1 A-V ratio.

Fig. 81-C is recorded from a patient with a ventricular-inhibited pacemaker, implanted because of a hemodynamically significant sinus bradycardia. The tracings indicate a good sensing function of the QRS blocking pacemaker. The occasional sinus beats are regularly sensed by the pacemaker, which is also promptly suppressed by CWS (bottom tracing), allowing for the exact measurement of the spontaneous sinus rate (F is a ventricular fusion beat).

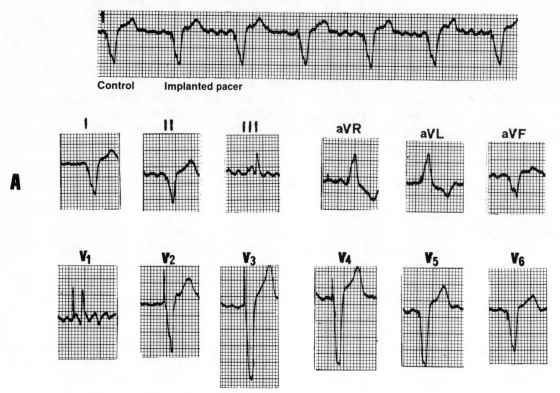

Fig. 82-A - Control L1 and 12 leads ECG in a patient with a QRS-inhibited pacemaker.

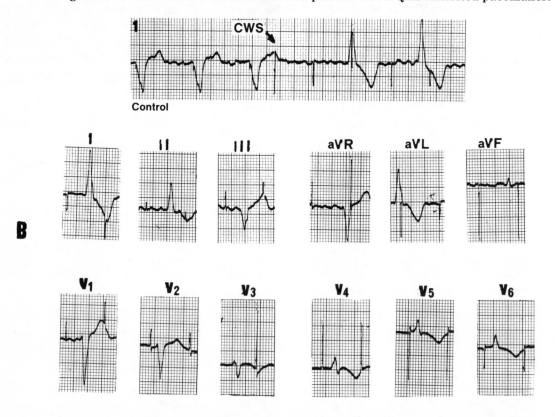

Fig. 82-B - CWS and QRS-inhibited pacemaker. The control L1 shows the beginning of a CWS and the suppression of the implanted pacemaker by external impulses. The complete 12 leads ECG is recorded during CWS and shows the patient's spontaneous beats.

C. *Morphological examination of the underlying spontaneous ECG.*

An important aspect of CWS is that, even in the presence of a QRS-inhibited permanent pacemaker, it is possible to record and evaluate a complete 12 leads ECG tracing. This permits a morphologic examination of spontaneous QRS's in patients with permanent pacemakers and offers a comparison with a complete ECG obtained before the implantation. Furthermore, since the results of CWS are easily reproducible, it is possible to obtain sequential tracings of the same patient even after long intervals of time.

It is well known that artificial pacing alters completely the morphology of QRS's and no information can be obtained about its own spontaneous ventricular potentials if the patient is being paced continously. It is obvious that the availability of bringing out spontaneous QRS's, in a patient with a permanent pacemaker, may be very useful in the diagnosis of coronary artery disease and myocardial infarctions and in the detection of underlying cardiac arrhythmias.

Fig. 82-A and 82-B show two groups of tracings. Figure A shows a control 12 leads ECG tracing of a patient, with a permanent QRS-inhibited "demand" pacemaker, whose pre-implantation tracing is not known. The fine baseline undulation is clearly indicative of an atrial fibrillation, while the ventricular rhythm is totally under control of a permanent pacemaker which has suppressed any spontaneous cardiac activity.

Tracing B is obtained during chest wall stimulation. In this case CWS offers a possibility to test the pacemaker sensing mechanism, to confirm the presence of an atrial fibrillation with a slow ventricular response, and to evaluate the morphology of spontaneous ventricular potentials in all the twelve routine electrocardiographic leads. However, it must be kept in mind that, while the QRS abnormalities of an acute myocardial infarction, revealed by CWS, have an unquestionably diagnostic value, the morphologic changes involving T waves and the ST segment do not necessarily indicate a pericardial or a coronary artery disease. In fact, it has been observed that prolonged electrical pacing, per se, may induce significant T wave and ST segment changes.

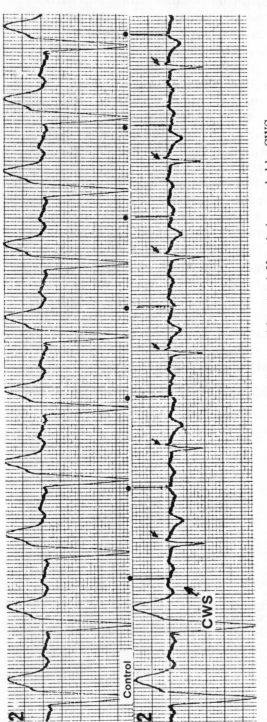

Fig. 83-A - CWS and QRS-inhibited pacemaker. An atrial flutter with a 4:1 A-V ratio is revealed by CWS.

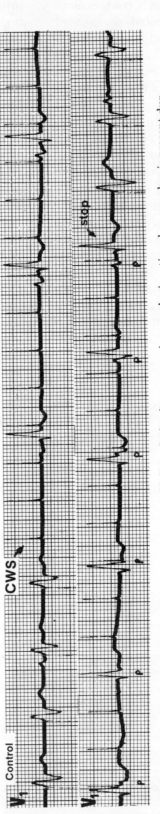

Fig. 83-B - CWS and QRS-inhibited pacemaker. An A-V dissociation between a sinus and a junctional pacemaker is present during CWS.

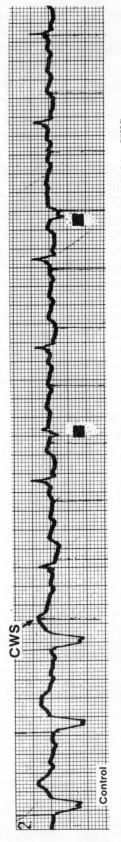

Fig. 83-C - CWS and QRS-inhibited pacemaker. An atrial flutter and multifocal ventricular extrasystoles are revealed by CWS, and confirm the clinical diagnosis of digitalis toxicity.

D. *Identification of underlying cardiac ar-rhythmias.*

The technique of CWS finds a useful clinical application also in the identification of spontaneous cardiac arrhythmias which are frequently present in patients with permanent pacemakers.

The upper tracing of fig. 83-A illustrates regular artificial pacing with good ventricular capture and a rate of 80/min. The isoelectric line separating two consecutive pacemaker beats is undulated and suggests the presence of an atrial flutter or fibrillation.

CWS is performed in the lower tracing and confirms the diagnosis of *atrial flutter with a stable 4:1 A-V ratio*. Note, that, in this patient, the suppression of the internal pacemaker is obtained through a low rate CWS (63/min.); the external potentials are coupled with the potentials of spontaneous QRS's liberated by CWS. They maintain the internal pacemaker continually suppressed and, in fact, the pacemaker senses potentials with a rate of 130/min.

The patient in fig. 83-B is already known (see page 84). What seems to be a underlying stable sinus rhythm, in symbiosis with that of ventricular-inhibited pacemaker, is instead a marked sinus bradycardia which rapidly develops into an A-V dissociation. This is confirmed by CWS which enables the emergence of a faster junctional pacemaker. Notice that, in the second tracing, although junctional QRS complexes are slightly faster than the sinus P waves, they are dissociated and move in and out of the junctional QRS's.

The CWS of fig. 83-C is performed in a patient with symptoms suggestive of digitalis toxicity. The ventricular rate is entirely controlled by an artificial pacemaker of the QRS-inhibited type. CWS reveals the presence of multifocal ventricular extrasystoles (dark square) during an atrial flutter with an A-V ratio of 4:1. This confirms the clinical diagnosis of digitalis toxicity.

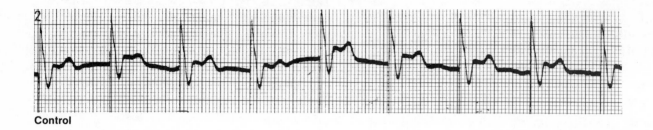

Control

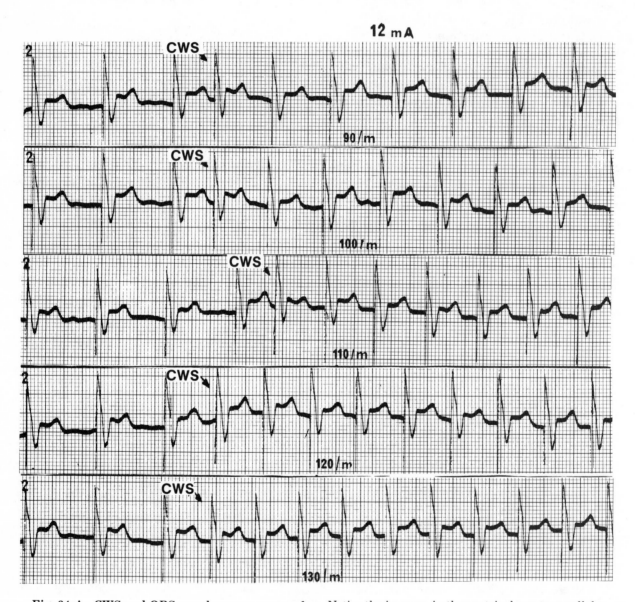

12 mA

CWS

CWS

90 / m

CWS

100 / m

CWS

110 / m

CWS

120 / m

CWS

130 / m

Fig. 84-A - CWS and QRS-synchronous pacemaker. Notice the increase in the ventricular rate parallel to an increase of the CWS rate.

CWS AND THE QRS-SYNCHRONOUS PACEMAKER

When a patient is a carrier of a *QRS-synchronous pacemaker,* the technique of chest wall stimulation permits the analysis of very important parameters of this type of "demand" unit. They are: a) identification of the type of stimulator used; b) evaluation of the pacemaker sensing function; c) evaluation of the pacing and synchronizing capacity to the maximum rate indicated by the manufacturer; d) identification of the refractory period.

All these parameters are clearly illustrated and summarized in the tracings of fig. 84-A. The control tracing shows a regular cardiac pacing (78/min.), with complete ventricular capture and absence of spontaneous activity. From the control tracing it is impossible: 1) to know the type of pacing unit; 2) to comment about the functional state of the pacemaker sensing mechanism, because of the absence of spontaneous cardiac potentials and, 3) to know about the maximum synchronizing capacity in the presence of fast spontaneous beats (if the unit in question is a QRS-synchronous type).

In the following tracings, a chest wall stimulation is performed at different rate levels, while the impulse intensity remains unchanged (12 mA). The arrows indicate the beginning of CWS and the pacemaker synchronization with the external signals.

The function of a QRS-synchronous pacer is such that it senses spontaneous cardiac potentials. It immediately delivers an impulse which falls within the absolute ventricular refractory period and does not compete with the patient's spontaneous rhythm (see page 52). The external chest wall stimuli are misinterpreted by the pacemaker as spontaneous cardiac potentials, and induce the delivery of a synchronized impulse. The artificial impulse does not find the cardiac muscle refractory and, is followed by ventricular capture.

The *response of a QRS-synchronous "de-mand" pacemaker to CWS is, therefore, characterized by an increase in the effective cardiac rate.* The pacing rate is in relation to the number of the external stimuli and to the maximum synchronization capacity of that particular type of pacemaker.

In the case of fig. 84-A, CWS is carried out up to a rate of 130/min.; the 1:1 ventricular response is, therefore, an "artifically induced ventricular tachycardia." By sensing the external potentials, the pacemaker indicates a definitely intact sensing function. Furthermore, it appears evident that in the presence of rapid spontaneous rates, the pacemaker would be able to synchronize up to 130 beats/min.

Occasionally, particular clinical situations are encountered in which it may be desirable to temporarily increase the cardiac rate, in relation to increased requirements (as in fever, hypotension, etc.). CWS may be usefully employed to increase the effective pacing rate in a patient with a "demand" QRS-triggered pacemaker for hours or even for days, without any discomfort for the patient.

Note that the CWS spikes are totally concealed by the almost simultaneous delivery of the implanted pacemaker spikes. Therefore, an automatic pacemaker beat cannot be differentiated from one synchronized with the chest wall stimuli. The CWS overdriving is recognized only by the prematurity of the "beats synchronized with CWS" when compared with pacemaker R-R intervals. In all tracings of fig. 84-A, for instance, the beat immediately preceding the QRS indicated by the arrow, is an automatic internal pacemaker beat. The direction of the spike and the morphology of the QRS is identical to that of the next beat which, however, has a shorter R-R interval. This signals the beginning of the increased ventricular rate, due to sensing and synchronization of the internal pacemaker with CWS.

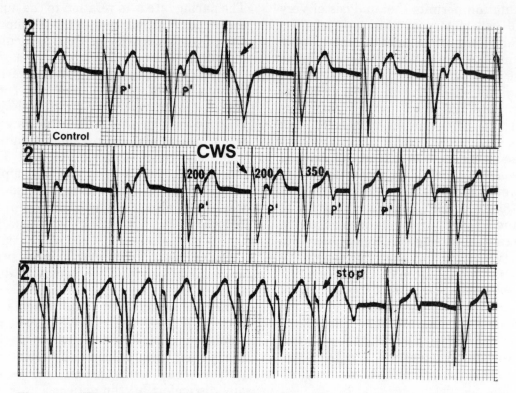

Fig. 85-A - CWS and QRS-synchronous pacemaker. The stimulation rate of the permanent pacemaker is increased through CWS. A delayed ventriculo-atrial conduction time may be noted (Q-P¹ interval).

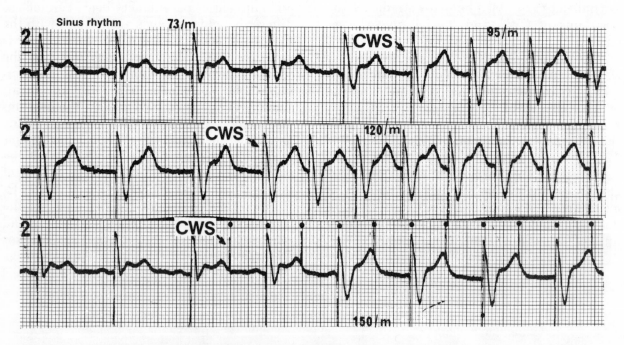

Fig. 85-B - CWS and QRS-synchronous pacemaker. The pacemaker synchronizes with external impulses up to a rate of 150/min. At this level a 2:1 "sensing block" is present and is determined by the pacemaker refractory period of 400 msec.

The impulses delivered on the thoracic wall influence the synchronizing mechanism of the "demand" QRS-synchronous pacemaker and induce an increase in the cardiac rate. Therefore, in particular clinical situations, the increase in ventricular rate through CWS may be usefully employed. The maximal synchronized rate is determined by the length of the pacemaker refractory period.

In tracings of fig. 85-A the CWS, performed with fast rates (115/min. and 145/min.), is perfectly synchronized with the implanted QRS-synchronous "demand" pacemaker and is followed by a ventricular response of 1:1. The control tracing shows P¹ waves (retrograde atrial depolarization) with a Q-P¹ interval of 200 msec. One ventricular extrasystole is also synchronized with the pacemaker (arrow). Simultaneous with the beginning of CWS, the Q-P¹ interval becomes progressively longer (200-350 msec. etc.) because of a delayed retrograde ventriculo-atrial conduction parallel to the increased ventricular rate. In the bottom tracing, P¹ waves are concealed within the following pacemaker spikes.

A good synchronization of a ventricular-triggered pacemaker with the QRS complexes of a sinus rhythm does not guarantee that an effective pacing, with good ventricular capture, would take over whenever the spontaneous rhythm will no longer be present. The CWS technique, using external impulses faster than the control sinus rate, is an easy method to test the stand-by mechanism of the pacemaker, in the presence of asystolic pauses that are longer than the escape pacemaker interval.

The first tracing of fig. 85-B shows a sinus rhythm (73/min.) synchronized with a QRS-triggered "demand" pacemaker. The CWS, performed at 95/min., and 120/min. in the top and middle tracings (arrows), takes over the slower sinus rhythm and controls the ventricular rhythm with a 1:1 response. In the bottom tracing, CWS is performed at 150/min. and only every other external impulse is followed by a ventricular response. Therefore, a *2:1 sensing block* is present between the chest wall stimuli and the maximum synchronizing capacity of the pacemaker. This is due to the presence of a refractory period of 400 msec. Every other impulse falls within the refractory period and is not sensed by the pacemaker which responds only to alternate external impulses. The ventricular rate is half the CWS rate (75/min.), but is still faster than the sinus rhythm of the control tracing.

In the presence of a QRS-synchronous pacemaker, the technique of CWS permits: a) suppression of the spontaneous rhythm; b) a ventricular overdriving at faster rates; c) a test of the synchronizing mechanism; d) a documentation of a good stimulating mechanism and, e) a determination of the pacemaker refractory period.

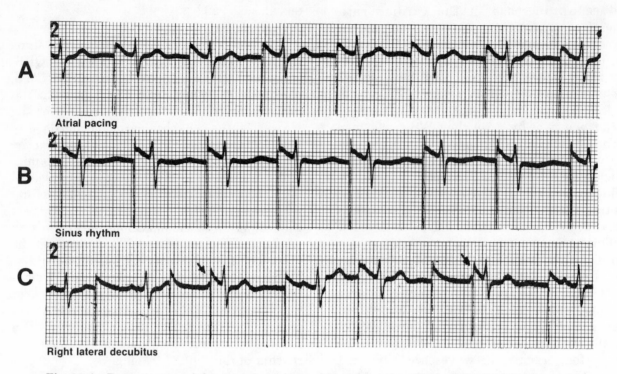

Fig. 86-A - Permanent atrial pacemaker. A) regular atrial pacing; B) sinus rhythm: the pacemaker spikes are synchronized with P waves; C) loss of sensing and stimulating functions.

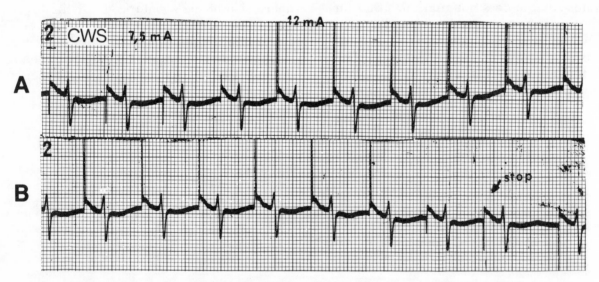

Fig. 86-B - CWS and permanent atrial pacemaker. The QRS-synchronous pacemaker is adapted to sense atrial signals and it is synchronized with CWS potentials. Therefore, the atrial pacing rate and, consequently, the ventricular rate are increased.

CWS AND THE QRS-SYNCHRONOUS PACEMAKER

The tracings of fig. 86-A and 86-B are recorded from the same patient of page 122. This is an attempt to perform a permanent atrial stimulation with an intracavitary atrial catheter connected to a "demand" QRS-synchronous type pacemaker. Instead of being synchronized with ventricular potentials, the pacemaker senses the P waves and delivers a spike into the atrial refractory period. When spontaneous atrial activity is not present, the pacemaker stimulates the atrium at a fixed rate.

Tracing A shows an atrial pacing at 75/min. with a good atrial capture (the spikes are sharply demarcated on the baseline). With the reappearance of a sinus rhythm, the impulses are delivered 20 msec. after the beginning of sinus P waves; they are not effective because they fall into the absolute atrial refractory phase (tracing B). The sinus rate is almost similar to the pacemaker automatic rate (about 75/min.) and tracing A and B seem almost identical. However, in tracing B, the pacemaker spikes fall *within* the P wave, whereas in tracing A, they *precede* the P waves.

Tracing C shows a complete loss of the capacity of sensing atrial signals; atrial capture is only occasional (only the impulses indicated by the arrows are synchronized with the P waves.) The pacemaker malfunction was due to the catheter instability in the atrial chamber and was particularly evident with the patient in a lateral decubitus.

CWS (95/min.) is then performed to analyze the behavior of the pacemaker which, it should be remembered, is of a QRS-synchronous type and modified to sense atrial signals and to capture the atria (fig. 86-B). The pacemaker immediately senses the chest wall potentials and it is synchronized with them. Therefore, the atrial rate increases because each synchronized chest wall impulse is followed by atrial capture.

The pacemaker behavior, therefore, is similar to that presented in pages 182 and 184. The difference, in this case, is that CWS influences the ventricular rate only indirectly through an increased atrial rate.

It is interesting to note that the amplitude of the chest wall spikes is the algebraic resultant of the implanted pacemaker spike and the external thoracic impulse amplitudes. Note the amplitude and polarity changes of the spikes, which signals the beginning and the end of CWS.

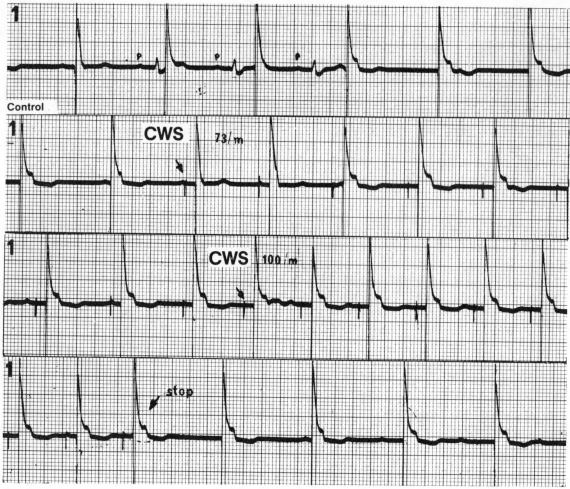

Fig. 87-A - CWS and P-wave synchronous pacemaker. The chest wall stimuli precede the implanted pacemaker spikes. The A-P ratio is normal and the pacemaker function is normal.

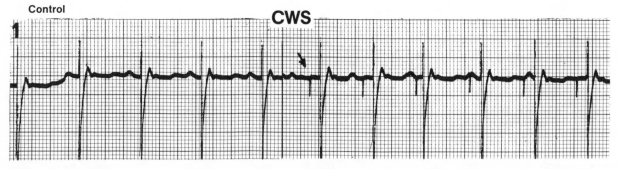

Fig. 87-B - CWS and P-wave synchronous pacemaker. The ventricular rate is guided externally with CWS.

CWS AND THE P-WAVE SYNCHRONOUS PACEMAKER

The P-wave synchronous pacemaker interprets external CWS signals as cardiac potentials coming from the atria and, if it works normally, it synchronizes with them. In this case, however, the chest wall spike precedes the permanent pacemaker impulse of a time interval equal to a normal A-P delay *(atria-pacemaker delay)*.

The control tracing of fig. 87-A shows a regular sinus rhythm, with low voltage P-waves (rate = 66/min.), dissociated and in competition with an otherwise regular pacemaker rhythm (60/min.). While the first three impulses are not effective, since they fall within the ventricular refractory period, the following three spikes capture the ventricles. This is seen by the change in the QRS morphology (which should not be confused with the voltage-decay curve of ineffective spikes). The patient has a P-wave synchronous pacemaker and, therefore, it is necessary to establish whether the lack of P-wave synchronization is due either to a low P-waves voltage or to a malfunction of the atria-pacemaker synchronizing mechanism.

CWS is performed in the following tracings with increasing stimulation rates (75/min. and 100/min.). The technique of CWS indicates a normal pacemaker sensing and synchronizing functions with a 1:1 response to external stimuli. It is also possible to measure the A-P delay (in this case = 0.14 sec.) and to increase the ventricular rate. This may come handy when faster cardiac rates are necessary. When CWS is discontinued (last tracing), the automatic permanent pacing reappears promptly.

Fig. 87-B shows a sinus rhythm recorded in a patient with a P-wave synchronous pacemaker. The sinus rate is 90/min. and each P wave is followed by a spike with good ventricular capture (the A-P delay is equal to 0.18 sec.). The ventricular rate of the patient is intentionally increased, using external thoracic stimuli with a rate of 100/min. The external impulses are interpreted by the pacemaker as coming from the atria and, since the A-P synchronism is normal, it responds 1:1 to the chest wall stimuli.

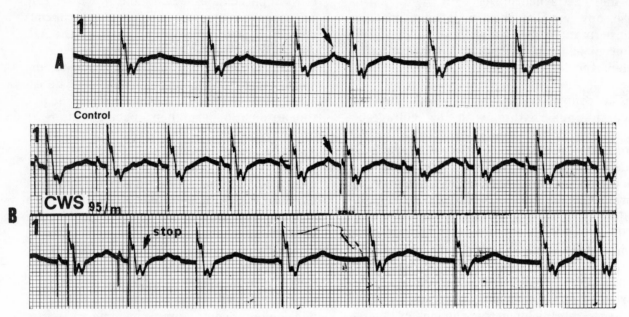

Fig. 88-A - CWS and P-wave synchronous pacemaker. The premature beat in the control tracing is a pacemaker beat synchronized with a P wave. In fact, CWS reveals a normal synchronizing mechanism.

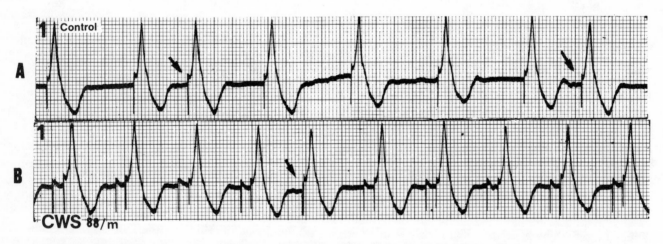

Fig. 88-B - **CWS and P-wave synchronous pacemaker.** Situation similar to that of fig. 88-A.

CWS AND THE P-WAVE SYNCHRONOUS PACEMAKER

In the presence of marked sinus bradycardias, the synchronism between spontaneous atrial beats and ventricular contractions induced by the pacemaker may be only sporadic (control tracing). Synchronized sinus beats appear as pacemaker premature beats especially when the P waves are not clearly visible. This may simulate a pacemaker malfunction. CWS is used, therefore, not only to identify the exact type of implanted pacemaker, but to document the presence of a normal atrio-pacemaker synchronism.

The control tracings (A) of both fig. 88-A and 88-B show an automatic fixed rate pacing, occasionally interrupted by premature pacemaker impulses with good ventricular capture (arrows). The pacemaker's behavior toward external chest wall impulses (B) indicates a normal synchronizing mechanism and a normal A-P ratio. During CWS, premature beats can also be observed (arrows). They are caused by occasional sinus impulses falling among the CWS cycles; the sinus impulse synchronizes with the pacemaker and stimulates the ventricles with a slight prematurity over the external stimulation rate.

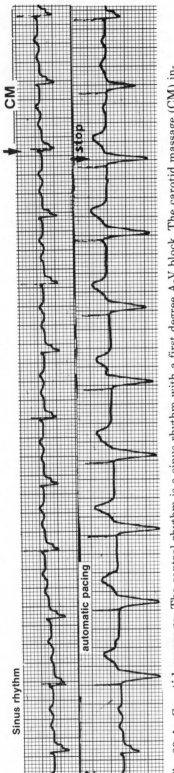

Fig. 89-A - Carotid massage. The control rhythm is a sinus rhythm with a first degree A-V block. The carotid massage (CM) increases the A-V block and allows for the emergence of an automatic QRS-inhibited pacemaker beat.

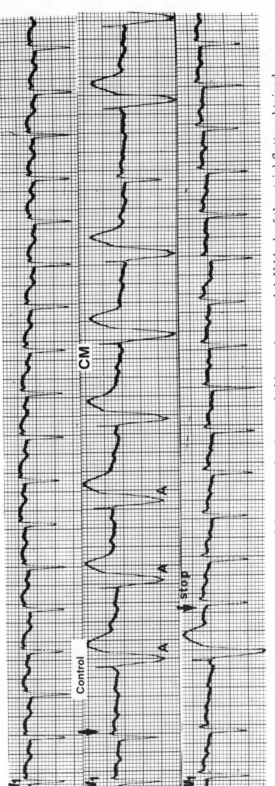

Fig. 89-B - Carotid massage. The presence of the pacemaker is revealed by an increased A-V block of the atrial flutter obtained with carotid massage (CM).

B. CAROTID MASSAGE

If a QRS-inhibited pacemaker is continuously suppressed by a spontaneous rhythm, with a rate faster than the automatic pacemaker rate, an evaluation of the pacemaker "demand" function can be obtained with a *carotid sinus massage*. This is done to document a good pacemaker ventricular capture, which could be "requested" by prolonged ventricular asystolic pauses. The usefulness of this technique may be limited by a poor pacemaker performance, during carotid sinus massage, and by the possibility of inducing dangerous and prolonged ventricular asystoles.

The presence of a sinus rhythm faster than the automatic pacemaker and with a first degree A-V block does not allow for a good evaluation of the pacing function (upper tracing of fig. 89-A). The presence of an artificial pacemaker is suggested by pseudo-fusion beats. The pressure over the carotid sinus (CM) slows down the sinus rate and increases the A-V block, enabling the escape of several automatic pacemaker beats with good ventricular capture (lower tracing). When the carotid massage is discontinued, the reappearance of the sinus rhythm is signaled by a true fusion beat (F).

An atrial flutter, with a 2:1 A-V ratio and a fast ventricular response, is present in the control tracing of fig. 89-B. The carotid massage, performed in the second tracing, determines a sudden increase in the A-V block and an asystolic pause longer than the pacemaker escape interval. This, in turn, permits the appearance of several pacemaker automatic beats (A). When the pressure over the carotid sinus is discontinued, the ventricular rhythm resumes a rate similar to control values.

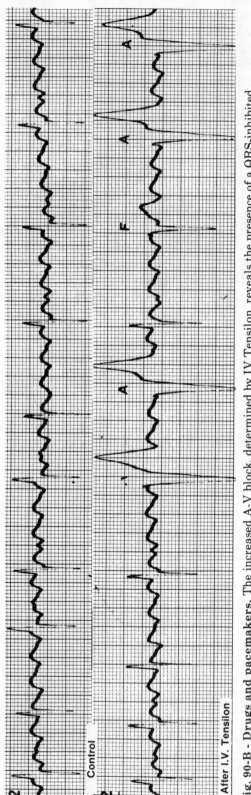

Fig. 90-B - **Drugs and pacemakers.** The increased A-V block, determined by IV Tensilon, reveals the presence of a QRS-inhibited "demand" pacemaker (beats A). The pacer protects the ventricles from the unstable ventricular response of the atrial flutter.

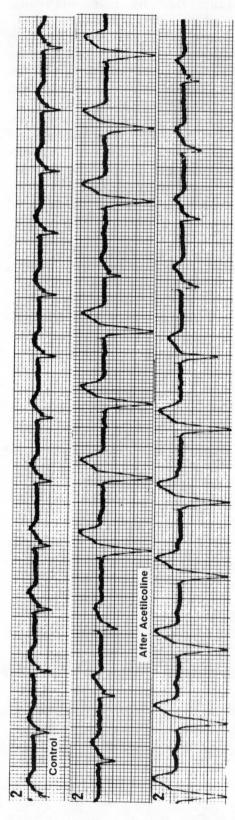

Fig. 90-C - **Drugs and pacemakers.** Acetilcoline reduces the rate of the spontaneous rhythm and sllows for the appearance of a QRS-blocking pacemaker.

C. DRUGS, RADIO-AUSCULTATION AND ARTIFICIAL PACEMAKERS

All pacemakers deliver short-wave radio signals. If, therefore, a small transistor radio is in the proximity of an implanted pacemaker generator, and one listens to the lowest frequency between broadcasting stations, an audible "click", synchronous with each pacemaker impulse (fig. 98), can be heard rotating the antenna over the generator. The *radio-auscultation* of a "demand" QRS-synchronous pacemaker, for example, may be used to separate an automatic from an impulse synchronized with a spontaneous QRS. The intensity of the latter is definitely lower.

The palpation of the peripheral pulse, associated with radio-auscultation, is a rapid method of diagnosing a pacemaker malfunction. A dissociation between a peripheral pulse and the radio "click" indicates a pacemaker malfunction.

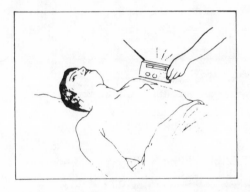

Fig. 90-A - Radio-auscultation of an artificial pacemaker

In the absence of electrocardiographic evidence of pacemaker activity, radio-auscultation may be the only way to determine the generator integrity, before proceeding to more complex explorations. The absence of a pacemaker click and of spikes on the surface ECG may indicate a pacemaker malfunction.

Radio-auscultation is also used for the final control of the battery pack before permanent implantation. Together with a stethoscope the radio-auscultation may be adopted in the routine examination of patients with permanent pacemakers.

Parasympathetic drugs may be used in evaluating the stimulating capacity of a QRS-inhibited pacemaker, particularly when the unit is continually suppressed by faster spontaneous rates. The mechanism of action and intrinsic risks in the use of these drugs are the same as those encountered with carotid sinus massage.

In fig. 90-B, the presence of a QRS-inhibited pacemaker, in a patient with atrial flutter and a variable A-V ratio, is diagnosed with an intravenous injection of *Tensilon*. The increased A-V block, caused by parasympathetic stimulation, enables several pacemaker automatic beats to emerge; this happens when the A-V ratio is long enough and reach the pacemaker stand-by interval (F is a fusion beat).

Acetylcholine is used in fig. 90-C, where the control tracing does not show any artificial rhythm. Numerous pacemaker automatic beats (80/min.) appear in the lower tracing and show a good ventricular capture. The drug, by reducing both the spontaneous rate and the conduction velocity through the A-V node brings out the QRS-inhibited pacemaker, otherwise continuously suppressed by the patient's spontaneous rhythm.

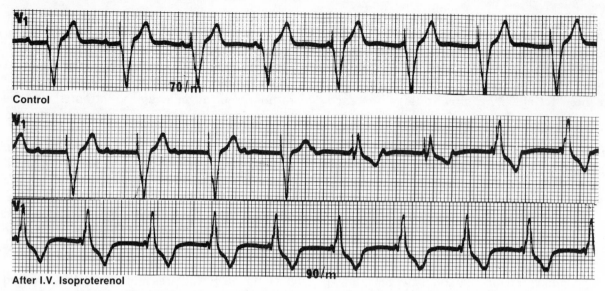

Fig. 91-A - Drugs and pacemakers. A slow infusion of Isoproterenol accelerates the rate of spontaneous impulses. This suppresses the pacemaker and documents a good sensing function.

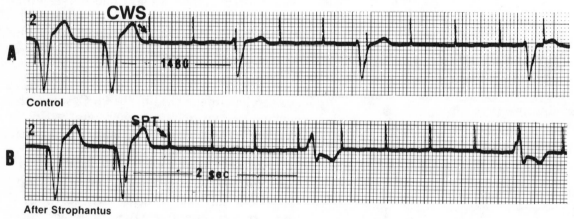

Fig. 91-B - Drugs and pacemakers. The asystolic pause induced by CWS is equal to 1480 msec. (A). Notice the prolongation of the asystolic pause (2 sec.) after I.V. Strophantus (B).

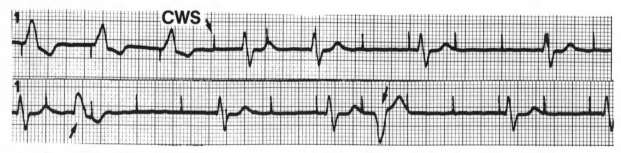

Fig. 91-C - Drugs and pacemakers. Ventricular extrasystoles (arrows) are present with the spontaneous rhythm liberated by CWS. In this patient they suggest an increased excitability secondary to Digitalis therapy.

C. DRUGS AND ARTIFICIAL PACEMAKERS

When a QRS-inhibited pacemaker is continuously pacing the ventricles, the behavior of its "demand" function may also be evaluated with the use of drugs which increase the rate of spontaneous foci suppressed by the artificial pacing. One of the drugs most commonly used in the past has been *Isoproterenol* which increases the automaticity of junctional and idio-ventricular spontaneous pacemakers.

The control tracing of fig. 91-A shows a regular artificial pacing, with good ventricular capture, in a patient with an A-V block. Spontaneous QRS complexes are not present and, therefore, it is difficult to recognize a good pacemaker sensing function. A slow infusion of *Isoproterenol* brings out a junctional rhythm with aberrant conduction (or an idio-ventricular rhythm). The spontaneous rhythm is faster than the automatic pacer rhythm (90/min.) and is able to suppress the pacemaker, indicating a normal "demand" function.

The intrinsic danger of this technique and the lack of reproducibility on one side, and the introduction of the easier, more effective and safe technique of CWS on the other side, have made the use of drugs obsolete in the evaluation of pacemaker function. CWS technique, which utilizes artificial instead of spontaneous cardiac potentials, offers a greater practicality and safety in obtaining the same type of information about the pacemaker QRS-blocking function (see page 171). Furthermore, CWS may be used in the evaluation of the action of drugs on spontaneous cardiac automaticity, conduction and excitability.

Tracings A and B of fig. 91-B were recorded from the same patient. Tracing A shows an atrial fibrillation, with a moderate degree of A-V block, in a patient with a ventricular-inhibited pacemaker, temporarily suppressed by CWS. The *asystolic interval* (interval from the last automatic pacemaker beat to the first spontaneous beat) is 1480 msec., the irregular ventricular rate indicates the presence of an atrial fibrillation.

Tracing B is recorded two hours after an intravenous injection of Strophantus. The artificial pacemaker is again suppressed by the chest wall stimuli, but the asystolic pause is now equal to 2 sec.; the slower QRS complexes are of idio-ventricular origin for the presence of a complete A-V block.

In figure 91-C, an increased ventricular excitability is revealed by suppressing a QRS-inhibited pacemaker with CWS, in a patient chronically treated with digitalis. Ventricular extrasystoles are indicated by the arrows.

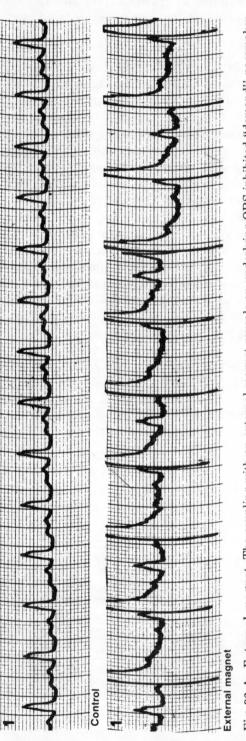

Fig. 92-A - **External magnet.** The coupling with an external magnet reveals an underlying QRS-inhibited "demand" pacemaker (tracing A) and the appearance of an automatic pacing (B).

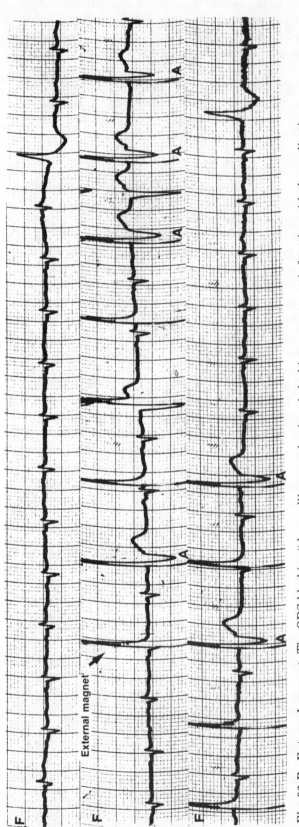

Fig. 92-B - **External magnet.** The QRS-blocking "demand" pacemaker is switched into an automatic function with the application of an external magnet over the generator.

D. EXTERNAL MAGNET

When examining a patient with a QRS-in-hibited pacemaker and before attempting a reduction of the spontaneous rate (with carotid massage or parasympathetic drugs), it is mandatory to test for the presence of a good pacemaker ventricular capture. This is done by a coupling with an *external magnet*. In fact, one of the characteristics of a QRS-inhibited pacemaker is that it can be switched from a demand into an automatic function (fixed rate) through coupling with an external magnet, applied on the skin over the generator and used as a switch. This is also true for the majority of QRS-synchronous pacemakers.

The cases presented in the left page show the application of an external magnet on two patients with a QRS-inhibited pacemaker.

In fig. 92-A, the sinus rhythm with L.B.B.B. of the control tracing (100/min.) suppresses the activity of an implanted QRS-inhibited pacemaker. The magnetic field, created on the cutaneous surface overlying the generator by an external magnet, immediately switches the artificial stimulation from a *demand* type into a *fixed rate* pacing; the pacemaker impulses, with a rate of 80/min., compete with the S-A node impulses.

A good ventricular capture from a QRS- inhibited pacemaker, switched into an automatic function through the use of an external magnet, is clearly demonstrated in beats "A" of fig. 92-B. All the other automatic impulses

fall into the ventricular refractory period of the preceding sinus beats and are not effective. An occasional ventricular extrasystole is also present.

Some of the QRS-inhibited pacemaker models may be directly activated by placing an antenna on the skin surface overlying the generator, and by connecting it to an external transmitter. The transmitter delivers bursts of variable radio-frequencies, up to a maximum of 120/min. Each radio-frequence burst triggers the delivery of a pacemaker impulse, synchronous with the external transmitter. This is an alternative method which makes it possible to overcome a spontaneous cardiac rate and to confirm a good pacemaker ventricular capture.

QRS-synchronous pacemakers, also, incorporate in their circuitry a magnet-switch whose function is to test the automatic pacemaker mechanism whenever a spontaneous cardiac rhythm is present. The pacemaker impulses are synchronized with the R waves of spontaneous beats and do not give information about their effectiveness (good ventricular capture) in case of necessity. The coupling with an external magnet switches the pacemaker from a *demand* into a *fixed rate mode* and the resulting competitive rhythm confirms the presence of a good pacemaker ventricular capture.

REFERENCES

Barold, S.S., Pupillo, G.A., Gaidula, J.J., et al.: *Chest wall Stimulation in the Evaluation of Patients with Implanted Ventricular Inhibited Pacemakers*, Brit. Heart J., 32:783-789, 1970.

Pupillo, Giovanni, A., and Linhart, Joseph, W.: *Chest-wall Stimulation and Phonocardiography in the Identification of the Pacemaker Heart Sound*, Annals of Internal Medicine, 73:3, 1970.

Trevino, Alfonso, J., Beller, Barry, M., Talley, Robert, C., Pupillo, Giovanni, A., and Linhart, Joseph, W.: *Chest-wall Stimulation: A Method of Demand QRS-blocking Pacemaker Suppression in the Study of Arrhythmias*, American Heart Journal, 81:1, 1971.

Furman, Seymour, and Escher, Doris, J.W.: *Principles and Techniques of Cardiac Pacing*, Harper and Row, New York, 1970.

Castellanos, A., Jr., Lemberg, L., Centurion, M.J., and Berkovits, B.V.: *Concealed Digitalis-induced Arrhythmias Unmasked by Electrical Stimulation of the Heart*, Amer. Heart J., 73:282, 1967.

Vasalle, M., Karis, J., and Hoffman, B.F.: *Toxic Effects of Ouabain on Purkinje Fibers and Ventricular Muscle Fibers*, Amer. J. Physiol., 203:433, 1962.

Walker, W.J., Elkins, J.T., and Wood, L.: *Effect of a Subthreshold Cardiac Pacemaker, Potassium in Restoring Myocardial Response to Med.*, 271:597, 1964. New Eng. J.

Castellanos, A., Jr., Maytin, O., Lemberg, L., et al.: *Ventricular-triggered Pacemaker Arrhythmias*, Brit. Heart J., 31:546-552, 1969.

Rubin, I.L., Arbeit, S.R., Gross, H.: *The Electrocardiographic Recognition of Pacemaker Function and Failure*, Ann. Intern. Med., 71:603-616, 1969.

Spritzer, R.C., Donoso, E., Gadboys, H.L., et al.: *Arrhythmias Induced by Pacemaking on Demand*, Amer. Heart J., 77:619-627, 1969.

Furman, S., Escher, D.J.W., Solomon, W.: *Standby Pacing for Multiple Cardiac Arrhythmias*, Ann. Thorac. Surg., 3:327-336, 1967.

Castellanos, A., Jr., Lemberg, L., Jude, J.R., et al.: *Implantable Demand Pacemaker*, Brit. Heart J., 30:29-33, 1968.

Furman, S., Escher, D.J.W.: *Ventricular Synchronous and Demand Pacing*, Amer. Heart J., 76:445-451, 1968.

Kastor, J.A., Berkovits, B.V., De Sanctis, R.W.: *Variations in Discharge Rate of Demand Pacemakers not Due to Malfunction*, Amer, J. Cardiol., 25:344-348, 1970.

Castellanos, A., Jr., Spence, M.: *Pacemaker Arrhythmias in Context*, Amer. J. Cardiol., 25:372-373, 1970.

Lister, J.W., Escher, D.J.W., Furman, S., et al.: *Heart Block: Method for Rapid Determination of Causes of Pacing Failure in Artificial Pacemaker Systems*, Amer. J. Cardiol., 18:64-72, 1966.

Gordon, A.J., Vagueiro, M.C., Barold, S.S.: *Endocardial Electrograms from Pacemaker Cathers*, Circulation, 38:82-89, 1968.

Parker, B., Furman, S., Escher, D.J.W.: *Input Signals to Pacemakers in a Hospital Environment*, Ann. N.Y. Acad. Sci., 167:823-834, 1969.

Furman, S., Escher, D.J.W., Parker, B., et al.: *Electronic Analysis for Pacemaker Failure*, Ann. Thorac. Surg., 8:57-65, 1969.

Furman, S., Escher, D.J.W.: *Choice of Cardiac Pacemaker*, Ann. N.Y. Acad. Sci., 167:577-570, 1969.

Samet, P., Hildner, F., Schoenfeld, C., et al.: *Effect of Chest Wall Stimulation on Cardiac Pacemaker Function (abstr)*, Circulation, 39-40: suppl. 3:176, 1969.

Samet, P., Center, S., Linhart, J.W., et al.: *Selected Current Aspects of Cardiac Pacing, Electrocardiographic Patterns*, Amer. J. Cardiol., 23:702-711, 1969.

King, G.R., Hamburger, A.C., Parsa, F., et al.: *Effect of Microwave Oven on Implanted Cardiac Pacemaker*, J.A.M.A., 212:1213, 1970.

Sowton, E.: *Detection of Impending Pacemaker Failure*, Israel J. Med. Sci., 3:260-269, 1967.

Siddons, H., Sowton, E.: *Cardiac Pacemakers*, Springfield, Ill., Charles C. Thomas, 1967, p. 152-154.

Bertrand, C.A., Zohman, L.R., Williams, M.H.: *Intracardiac Electrocardiography in Man*, Amer. J. Med., 26:534-542, 1959.

Charterjee, K., Sutton, R., Davis, J.G.: *Low Intracardiac Potentials in Myocardial Infarction as a Cause of Failure of Inhibition of Demand Pacemakers*, Lancet, 1:511, 1968.

Barold, S.S., Gaidula, J.J.: *Failure of Demand Pacemaker from Low Voltage Bipolar Ventricular Electrograms*, J.A.M.A., 215:923-926, 1971.

Bilitch, M., Lau, F.Y.K., Cosby, R.S.: « *Demand » Pacemaker Inhibition by Radiofrequency Signals (abstr)*, Circulation, 35: suppl. 2:68, 1967.

Bilitch, M.: *Ventricular Fibrillation and Pacing*, Ann. N.Y. Acad. Sci., 167:934-940, 1969.

Pickers, B.A., Goldberg, M.J.: *Inhibition of a Demand Pacemaker and Interference with Monitoring Equipment by Radiofrequency Transmissions*, Brit. Med. J., 2:504-506, 1969.

Furman, S., Parker, B., Krauthamer, M., et al.: *The Influence of Electromagnetic Environment on the Performance of Artificial Cardiac Pacemakers*, Ann. Thorac. Surg., 6:90-95, 1968.

Wajszczuk, W.J., Mowry, F.M., Dugan, N.L.: *Deactivation of Demand Pacemaker by Transurethral Electrocautery*, New Eng. J. Med., 280:34-35, 1969.

Barold, S., Serge, Gaidula, John, J.: *Evaluation of Normal and Abnormal Sensing Functions of Demand Pacemakers*, Amer. J. Cardiol., 28:201, 1971.

Chapter IX

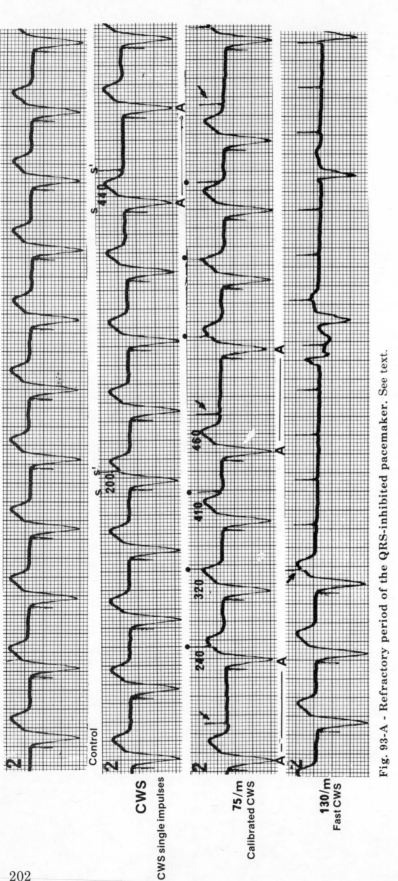

Control

CWS
CWS single impulses

75/m
Calibrated CWS

130/m
Fast CWS

Fig. 93-A - Refractory period of the QRS-inhibited pacemaker. See text.

Fig. 93-B - Refractory period of the QRS-inhibited pacemaker. See text.

THE REFRACTORY PERIOD OF ARTIFICIAL PACEMAKERS

The refractory period of an artificial pacemaker is that interval of time during which the pacemaker does not record electrical signals. The clinical importance of a refractory period involves only pacemakers with a sensing mechanism and, therefore, only the "demand" pacemakers of the QRS-synchronous or QRS-inhibited type and the P-wave synchronous pacemaker. Furthermore, when using "demand" QRS-inhibited pacemakers it is possible to separate a refractory period which follows the delivery of an automatic impulse *(delivery refractory period)* from that following the sensing of a spontaneous QRS *(sensing refractory period)*. The *refractory period* of a "demand" pacemaker may be easily measured from a surface ECG by using the CWS technique (see page 169).

A. The refractory period of the QRS-inhibited "demand" pacemaker

In this type of unit the refractory period has been introduced for the following reasons: a) the pacemaker must not be disturbed by its own QRS complexes; b) the impulse must not be able to re-enter the generator amplifier; c) the pacemaker must not sense high amplitude T or P waves and, d) the pacemaker must not sense, at least for a certain interval of time, electrical signals of cardiac or extra-cardiac origin.

A CWS may be performed by using single external impulses, suitably calibrated and delivered at critical time intervals from the preceding pacemaker automatic beats, or by delivering chest wall stimuli with a rate slower than the basic automatic pacemaker rate. A fast CWS would keep the implanted pacemaker continuously suppressed.

A classical example of identification of a ventricular-inhibited pacemaker refractory period is presented in fig. 93-A. The control tracing shows a regular automatic pacing with a rate of 80/min.; spontaneous beats are not present and, therefore, no data is available about the pacemaker sensing mechanism. In the second tracing, CWS is performed with two single stimuli (arrows) delivered after S-S[1] intervals of different length (interval of time between the permanent pacemaker spike and that of CWS).

The first external impulse (S-S[1] interval = 200 msec.) is not sensed and does not influence the automatic time-table of the permanent pacemaker. The second external impulse falls 440 msec. after the pacemaker automatic impulse, and is sensed; therefore, the impulse inhibits the permanent pacemaker and starts a new recharging cycle (the A-A interval of the sensed stimulus is longer than the automatic A-A intervals).

When CWS is performed with a rate slower than the pacemaker automatic rate (third tracing), it permits the measurement of the exact length of the pacemaker refractory period. In fact, the rate of CWS is suitably calibrated (75/min.) in such a way that the external impulses fall at increasing distance from the preceding pacemaker impulse (240 msec. . . . . . 460 msec.). Only when the chest wall impulse falls after an S-S[1] interval of 460 msec. does it suppress the permanent pacemaker. The S-S[1] interval of 460 msec. represents, therefore, the maximal refractory period length for that type of stimulator. Three stimuli are sensed (arrows) and determine A-A intervals longer than the basic A-A intervals. The ineffective chest wall impulses are indicated by dots. Therefore, from the analysis of the second and third tracings, it appears that the maximal length of the pacemaker refractory period is located somewhere between 410 and 440 msec. after the delivery of an automatic impulse.

The last tracing records a fast CWS (130/min.) with continuous suppression of the permanent pacemaker. It also shows the emergence of an idio-ventricular rhythm.

Tracing A of fig. 93-B shows a QRS-inhibited pacemaker rhythm interrupted by spontaneous QRS's (arrows) and by an external stimulus of a CWS. The spontaneous beats and the single external impulse are sensed by the internal pacemaker. Note that the A-A intervals, which contain both the spontaneous and the artificial impulses, have different lengths. This is due to the summation of the pacemaker escape interval and the variable coupling intervals of the QRS's, and/or CWS impulse, with the preceding pacemaker automatic beat.

A similar finding is shown in tracing B where CWS is performed at a slow rate (48/min.). Only the first impulse is not effective (S-S[1] interval = 400 msec.), while all the others inactivate the permanent pacemaker. Since the chest wall stimuli fall in different areas of the pacemaker recharging cycle, the interval between two successive pacemaker beats (A-A intervals) may be of different length. This does not indicate a pacemaker malfunction, but a sensing of impulses which fall in different areas of the recharging cycle.

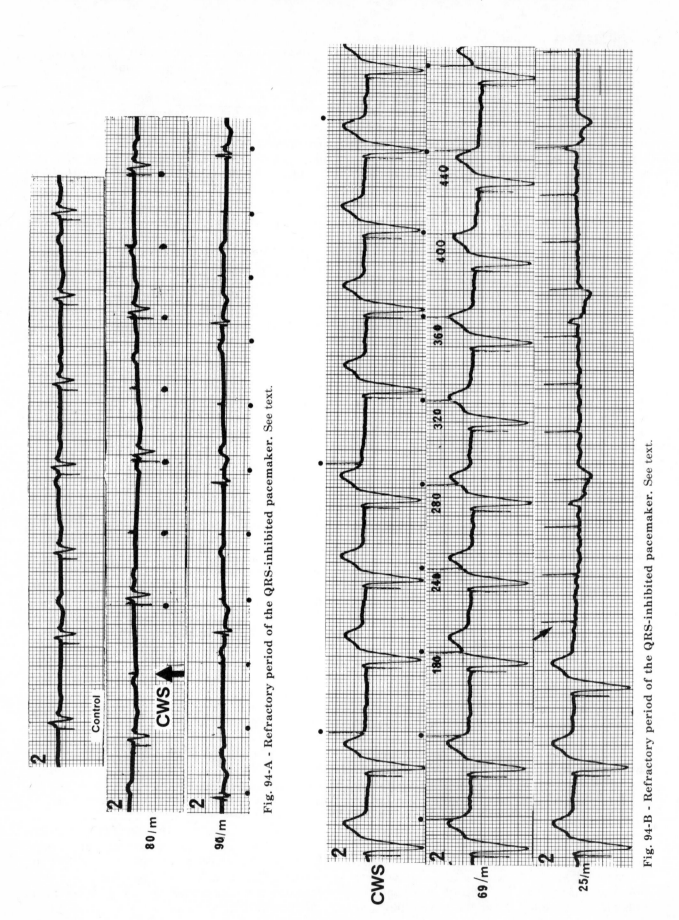

Fig. 94-A - Refractory period of the QRS-inhibited pacemaker. See text.

Fig. 94-B - Refractory period of the QRS-inhibited pacemaker. See text.

A. The refractory period of the QRS-inhibited "demand" pacemaker

When a CWS is performed with a rate calibrated to the pacemaker automatic interval, it is possible to suppress the implanted stimulator with alternate external impulses and to reduce in half the effective pacing rate. For this to happen it is necessary that the external stimuli fall within the pacemaker *refractory period*.

The control tracing of fig. 94-A shows a regular pacing of 66/min. A CWS is performed in the second tracing with a rate of 80/min. Every other stimulus falls within the pacemaker refractory period, a few msecs. after the pacemaker spike and, therefore, is not effective. The following stimulus suppresses the pacemaker and reduces in half the effective stimulation rate (33/min.).

The bottom tracing shows a CWS performed with a faster rate (90/min.). The stimuli continuously suppress the internal pacemaker while a sinus rhythm, with a complete A-V block and a subsidiary junctional pacemaker is recorded in L2.

In fig. 94-B CWS is again used in the three different modalities: single stimulus (upper tracing); continuous stimulation with a rate slower than the automatic pacemaker rate (middle tracing); and fast CWS (lower tracing).

The refractory period can be measured in the middle tracing. It extends up to 400 msec. after the delivery of an automatic impulse. In fact, the stimulus, with a S-S[1] interval of 440 msec., is sensed by the pacemaker.

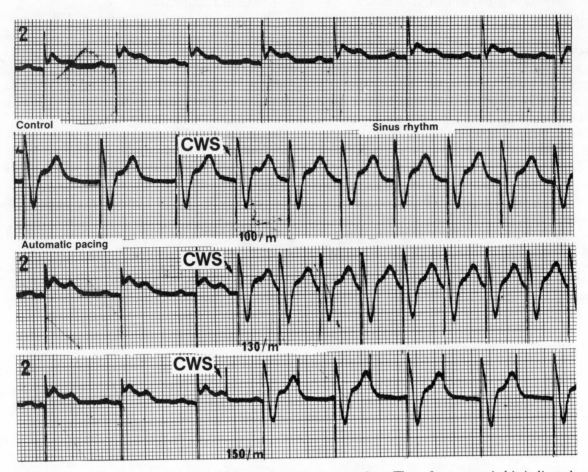

Fig. 95-A - Refractory period of a QRS-synchronous pacemaker. The refractory period is indicated by the 2:1 synchronization with a CWS rate of 150/min. and is equal to 400 msec.

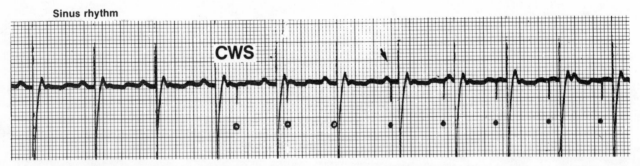

Fig. 95-B - Refractory period of a P-wave synchronous pacemaker. The first three impulses of a CWS are not synchronized with the pacemaker since they fall within the refractory period. The arrow indicates the pacemaker capture by the external impulses.

THE REFRACTORY PERIOD OF ARTIFICIAL PACEMAKERS

B. The refractory period of the QRS-synchronous "demand" pacemaker

The refractory period of the QRS-synchronous pacemaker determines its maximal synchronizing rate with spontaneous cardiac signals (see page 64). This is calculated from the formula:

$$\frac{60}{\text{Maximal Pacemaker Rate}} = \text{Pacemaker Refractory Period in Seconds}$$

Therefore, a pacemaker with a refractory period of 400 msec. (0.40 sec.) has a maximal synchronizing rate of 150/min. Since this type of unit does not have a delivery and sensing refractory periods, (see the QRS-inhibited pacemaker), it continuously delivers impulses either in the presence or in the absence of spontaneous cardiac activity.

The ideal refractory period for this type of pacemaker is still a matter of discussion. Since it is rare to find a premature spontaneous beat appearing within 300-350 msecs. after a pacemaker automatic beat, the maximal length of the refractory period must be around 380 msecs. A shorter refractory period (for ex. 100 msecs.) could enable the sensing of QRS's determined by the pacemaker spikes and induce a change in the pacemaker delivery rate. On the other hand, if the refractory period is too long (for ex. 500 msecs.), one could run the risk of not sensing spontaneous ventricular potentials (see page 97).

Fig. 95-A shows the identification of a QRS-synchronous "demand" pacemaker refractory period with the use of chest wall stimulation. The control tracing shows a sinus rhythm with QRS complexes that are normally synchronized with the pacemaker. Notice the spikes within the spontaneous QRS's.

Observe from the first three beats (rate = 73/min.) in the second tracing, that the rhythm of the patient is determined by the pacemaker in automatic function. A CWS is initiated (arrows) with a rate of 100/min.; the pacemaker responds promptly to CWS with an increase in the effective pacing rate (100/min.). The third tracing records a CWS performed with a rate of 130/min. and is still followed by a ventricular response of 1:1. When the external stimulation reaches a rate of 150/min. (bottom tracing), only every other external impulse is sensed and followed by ventricular capture; the other impulse falls within the refractory period (whose maximal length is, therefore, equal to 400 msec.).

C. The refractory period of the P-wave synchronous pacemaker

With CWS it is also possible to identify a refractory period of a P-wave synchronous pacemaker. This is shown in fig. 95-B where the first three external stimuli (indicated with clear circles) are not sensed by the atrial electrode and are not synchronized with the pacemaker. They fall at time intervals of 220, 120, 20 msecs. from the delivery of the preceding pacemaker impulse and, therefore, within the pacer refractory period. The following impulses, instead, are interpreted as atrial signals because they synchronize with the internal pacemaker, as it appears from the increased ventricular rate and the fixed A-P delay.

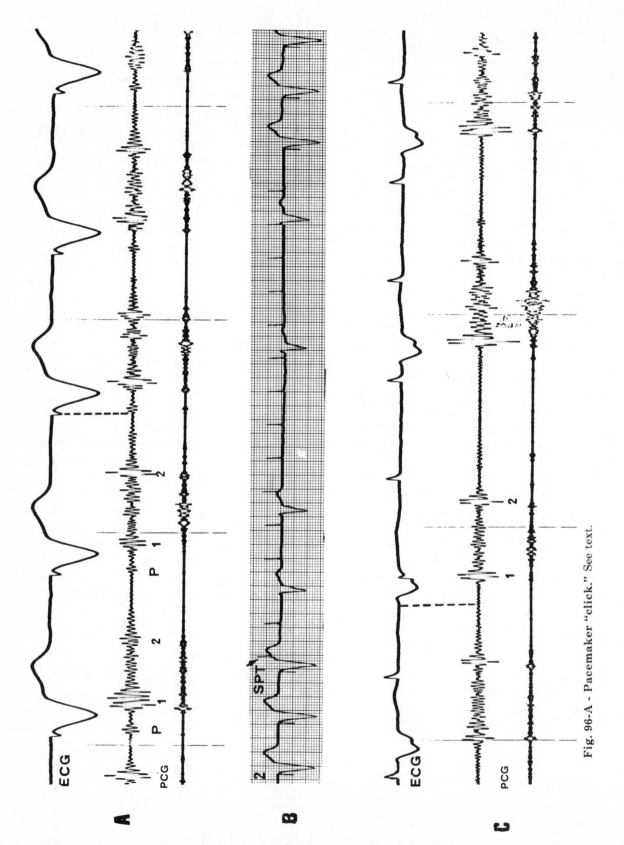

Fig. 96-A - Pacemaker "click." See text.

"PACEMAKER CLICK"

A new ascoltatory phenomenon, occasionally found in the clinical examination of patients with artificial pacemakers, is the so called "pacemaker click". It is a presystolic finding occasionally associated with rhythmic contractions of several muscular groups (pectoral, intercostal, and hemidiaphragm) and which typically occurs 6 msec. after a pacemaker spike.

The *pacemaker click* is usually a high frequency phenomenon. It has a metallic character and it always precedes the first heart sound. During auscultation of a patient with an artificial pacemaker one must search for a pacemaker click. Because of its particular position within the cardiac cycle, attention must be paid not to confuse the "click" with a split first sound or with a S4 sound.

Muscular contractions may, at times, be seen and palpated simultaneous to a pacemaker click. The apexcardiogram records a rapid and premature outward movement of the chest wall coincident with the click.

Due to a propagation of electrical current from the tip of the stimulating catheter to neighbor muscular groups, the extracardiac origin of the click has been proved by: a) the recording of an ascoltatory phenomenon, similar to a pacemaker click, with isolated stimulations of the pectoral muscle; b) the absence of a click with intracavitary phonocardiograms; c) the absence of a premature elevation of the right ventricular pressure, coincident with the outward motion on the apexcardiogram; and, d) the suppression of the click with neuromuscular blocking agents. agents.

When a pacemaker click is caused by a "demand" QRS-inhibited pacemaker, it can be easily identified through the use of CWS associated with a phonocardiographic recording. If a good residual cardiac rhythm is present, CWS can also temporarily suppress the uncomfortable muscular contractions, sometimes associated with a *pacemaker click*.

Tracing A of fig. 96-A is a phonocardiographic recording of a patient with a QRS-inhibited pacemaker in automatic function. The routine clinical examination had shown the presence of an extracardiac sound located in the left fifth intercostal space at the parasternal line. The extra sound was better heard in the left lateral decubitus and it regularly preceded the first heart sound by 0.12 sec.

The ECG recording shows a regular pacing with a rate of 78/min. The two phonocardiographic tracings, simultaneously recorded, show a systo-diastolic murmur of a concomitant aortic valvular disease and, at the same time, identify a *pacemaker click* almost simultaneous with the pacemaker spike (dashes).

Tracing B shows a CWS which promptly suppresses the pacemaker and reveals an atrial fibrillation with a slow ventricular rate. Therefore, once the presence of a presystolic sound is excluded because of atrial fibrillation, the recording of a phonocardiogram, coupled with CWS (tracing C), easily identifies the presence of a pacemaker click. In fact, the phonocardiogram obtained during CWS (135/min.) clearly shows the disappearance of the presystolic click with the emergence of spontaneous QRS's.

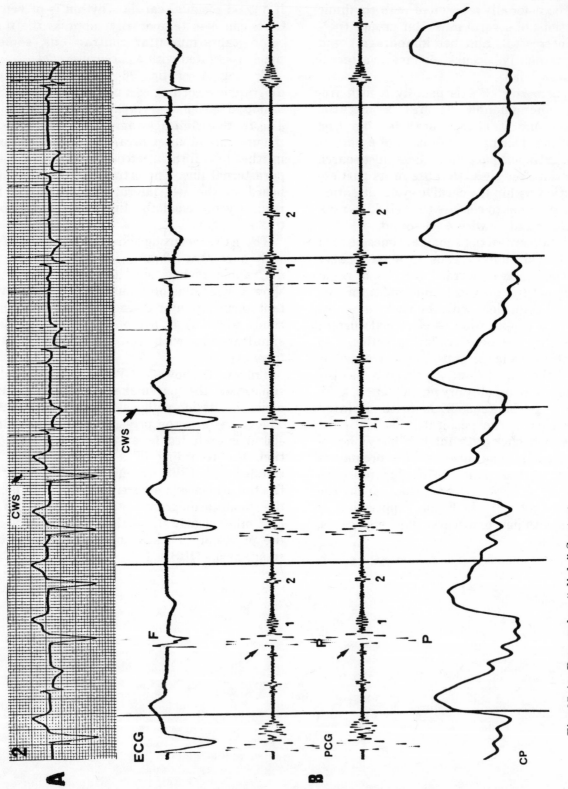

Fig. 97-A - Pacemaker "click." See text.

"PACEMAKER CLICK"

A *presystolic click of a QRS-inhibited pacemaker* is presented in fig. 97-A. In this patient, the auscultatory finding was associated with uncomfortable contractions of the left hemidiaphragm, when the stimulating electrode was in a right apical location. The *pacemaker click* and the troublesome "artificial hiccup" were suppressed with the application of a continuous CWS, until the stimulating catheter was repositioned.

Tracing A exhibits a control ECG, recorded to test the response of the internal pacemaker to CWS and to document the presence of an adequate spontaneous rhythm, before the application of a prolonged CWS. Note that the pacemaker promptly responds to the external impulses and a sinus rhythm, moderately bradycardic, immediately reappears.

Tracing B shows the simultaneous ECG phonocardiogram (PCG) and carotid pulse (CP) recording; they document the presence of a pacemaker presystolic click. Observe that the phonocardiogram records a high frequence phenomenon, faster than the first and second heart sounds, and coincident with a pacemaker spike (the click is present also during a ventricular fusion beat). With the beginning of CWS and the suppression of the permanent pacemaker, the pacemaker click immediately disappears, (the dash line indicates where the pacemaker click should fall) while the first and second heart sounds remain unchanged. (Notice the higher amplitude of the carotid pulse during the slower sinus rhythm.)

SHAPE	MANUFACTURER	TYPES			
	CORDIS	VENTRICOR ATRICOR		ECTOCOR STANICOR	
	MEDTRONIC	BIPOLAR		UNIPOLAR	
		5912	5950	5913	5951
		XYTRON - RA 5954	XYTRON - HT 5960	5951 AD	
		XYREL 5972	9000	XYTRON - RA 5955	XYREL 5973
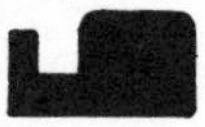	GENERAL ELECTRIC	QRS - INHIBITED PACEMAKER 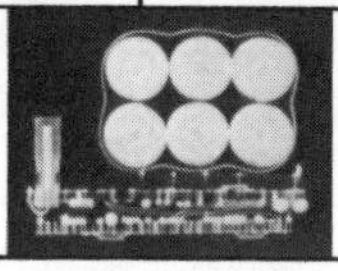			
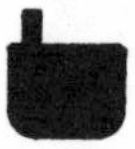	CARDIAC PACEMAKERS	MINILITH 501/601 MINILITH 503/603		MINILITH 504/604 MINILITH 508/608	
	CORATOMIC	L - 500 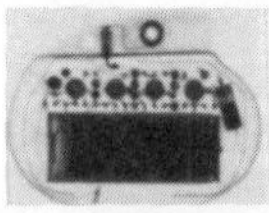		C - 101 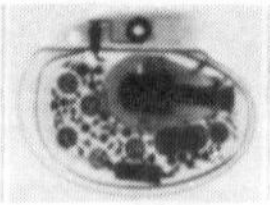	
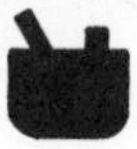	VITATRON	S6121/6221 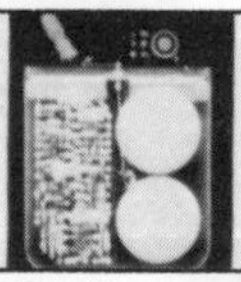			
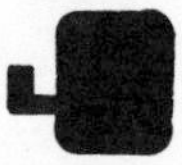	EDWARDS	PROLITH 21 S/21 U 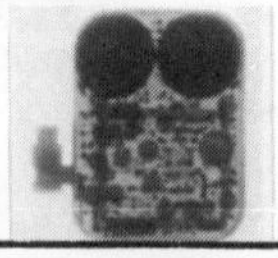		MICROPULSE 20 S/20 U 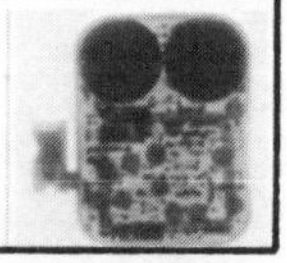	

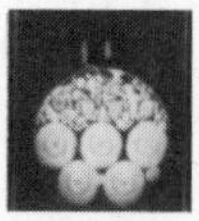

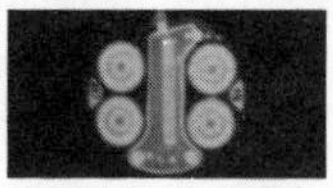

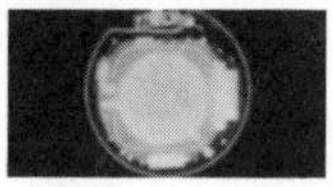

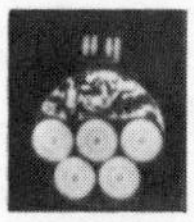

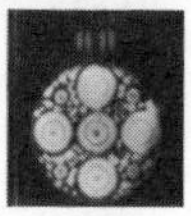

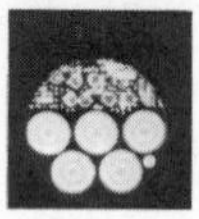

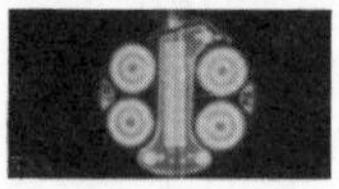

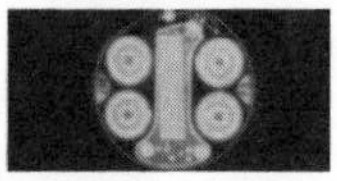

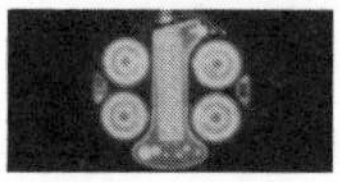

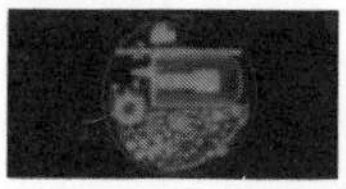

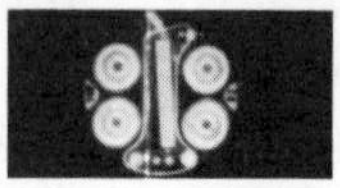

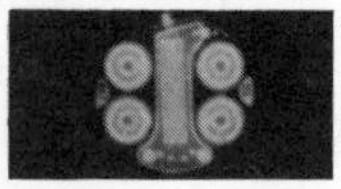

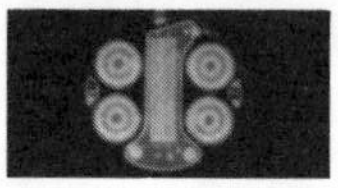

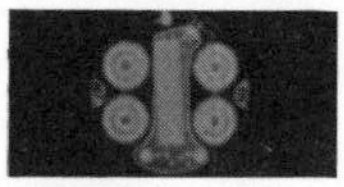

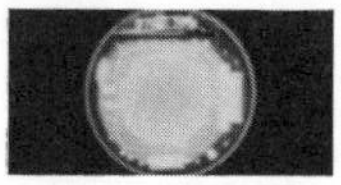

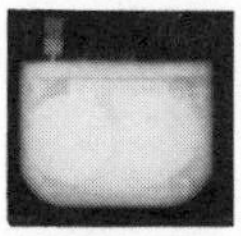

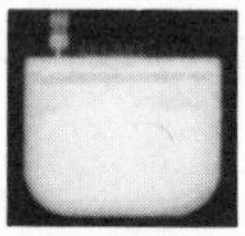

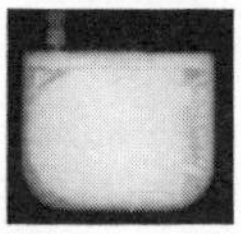

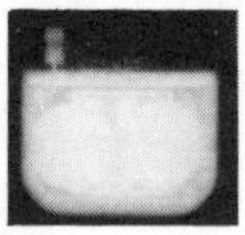

Fig. 98-A - Radiologic identification of the most commonly used artificial pacemaker. See text.

RADIOLOGICAL INDENTIFICATION OF THE MOST COMMONLY USED ARTIFICIAL PACEMAKERS

Patients with permanent artificial pacemakers, may present themselves in emergency situations. It is, therefore, necessary for the physician to have a fast and reliable method for an immediate identification of the type of implanted unit.

One of the first tests that must be performed together with an ECG tracing is the X-ray examination of the area where the generator has been implanted. This must be performed using projections perpendicular to the unit with high penetration, and at an exposure approximately twice the normal for the body area where the unit is implanted.

The radiographic appearance of the generator, the analysis of its shape, number and position of the batteries and of other electronic components, permits the identification of most types of stimulators in use. Each brand of pacemakers has a distinctive shape and characteristic which can be viewed in examination of an X-ray film of the unit. The major brands of electronic pacemakers are not interchangeable and some units require subdifferentiation according to type. The chart on the opposite page was developed for an accurate rapid identification of pacemakers.

Particular importance has been placed on the radiological diagnosis of battery discharge. The external wall and the internal ring of the mercury cells are radiopaque and contain a thin, radio-transparent, electrolitic ring. With battery exhaustion, mercury filled components move toward the electrolitic zone and this area becomes progressively radiopaque till it is totally covered by a uniform density. This indicates that the mercury cells are totally exhausted.

These radiographic changes are easily recognized if a generator is placed directly on a radiographic cassette. They are, however, very difficult to observe in a patient with an implanted pacemaker, since it is impossible to obtain an X-ray plate with the mercury cells perfectly perpendicular to the radiographic film plane.

In fig. 98-A the radiologic appearance of the most common artificial pacemakers in use are reproduced. The radiologic gross appearance of the battery pack is indicated to the left of the manufacturer's name.

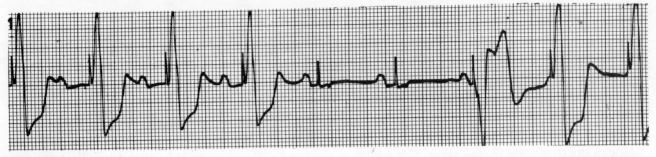

Fig. 99-A

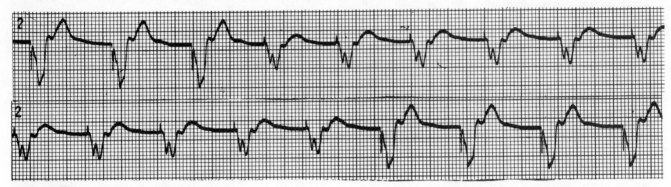

Fig. 99-B

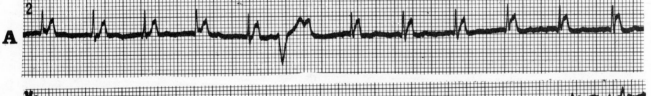

A

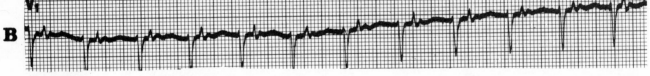

B

Fig. 99-C

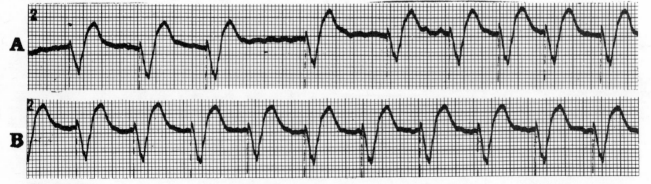

A

B

Fig. 99-D

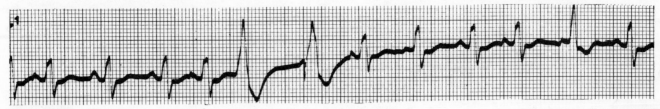

Fig. 100-A

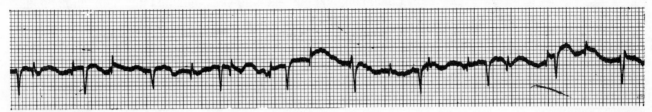

Fig. 100-B

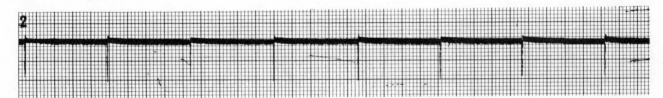

Fig. 100-C

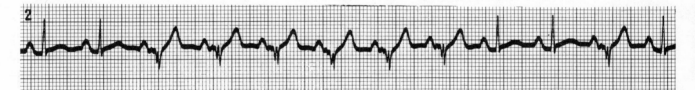

Fig. 100-D

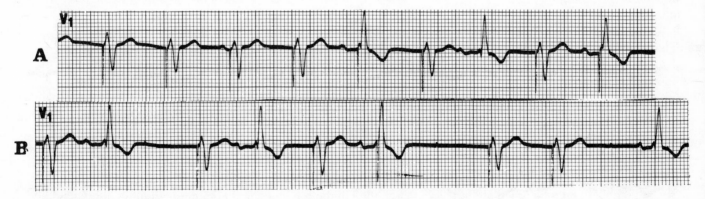

Fig. 100-E

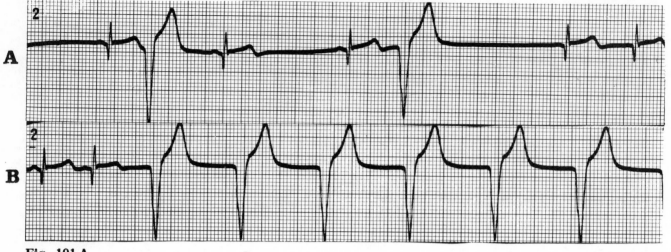

Fig. 101-A

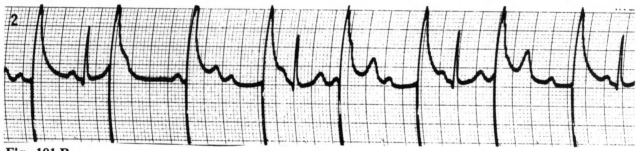

Fig. 101-B

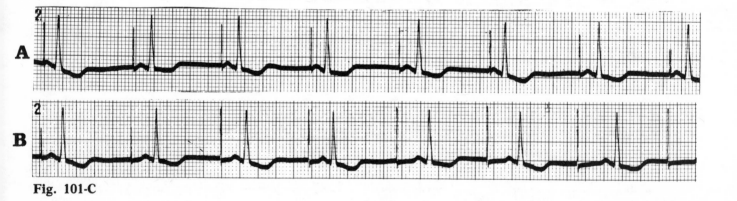

Fig. 101-C

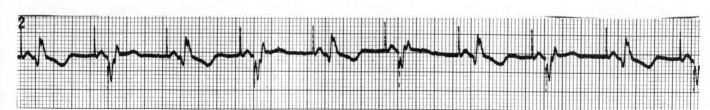

Fig. 101-D

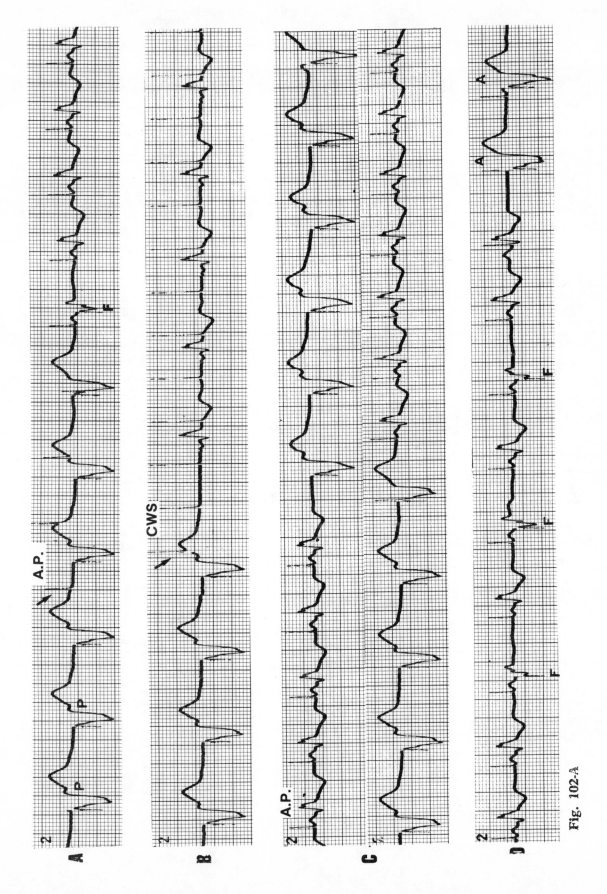

Fig. 102-A

217

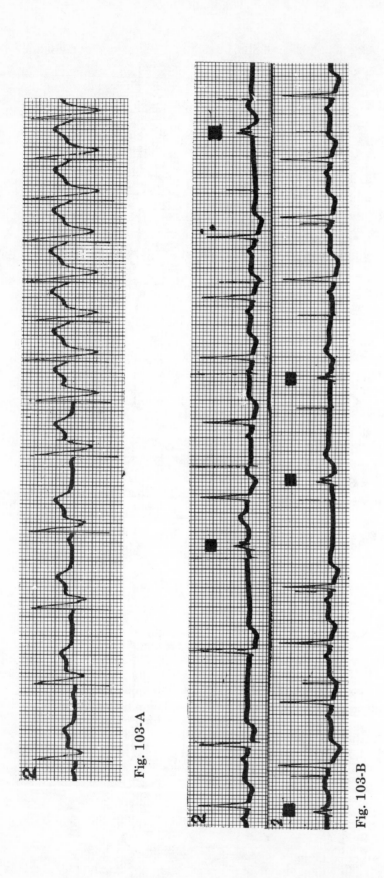

Fig. 103-A

Fig. 103-B

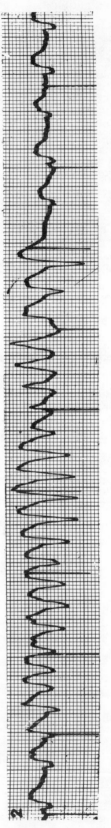

Fig. 103-C

Fig. 99-A: *Although they appear to be, they are not spontaneous QRS complexes.* The two P-waves in the middle of the tracing are followed by pacemaker spikes which resemble spontaneous QRS's. The tracing may suggest a QRS-inhibited pacemaker; it shows, however, a malfunctioning asynchronous pacemaker. The pacemaker spikes are not followed by a QRS and, therefore, do not capture the ventricles. The next beat is a ventricular escape beat.

Fig. 99-B: A reduction of the QRS amplitude does not necessarily mean pacemaker malfunction. It may be present, especially in lead 3, during respiratory cycles. Notice the P^I waves? Now try to explain the different polarity of the pacemaker spikes!

Fig. 99-C: What appears as a spike is followed by what appears as a QRS. This suggests a QRS-inhibited pacemaker (tracing A). There is also an extrasystole without a spike. The diagnosis is: sinus rhythm with a first degree A-V block and a very prolonged P-R interval (tracing B)!!

Fig. 99-D: No, it is not a malfunctioning pacemaker. There is an absolutely unstable atrial rhythm (tachycardia-fibrillation-flutter). The *P-wave synchronous pacemaker* does its best to be synchronized with the atrial activity or to work in an automatic fashion. When a sinus rhythm is re-established (B), the pacemaker works well.

Fig. 100-A: Atrial and ventricular extrasystoles. But there is also an automatic pacemaker beat. What type of pacer?

Fig. 100-B: Don't ever confuse a fetal ECG with that of an artificial pacemaker.

Fig. 100-C: The operation was successful but the patient . . .

Fig. 100-D: Intermittent Wolff-Parkinson-White. It does not have anything to do with a pacemaker but the simulation is perfect.

Fig. 100-E: In tracing A everything is fine. In tracing B prolonged asystolic pauses are present. Have you heard about CWS? With a magnifying lens it is easy to recognize the chest wall stimuli which suppress the implanted pacemaker.

Fig. 101-A: The simulation of a ventricular tachycardia is perfect (B), especially in the presence of ventricular extrasystoles (A) and almost invisible bipolar spikes.

Fig. 101-B: Can you separate the ineffective spikes from those with ventricular capture? It is almost impossible. The prerequisite for a good ECG tracing is a good ECG machine.

Fig. 101-C: It is not a malfunctioning atrial pacemaker (B). It is not even an atrial pacemaker (A). The ineffective stimuli are those of an asynchronous pacemaker, occasionally falling before sinus P-waves. (The sinus rate and that of the pacemaker are almost equal).

Fig. 101-D: This tracing is quite difficult. It may be defined as an artificial Wolff-Parkinson-White. To decipher the tracing, it is advisable to analyze the next figure.

Fig. 102-A: Tracing A = the initial ventricular rhythm (68/min.) is determined by a permanent ventricular pacemaker. The arrow indicates impulses with different polarity and with a slightly faster rate (85/min.). Although they suggest a chest wall stimulation (CWS), this is not the case. The first four impulses are not effective; starting from the sixth positive impulse, each spike is followed by a P-wave and by a QRS complex with a normal morphology. The patient, therefore, has a QRS-inhibited pacemaker working at a fixed, automatic, rate and also has a second catheter located in the right atrium. Since the atrial stimulation is slightly faster than the ventricular pacing rate, each QRS's potentials inhibit the permanent pacemaker and the cardiac rhythm is, therefore, guided by the atrium. The first four impulses do not capture the atrium because they find it refractory due to retrograde atrial depolarization (P^1) by the permanent pacemaker impulses. The beat indicated with F is a ventricular fusion beat. The ventricles are still partly activated by the permanent ventricular pacemaker and partly by the atrial impulse.

B = same patient. This time, the pacemaker is inactivated by a chest wall stimulation. CWS liberates the patient spontaneous rhythm. (Notice that the QRS morphology of spontaneous beats is identical to that of the pacing beats of tracing A.)

C = same patient. At the beginning, the cardiac rhythm is under control of atrial impulses; when atrial pacing is discontinued, the ventricles are then activated by the ventricular pacemaker and vice-versa (second tracing).

D = same patient. A.P. = atrial impulses which capture both atria and ventricles; A = automatic ventricular impulses of the permanent pacemaker; F = ventricular fusion beat (the ventricles are partially activated by the artificial impulse coming from the atria and partially from the ventricular artificial impulse).

Fig. 103-A: It is not a "runaway pacemaker"; the ventricular pacing suddenly becomes rapid because of pacemaker synchronization with chest wall stimuli (CWS). The pacemaker is of the QRS-synchronous type. Notice that the first of the external impulses falls 200 msec. after the pacemaker automatic impulse and, therefore, is not effective (pacemaker refractory period equals 400 msec.). The ventricular rate is guided by the chest wall stimuli.

Fig. 103-B: The tracing is recorded from a patient with a permanent pacemaker and with an intracavitary catheter dislodged from the right ventricular apex into the supraclavicular area. Each pacemaker impulse was closely associated with muscular contractions of the surrounding areas and with a "pacemaker click". The tracing was recorded after the insertion of a second catheter into the right ventricular chamber and connected to an external unit of the QRS-inhibited type. Analysis of the continuous tracing shows that the patient has a normal sinus rhythm slightly irregular, probably caused by the presence of a "sino-atrial Wenckebach". The Wenckebach sequences are followed by asystolic pauses. They are terminated by pacemaker escape beats (indicated by dark squares). All the other spikes do not have any functional significance. They only disturb the ECG recording and they are caused by the tip of the catheter stimulating the shoulder muscles.

Fig. 103-C: Ventricular fibrillation and ineffective pacing. Many cases have been reported in which ventricular fibrillation is not signaled by the monitors in the Coronary Care Units; the regular pacemaker impulses would interfere with the recording of the arrhythmia and would prevent the setting off of the alarm signals.

REFERENCES

Pupillo, Giovanni, A., and Linhart, Joseph, W.: *Chest-wall Stimulation and Phonocardiography in the Identification of the Pacemaker Heart Sound*, Annals of Internal Medicine, 73:3, 1970.

Barold, S.S., Pupillo, G.A., Gaidula, J.J., et al.: *Chest wall Stimulation in the Evaluation of Patients with Implanted Ventricular-inhibited Demand Pacemakers*, Brit. Heart J., 32:783-789, 1970.

Walter, William, H., Lieutenant Colonel and Wenger, Nanette, K.: *Radiographic Identification of Commonly Used Implanted Pacemakers*, New Eng. J. Med., 281:1230-1231, 1969.

Barold, S., Serge: *Clinical Significance of Pacemaker Refractory Periods*, Amer. J. Cardiol., 28:237, 1971.

Castellanos, A., Jr., Lemberg, L.: *Electrophysiology of Pacing and Cardioversion*, New York, Appleton-Century-Crofts, 1969, p. 46-61.

Parsonnet, V.: *A Decade of Permanent Pacing of the Heart*, Cardiovasc. Clin., 2:182-199, 1970.

Zipes, D.P., McIntosh, H.D.: *Pacemaker-induced Arrhythmias*. In *Cardiac and Vascular Diseases* (Conn, H.L., Horwitz, O., ed.). Philadelphis, Lea & Febiger, 1971, p. 366-372.

Keller, J.W.: *Panel Discussion. Advances in Cardiac Pacemakers*, Ann. N.Y. Acad. Sci., 167:1-902, 1969.

Keller, J.W.: *Atrial and Ventricular Synchrony: The Engineering-Physiology Interface*, In Ref. 4, p. 869-885.

Barold, S.S., Gaidula, J.J.: *Evaluation of Normal and Abnormal Sensing Functions of Demand Pacemakers*, Amer. J. Cardiol., 28:201-213, 1971.

Kastor, J.A., Berkovits, B.V., De Sanctis, R.W.: *Variations in Discharge Rate of Demand Pacemakers Not Due to Malfunction*, Amer. J. Cardiol., 24:344-348, 1970.

Bilitch, M.: *Ventricular Fibrillation and Pacing*. In Ref. 4, p. 934-940.

Castellanos, A., Jr., Maytin, O., Lemberg, L., et al.: *Pacemaker-induced Cardiac Rhythm Disturbances*. In Ref. 4, p. 903-910.

Friedberg, H.D.: *Syncope During Standby Cardiac Pacing*, Brit. Heart J., 31:281-284, 1969.

Barold, S.S., Gaidula, J.J., Banner, R.L. et al.: *Interpretation of Complex Demand Pacemaker Arrhythmias*, Brit. Heart J., in press.

Barold, S.S., Gaidula, J.J.: *Pacemaker Refractory Periods (letter to the editor)*. New Eng. J. Med., 284:220-221, 1971.

Barold, S.S., Gaidula, J.J., Lyon, J.L., et al.: *Irregular Recycling of Demand Pacemakers from Borderline Electrographic Signals*, Amer. Heart J., in press.

Kramer, D.H., Moss, A.J.: *Permanent Pervenous Atrial Pacing from the Coronary Vein*, Circulation, 42: 427-436, 1970.

Harris, A.: *Pacemaker « Heart Sound »*, Brit. Heart J., 29·608-615, 1967.

Nager, F., Buhlmann, A., Schaub, F., et al.: *Auskultatoresche und kardiographische Befunde bei Patienten mit implantientem elektrischem Schrittmacher*, Klin Wschr, 43:1232-1237, 1965.

Murdock, M.I., Meyers, B.A., Bacos, J.M.: *Auscultatory Clicks Produced by Pacemaker Catheters*, Ann. Intern. Med., 68:1320-1322, 1968.

Furman, S., Escher, D.J.W., Parker, B., et al.: *Electronic Analysis for Pacemaker Failure*, Ann. Thorac. Surg., 8:57-65, 1969.

Smyth, N.P.D.: *Cardiac Pacemaking*, Ibid., pp. 166-190.

Samet, P., Hildner, F., Schoenfeld, C., et al.: *Effect of Chest wall Stimulation on Cardiac Pacemaker Function (abstract)*, Circulation (suppl. III), 40:176, 1969.

Sowton, E., Leatham, A., Carson, P.: *The Suppression of Arrhythmia by Artificial Pacing*, Lancet, 2:1098-1100, 1964.

Chapter X

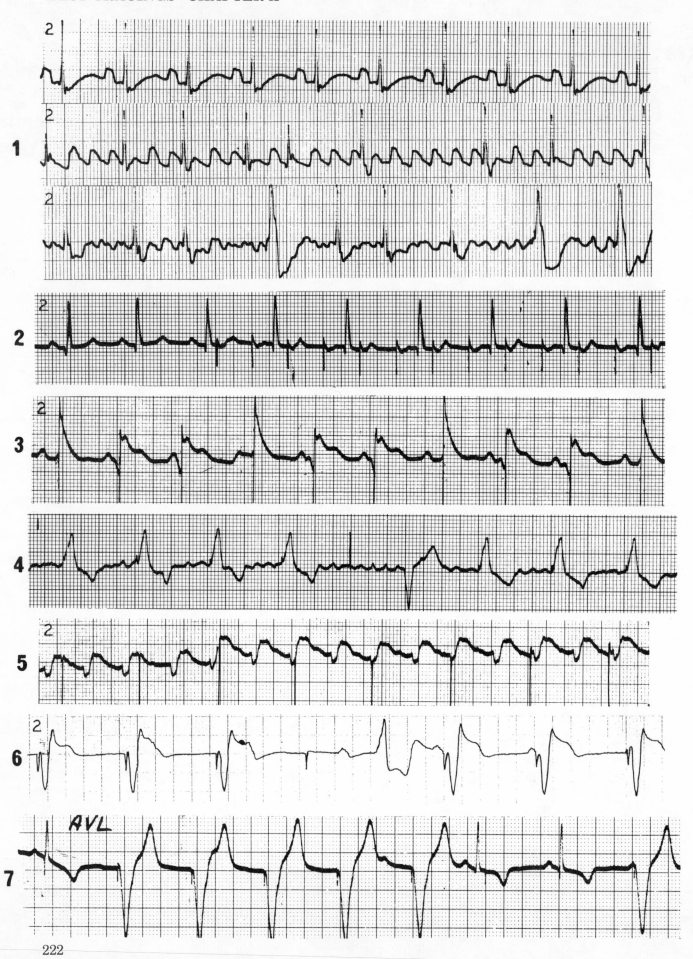

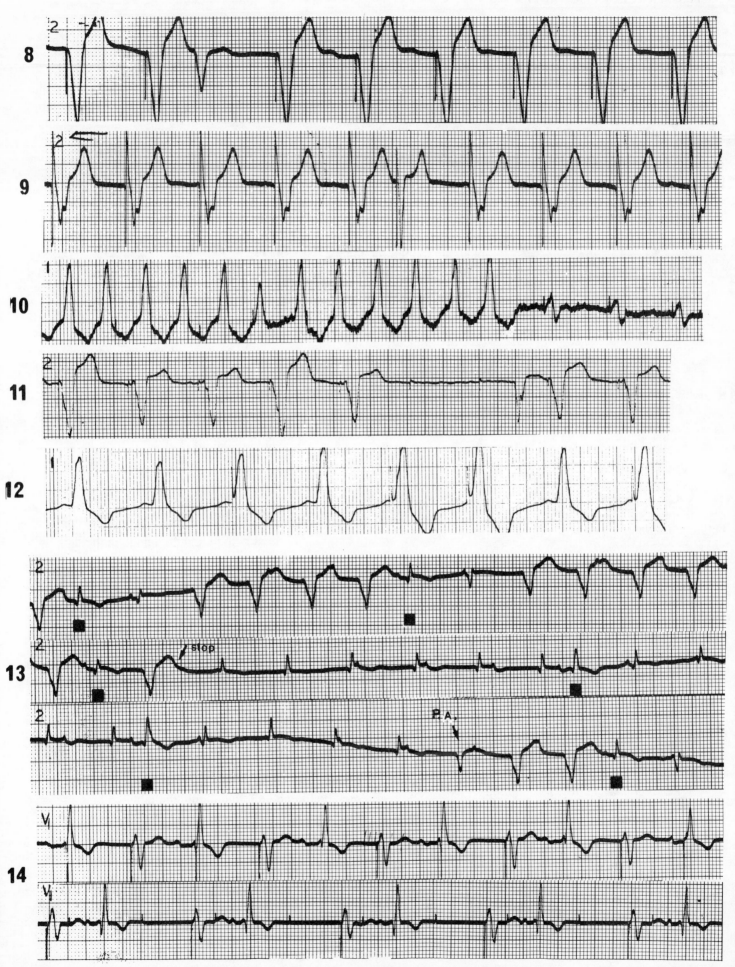

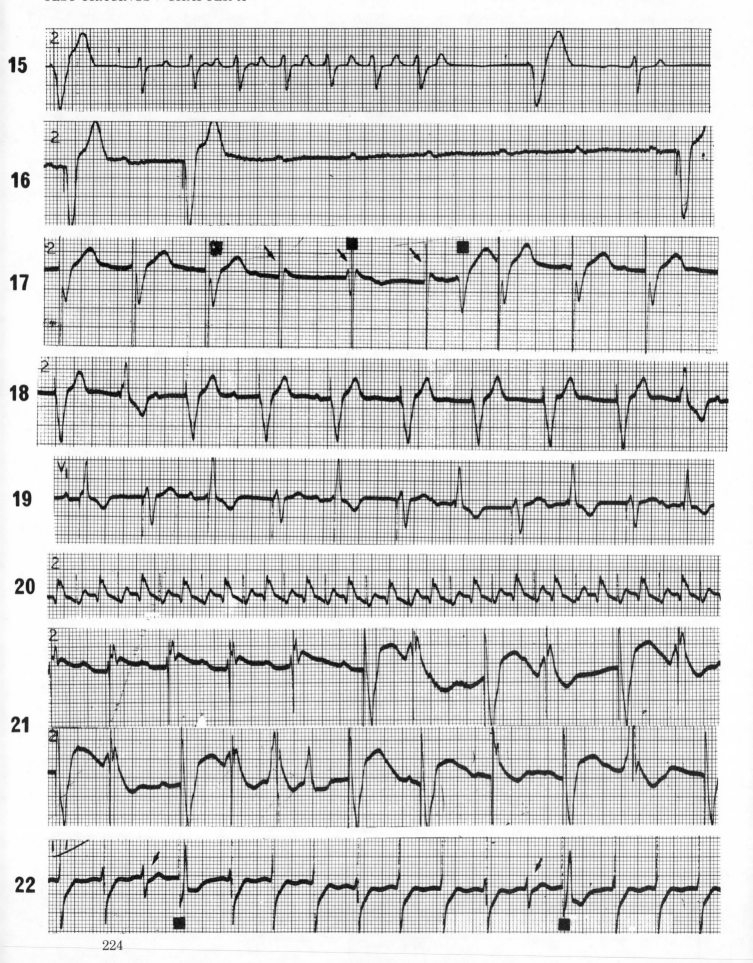

15

16

17

18

19

20

21

22

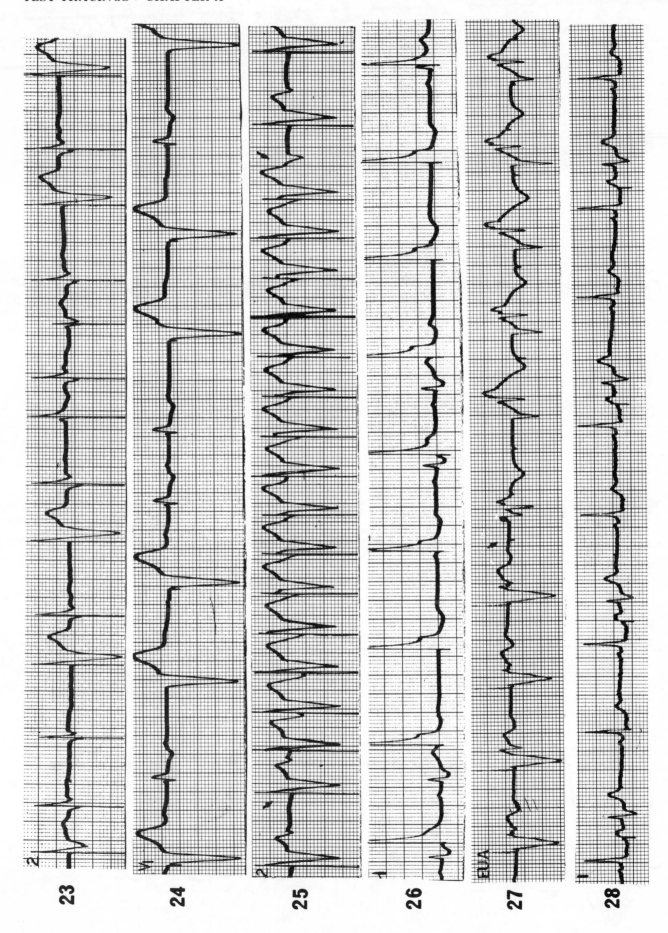

23

24

25

26

27

28

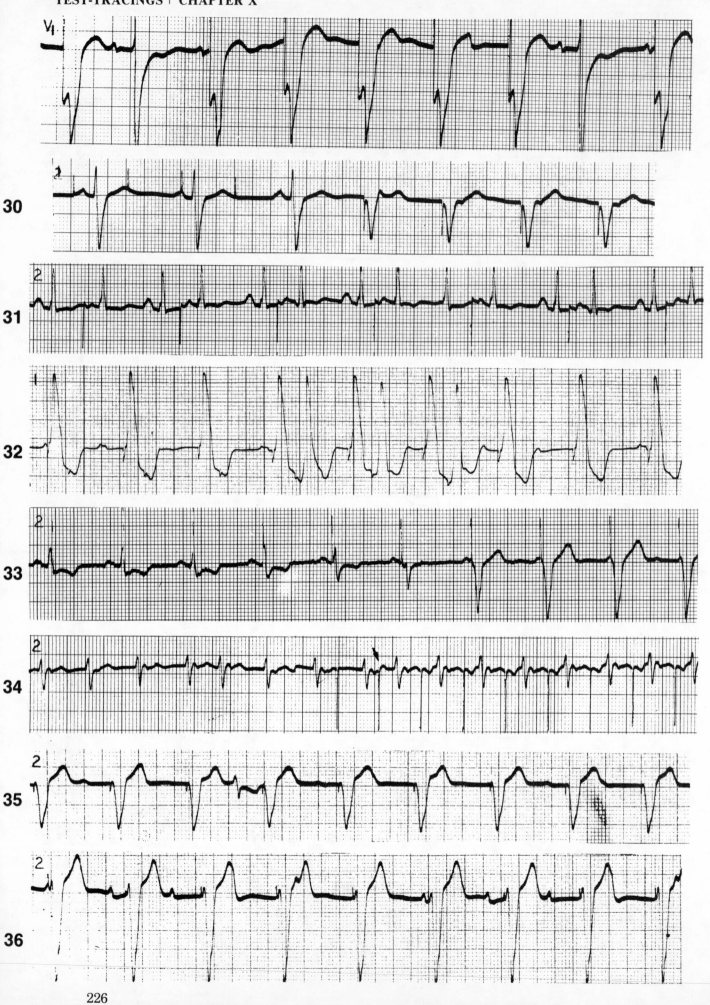

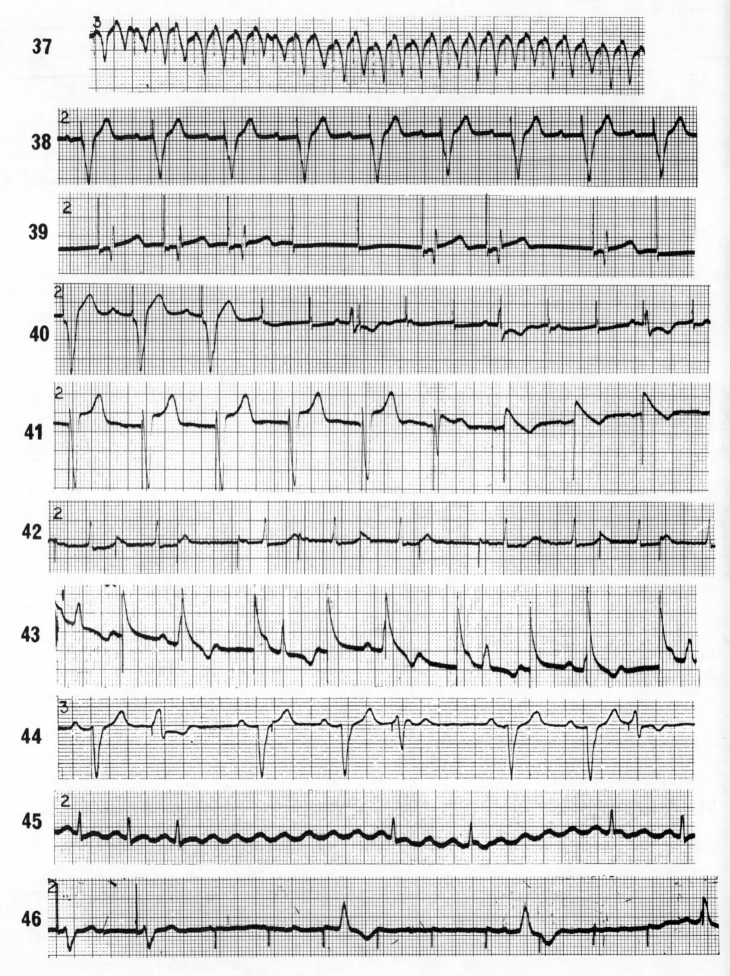

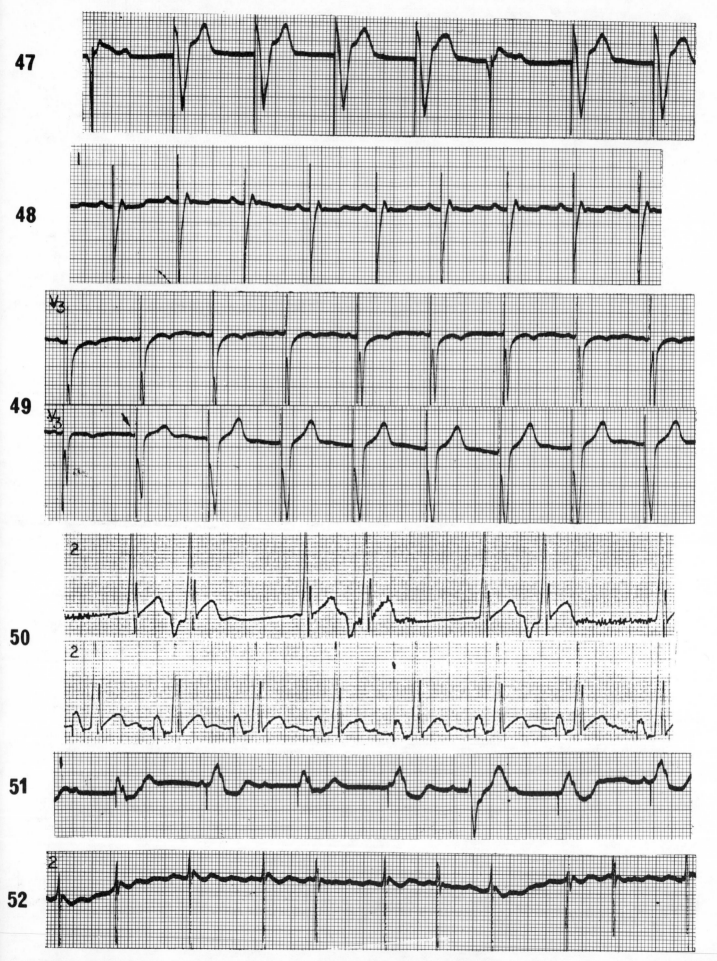

1. **QRS-inhibited "demand" pacemaker.** As is evident from the tracings, the pacemaker has been used to control the unstable ventricular rhythm associated with a variable atrial rhythm. The first tracing shows the patient in a sinus rhythm; the second tracing shows an atrial flutter with a high degree of A-V block; a QRS-inhibited pacemaker is present in the third tracing and controls the irregular ventricular response of an atrial fibrillation. The fourth and eighth QRS's are automatic pacemaker beats appearing at the end of a one second escape interval. The last QRS is a ventricular fusion beat. The spikes are barely visible because of a bipolar stimulation.

2. **Atrial pacing.** The first three beats are of sinus origin. An atrial pacing, with a rate of 150/min., induces a 2:1 A-V block.

3. **QRS-synchronous "demand" pacemaker.** The rhythm is sinus with a tendency to A-V dissociation. The first, fourth, seventh, and last QRS are caused by sinus impulses, which are conducted to the ventricles and synchronized with the pacemaker. The other QRS's are of a junctional origin and dissociated from the P waves. (Notice the variable P-R intervals.) The pacemaker is normally synchronized both with sinus QRS's and with junctional beats (good sensing function).

4. **Chest wall stimulation.** The single external impulse (in the middle of the tracing) temporarily suppresses the QRS-inhibited pacemaker and reveals a spontaneous ventricular activity. (The negative QRS is a spontaneous beat.) The atria are fibrillating and the ventricular rhythm is otherwise under the automatic control of the pacemaker.

5. **Ventricular tachycardia and ineffective pacing.** The pacemaker does not sense ventricular signals and delivers ineffective, fixed rate, impulses.

6. **Pacemaker malfunction.** The fourth artificial impulse is not followed by a QRS and allows for the escape of an idio-ventricular beat.

7. **Competition between a sinus rhythm and an asynchronous pacemaker.** The spike immediately following a sinus QRS is ineffective. The central sequence is totally under control of an asynchronous pacemaker. The rhythm may also be defined as pacemaker iatrogenic parasystole.

8. **QRS-inhibited "demand" pacemaker.** The QRS-inhibited nature of the pacemaker is revealed by the ventricular extrasystole (third QRS) which temporarily suppress the otherwise regular pacing.

9. **QRS-synchronous "demand" pacemaker.** The type of stimulation is revealed by the premature beat in the center of the tracing. The sinus QRS is synchronized with the pacemaker. All the others are automatic pacemaker beats.

10. **Stand-by pacemaker and ventricular tachycardia.** During the tachycardia, ineffective pacemaker spikes are present. With the cessation of the arrhythmia, the ventricular rhythm is promptly re-established by a regular pacing with good ventricular capture (last three QRS's).

11. **Pacemaker malfunction.** The ineffective stimuli allows for the emergence of an idio-ventricular beat. The following pacemaker spike captures the ventricles, probably because it falls within the supernormal ventricular excitability phase.

12. **Pacemaker malfunction.** The stimulation is intermittent and a sinus rhythm is present with a complete left bundle branch block. Notice the extraordinary similarity between a pacemaker QRS (right ventricular pacing) and a sinus QRS with left bundle branch block.

13. **Escape beats with ventricular capture.** The first tracing shows a QRS-inhibited pacemaker, in the presence of a sinus rhythm, occasionally crossing the A-V junction and determining *escape capture beats* (dark squares). Ventricular fusion beats are present (F). The stimulation is intentionally interrupted in the second tracing (arrow). The spontaneous rhythm appears to be an A-V dissociation between a junctional and a sinus rhythm. When P waves fall far enough from preceding QRS's, they cross the A-V junction and determine escape capture beats (dark squares). The spikes are almost invisible (bipolar pacing) and the artificial stimulation is resumed in the last tracing.

14. **Chest wall stimulation.** The upper tracing shows automatic pacemaker beats alternating with sinus beats. (note the variable P-R intervals of sinus beats due to "concealed penetration" of the artificial impulses into the A-V junction.) The middle tracing records a chest wall stimulation (75/min.) with alternate stimuli suppressing the pacemaker; every other chest wall impulse always falls within the pacemaker refractory period. This determines a reduction of the ventricular rate (ventricular bigeminy) and permits the measurement of the P-R interval of sinus beats (0.16 secs.).

15. **"Sick S-A node syndrome" and QRS-inhibited pacemaker.** The atrial tachyarrhythmia is followed by a prolonged asystolic pause, promptly terminated by a QRS-inhibited pacemaker escape beat. The stand-by interval is quite prolonged (1200 msecs.).

16. **"Overdrive suppression".** The sudden discontinuance of artificial pacing is not followed by spontaneous ventricular activity. A sinus rhythm is present (75/min.) with P waves blocked within the A-V junction. After an asystolic pause of 5.5 sec., the artificial pacing is re-activated with a good ventricular capture.

17. **QRS-synchronous pacemaker malfunction.** The first and last three beats are automatic pacemaker beats. The three spikes in the middle of the tracing are ineffective. A sinus rhythm is present (find the P-waves), with a complete A-V block and a slow idioventricular rhythm (dark squares). The voltage-decay curves simulate a pacemaker synchronization with non existing QRS's (arrows).

18. **QRS-inhibited pacemaker.** The pacemaker is suppressed by the second and last QRS, of junctional origin and with aberrant conduction; otherwise, it paces at a fixed rate and is dissociated with the slower sinus rhythm (P-P interval).

19. **"Concealed A-V conduction".** The retrograde penetration of the pacemaker impulses in the A-V junction is documented by the changing P-R intervals of sinus beats alternating with pacemaker beats. The first three sinus beats show the "pseudo-fusion phenomenon".

20. **Overdrive atrial pacing.** Artificial impulses (135/min.) precede P^1 waves. The A-V conduction is good, even in the presence of an elevated atrial rate, and determines a 1:1 ventricular response.

21. **QRS-synchronous "demand" pacemaker.** The first five QRS's are of sinus origin and are normally synchronized with the pacemaker. (Notice the presence of a prolonged P-R interval.) The following pause, due to an increase in the A-V block, is terminated by an automatic pacemaker beat. This is followed by a bigeminal rhythm with "couplets" formed by automatic beats and ventricular extrasystoles. In the second tracing a burst of ventricular extrasystoles appears; two of them are normally synchronized with the pacemaker, while the one indicated by the arrow is not "sensed" because it falls within the pacemaker refractory period (320 msecs. from the preceding stimulus). Both the sensing and the stimulating mechanisms are in perfect working conditions.

22. **Atrial flutter and QRS-synchronous pacemaker.** The beats indicated by dark squares are pacemaker automatic beats, delivered at the end of a stand-by interval of 800 msecs. from the preceding spontaneous QRS (arrows). The ventricular rate is fast and reaches the maximal synchronization limit for this type of pacemaker. To be certain of a sensing mechanism malfunction, the pacemaker must be evaluated at slower spontaneous rates.

23. **QRS-synchronous "demand" pacemaker.** The demand stimulator is in a perfect symbiosis with the irregular ventricular rhythm of the atrial fibrillation. Automatic beats are present and all spontaneous QRS's are synchronized with the pacemaker.

24. **QRS-inhibited "demand" pacemaker.** A sinus rhythm, with a delayed A-V conduction of a Wenkebach type, is present in symbiosis with a QRS-inhibited pacemaker. Automatic pacemaker beats terminate the asystolic pauses following blocked P waves.

25. **Chest wall stimulation and QRS-synchronous pacemaker.** The two arrows indicate the beginning and the end of a CWS (140/min.). The external impulses are sensed by the pacemaker which responds 1:1, determining an increase in the ventricular pacing rate.

26. **Iatrogenic parasystole from an asynchronous pacemaker.** The first, fifth, and last artificial impulses are not effective because they fall in the ventricular absolute refractory phase following the sinus beats. The spikes which capture the ventricles compete with the sinus rhythm.

27. **Chest wall stimulation and atrial electrogram**. The unipolar recording is performed into the atrial chamber. The first four beats are pacemaker induced. (Notice P^1 waves following each QRS, indicating a retrograde atrial activation.) The arrow shows the beginning of the chest wall stimulation which immediately suppresses the QRS-inhibited pacemaker, allowing for the emergence of a sinus rhythm. The chest wall impulses appear as small spikes on the atrial electrogram (rate = about 60/min.); the atrial waves are clearly distinct and precede the ventricular activation waves.

28. **Atrial pacing.** The atrial impulses, with a rate of about 53/min., capture the atria only alternatively and determine a bigeminal type of rhythm. The QRS complexes which follow the P^1 waves are slightly aberrant (right bundle branch block type) because of the prematurity of the impulses which, when crossing the A-V junction, find the right bundle still refractory. The ineffective impulses are almost concealed within the sinus QRS complexes.

29. **QRS-synchronous "demand" pacemaker**. Only the second and eighth QRS's are of sinus origin and are synchronized with the pacemaker. (Notice the presence of sinus P waves and the QRS aberration secondary to the voltage decay curve.) All the others are automatic pacemaker beats.

30. **Chest wall stimulation**. The tracing records the ending of a CWS which suppresses a QRS-inhibited pacemaker and reveals a sinus rhythm with a right bundle branch block. Notice that each automatic pacemaker QRS is followed by a small negative deflection, indicating a retrograde atrial activation (P^1).

31. **Atrial pacing**. The artificial impulses, alternating with those of sinus origin, result in an "atrial bigeminy".

32. **"Echo beats"**. The first six QRS's, caused by automatic pacemaker impulses, show P^1 waves partially hidden within the ST segment. The three *"couplets"* in the center of the tracing are caused by the re-entry of retrograde impulses into the ventricles. The "echo beats" simulate ventricular extrasystoles. Notice the absence of P^1 waves within the last three automatic pacemaker beats.

33. **Ventricular pseudo-fusion and ventricular fusion**. The pacemaker is of the QRS-inhibited type. The first four QRS's are of sinus origin but they still show pacemaker spikes on the peak of the R-wave. The fifth, sixth and seventh QRS are ventricular fusion beats while the last three QRS's are pacemaker automatic beats.

34. **Overdrive atrial pacing**. The tracing starts with an A-V dissociation between a sinus rhythm and a faster junctional rhythm. The ventricular rate, irregular for the presence of "escape capture beats," is stabilized with a faster overdrive atrial pacing. (The arrow indicates the beginning of atrial capture.)

35. **Asynchronous pacemaker**. The stimulation is regular and is not disturbed by the sinus beat sandwiched between two pacemaker QRS's.

36. **Atrial-pacemaker dissociation**. The stimulation is due to an asynchronous pacemaker which controls the ventricular activation. P waves are blocked in the A-V junction and the sinus rhythm is dissociated from that of the pacemaker.

37. **"Runaway pacemaker"**. The rapid stimulation is followed by a 1:1 ventricular response and determines a ventricular tachycardia.

38. **QRS-inhibited "demand" pacemaker**. The presence of P waves before each QRS would suggest a P-wave synchronous pacemaker. However, the variable P-R intervals rule out a pacemaker synchronization with atrial potentials (see tracing n. 18).

39. **Ineffective atrial pacing**. Atrial capture is not constant. The fourth, fifth and last pacemaker spikes are ineffective and are not followed by spontaneous atrial activity.

40. **Chest wall stimulation**. The pacemaker is a QRS-inhibited type. The external impulses enable the reappearance of a sinus rhythm with a second degree A-V block.

41. **"Concertina effect"**. From a regular automatic pacing of 71/min. (QRS-synchronous pacemaker) and through a ventricular fusion beat, the cardiac rhythm changes into a sinus mechanism synchronized with the pacemaker (80/min.).

42. **Atrial pacing.** The atrial impulses (rate = 90/min.) show an abnormal A-V conduction. In fact, sequences of second degree A-V block, with Wenkebach periods, are present in the tracing.

43. **QRS-synchronous "demand" pacemaker malfunction.** The pacemaker has not lost the capacity of synchronization with sinus QRS's, but does not capture the ventricles (abnormal pacing function). The "non-sensed" QRS falls within the pacemaker refractory period.

44. **Iatrogenic asynchronous pacemaker parasystole.** Only one of every other impulse captures the ventricles, while the other falls within the absolute ventricular refractory period of the spontaneous beat. Notice that sinus P waves follow immediately after each pacemaker beat and are blocked within the A-V junction (which is refractory because of the concealed retrograde penetration of the artificial impulse).

45. **Atrial flutter.** The A-V block is variable and, occasionally, is of such a high degree as to determine asystolic pauses of about 2 secs. In patients refractory to drugs and cardioversion, a "demand" pacemaker may be the only alternative to maintain a stable ventricular rhythm.

46. **Chest wall stimulation.** The suppression of a QRS-inhibited pacemaker indicates a good sensing function and reveals a markedly bradycardic idio-ventricular rhythm.

47. **QRS-synchronous "demand" pacemaker.** The nature of the stimulator is indicated by the two ventricular extrasystoles which synchronize with the ventricular-triggered pacemaker.

48. **P-wave synchronous pacemaker.** Each spike captures the ventricles and is preceded by a P wave with a constant P-S interval (P-stimulus).

49. **QRS-synchronous "demand" pacemaker.** Notice the extraordinary similarity of the top tracing with that of the preceding figure. Again, in this case the spike is preceded by a P wave with a constant P-S interval. The impulse, however, does not capture the ventricles because it is synchronized with sinus QRS's. In the bottom tracing, the sinus rhythm is replaced by an automatic pacemaker rhythm with good ventricular capture. The arrow indicates the transition between the two rhythms, which occurs through a ventricular fusion beat.

50. **Overdrive atrial pacing.** The top tracing shows a slow junctional rhythm with impulses activating the atria in a retrograde fashion (P¹) and returning to the ventricles (echo beats). The ventricular rate is somewhat slow and the bigeminal rhythm, determined by the presence of echo beats, is stabilized with atrial pacing. The faster atrial rate (overdrive atrial pacing) controls the ventricular rhythm and suppresses the echo beats.

51. **Escape capture beats and QRS-inhibited "demand" pacemaker.** The only spontaneous QRS present in the tracing is that of a sinus beat able to cross the A-V junction and to capture the ventricles. All other P waves are dissociated from the automatic pacemaker rhythm.

52. **Atrial fibrillation and QRS-synchronous "demand" pacemaker.** Each QRS of the atrial fibrillation is synchronized with the pacemaker. Notice the spike falling 20 msec. after the beginning of the spontaneous ventricular depolarization.